THE
ESTROGEN
ALTERNATIVE

THE
ESTROGEN
ALTERNATIVE

A GUIDE TO NATURAL
HORMONAL BALANCE

Fourth Edition

Raquel Martin
and Judi Gerstung, D.C.

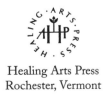

Healing Arts Press
Rochester, Vermont

Healing Arts Press
One Park Street
Rochester, Vermont 05767
www.InnerTraditions.com

Healing Arts Press is a division of Inner Traditions International

Note to the reader: This book is intended as an informational guide. The remedies, approaches, and techniques described herein are meant to supplement, and not to be a substitute for, professional medical care or treatment. They should not be used to treat a serious ailment without prior consultation with a qualified health care professional.

The Library of Congress has catalogued a previous edition of this title as follows:

Martin, Raquel.
    The estrogen alternative : natural hormone therapy with botanical progesterone /
Raquel Martin, with Judi Gerstung.
        p. cm.
    Includes bibliographical references and index.
    ISBN 0-89281-893-X
        1. Progesterone—Therapeutic use. 2. Generative organs, Female—Diseases—
Alternative treatment. 3. Menopause—Complications—Alternative treatment. 4. Plant
hormones—Therapeutic use. 5. Generative organs, Female—Diseases—Hormone therapy.
I. Gerstung, Judi. II. Title.
RG129.P66 M373 2000
618.1'06—dc21
                                                                99-089914

ISBN of fourth edition: 1-59477-033-6

Printed and bound in the United States at Lake Book Manufacturing, Inc.

10 9 8 7 6 5 4 3 2

Text design and layout by Kristin Camp Sperber

This book was typeset in Adobe Caslon, with Bauer Bodoni and Gill Sans as display typefaces

Contents

Foreword to the
Third Edition

Raquel Martin and her coauthor, Dr. Judi Gerstung, have performed a tremendous service to the women of America by writing *The Estrogen Alternative*. I believe all women will greatly benefit from reading this well-written and resource-laden book. I am sure many will identify with Raquel's experiences and frustration as she wanders through the maze of traditional medical therapy seeking relief for her menopausal symptoms.

It has been my observation that when women are presented with the information in this book, it makes sense to them and provides encouragement for change. As the authors point out, not only are the hot flashes, irregular menses, and emotional upsets relieved by natural hormone therapy, but also such conditions as insomnia, weight gain, dry skin, fatigue, osteoporosis, thinning hair, and depression. Unfortunately, the symptoms on this list, often wrongly attributed to estrogen deficiency rather than estrogen dominance, are treated by allopathic medicine with even more estrogen. This can lead to worsening of symptoms, increased bleeding, or the often unnecessary hysterectomy.

Not recognizing that many of these problems could be eliminated or controlled by Nature's counterbalance to estrogen, natural progesterone, the physician may deal with the other notable symptoms created by estrogen dominance as separate maladies, resulting in individual testing and treatment for each complaint. Depression is treated as a Prozac deficiency, water retention with a diuretic, weight gain with appetite suppressants, whereas the solution can be as simple as counteracting estrogen overload with what the patient is no longer able to produce on her own—namely, progesterone.

Women today need a book like this to understand what is happening to their bodies during pre-, peri-, and postmenopause and to recognize the symptoms of estrogen dominance and anovulation that are so prevalent. It is a tremendous resource to any practitioner such as myself to recommend to this patients. It is a valuable teaching tool as I try to educate my patients about the many hormonal changes that are taking place. With this knowledge, women can make informed choices, not only about natural hormone therapy but also about exercise, diet, and vitamin and mineral supplementation. *The Estrogen Alternative* fulfills this need. Otherwise, my patients are at the mercy of the pharmaceutical industry and their dollars that are pumped into women's magazines and other advertising media.

John T. Hart, M.D.

Foreword to the Second Edition

The 1990s have brought about considerable changes in health care in this country. Many of these changes result from the emergence of managed care organizations in an attempt to reduce medical costs. This approach, unfortunately, has brought with it limitations and restrictions on health care delivery. Many consumers are now turning to more user-friendly complementary and alternative care in which individuals take an active part in the decisions necessary to maintain optimum health.

Expanding knowledge of the usefulness of such complementary care is supported by the Dietary Supplement Health and Education Act of 1994. A major aspect of this includes the greater use of plant chemicals (phytochemicals) as dietary supplements or "medicinals," which in many cases may replace synthetic pharmaceuticals.

As women become more and more involved in decisions about hormone replacement therapy (HRT), *The Estrogen Alternative* serves a vital need. It is very timely and addresses this increasingly complex problem. The dilemma of HRT today stems largely from the many inconclusive and contradictory studies published by traditional medical institutions.

The woman who chooses to be an active participant in decisions regarding hormone therapy must first heed the authors' reminder that we still have a lot to learn. With that in mind, they have presented an extensive amount of information on HRT, with emphasis on the use of natural progesterone. The decisions a woman makes must include consideration of risk versus benefit, a vital factor in all health care choices. It's not an easy task, and unfortunately, the focus of most scientific studies has been only synthetic preparations. This book addresses the many aspects of HRT, whether natural or synthetic, that we need to consider. On one hand, benefits include a reduction in both osteoporosis (progesterone decreases the risk of bone fractures and vertebral body collapse) and vascular disease (it also decreases the risk of heart attacks and stroke). On the other hand is increased risk of breast and endometrial cancer with traditional HRT. A woman's quality of life, as well as her longevity, are influenced by her decisions about hormone therapy. Yet much of the information that reaches the general public provides inconclusive data on which to base proper decisions.

The Estrogen Alternative examines the benefits of natural progesterone therapy for women of all ages. The authors' shared experiences make it even more appealing. They provide educational support for women who wish to participate in decisions about their own care. They also present a challenge to the physicians who, it is hoped, will become more receptive to patients considering a more natural approach.

I. Sylvia Crawley, M.D.
Chair, Medical Education Committee
American Nutraceutical Association

Foreword to the First Edition

Many good books have been written about natural health alternatives, a large number of them by health care professionals. Raquel Martin's well-written book is unique, however, in that it comes to us from a layperson—a consumer of health care, if you will. As a woman, she herself has had to cope with many of the problems described here. As a knowledgeable health activist and author of *Today's Health Alternative*, she has investigated the options open to her and examined those that were most effective. As a dedicated writer, she has researched her subject, gathered the important facts from scientific journals and the medical literature about the benefits of natural foods and hormones, and, finally, collaborated with health care professionals to put it all together into an accurate and highly readable text.

This book will be important to women around the world who have been bombarded with chemical therapies. They have been on a physiological roller coaster, and it's time for them to have safe and effective solutions. Raquel Martin is an inspiring role model for all the women who are not getting the help they need. She urges them to seek out the answers for themselves, sort out for themselves the good from the bad, and find out what works and what doesn't—in short, to take charge of their own health care, be more informed about prescription and over-the-counter pharmaceuticals, and ask the right questions of their doctors.

My grandfather founded a pharmaceutical company more than a century ago. In the old days he and my father manufactured herbal products and other concentrates of botanical origin for physicians all over the country. As medicine began to change and drug companies decided to patent and market synthetic products instead, the natural remedies became scarce. I chose to carry on the family tradition by creating natural products that make a difference.

More than twenty years of studying phytogenins led me to effective natural sources for a number of hormones. Along the way I became impressed with the efficacy of the wild yam. I have devoted a lot of time to studying the yam and identifying the characteristics and bioavailability of different species. Wild yams are an unbelievably effective resource for natural hormone therapy if you select the right species and extraction methods. Let's hope that in the future these products will be standardized and properly labeled, so the consumer can know what she is getting.

When I learned about the effort that Raquel Martin has expended to find out everything she could from medical reports, medical doctors, natural health care practitioners, pharmacies, manufacturers, and other studies on the effectiveness of the wild yam, and in particular phytogenin markers from specific species, I was intrigued. The anecdotal evidence from women who have been helped affirms the value of this botanical supplement.

I feel it is an honor to be part of this work, which brings a wealth of good information to the table for our consideration. Many doctors have written books that are biased toward drugs, and naturalists have written books slanted toward herbs. But this team of authors has addressed a subject of vital importance to women in a simple, straightforward manner—without bias, and with a lot of very useful information.

It's refreshing to read a book written from the soul. Perhaps someday the author's song will become a full chorus. Forget about the science for a moment; zero in on the message: Women have a choice! Take control of your health! Read the book, study the alternatives, ask questions, and above all, think for yourself.

James Jamieson
Pharmacologist

Acknowledgments

This book was achieved through unmatched creative teamwork, where everyone's goal was the same: to raise public consciousness about disease prevention by exploring our choices and documenting the remarkable health benefits of natural alternatives. To Judi Gerstung, D.C., I owe untold thanks for the long hours she devoted to this undertaking—time away from her other jobs as chiropractor, radiologist, teacher, and lecturer. Her comprehensive background in the health care field has been invaluable. She assisted me in the organization of rapidly changing information and with editing throughout the project, making clarifying revisions in a logical and orderly way. Her desire to bring this immensely important subject to the attention of women worldwide and her special interest in the detection and prevention of osteoporosis guided me through tough and discouraging moments as we worked to reach our goal.

And my thanks to Glenn and Judy Parnham; Tom Flynn; and Irene Inglis, a longtime friend, for her support and partnership in our mutual quest for safe alternatives to drugs. The ideal combination of her training as a registered nurse with her interest in natural means of healing helped me transform medical terminology into practical knowledge. She was truly God-sent with her assistance in proofreading and meeting necessary deadlines.

Appreciation goes to Laurie Skiba, writer and writing consultant, who contributed essential insight to some of the more difficult and technical chapters in the book's early stages. She generously shared her professional talent and experience, sacrificing time from her freelance work and the writing of her own books. Her critical analysis spurred me to deepen my investigation. I gained much from her intelligent, thought-provoking editorial comments.

Thank you to Marcia Jones, Director of the PMS and Menopause Center at Dixie Health, Inc., for her advice on the manuscript, for contributing new reference material, and for her many introductions to health care advocates. Through her enthusiasm to get the facts out to women, I was introduced to Coeli Carr. I am sincerely grateful to both Coeli and Marcia for their generous counsel, as they guided me in my attempt to educate and motivate women toward a better quality of life.

Special thanks to Katharina Dalton, M.D.; Wallace Simons, R.Ph. (Women's International Pharmacy); Scott Stamper, R.Ph. (Women's Health America Group); Mark H. Mandel, R.Ph. (Snyder-Mark Drugs Roselle); Ole Krarp; Sam Georgiou, R.Ph. (Professional Arts Pharmacy); Brad Sorenson; and James Jamieson, pharmacologist, for supplying pertinent research data and documentation and helping me better appreciate the importance of natural HRT; and to Stuart and Jane Burke for testimonials that added a personal touch to this story. And thanks to Jay G. Fromer, Ray Silverman, Sasha Silverman, Debbie Dombrowski, Charis Dike, David Bundrick, Karla Emling, Beverly Kapple, Patricia Gibson, William C. Amala, D.C., DIIACT, FIACT, and Robert A. Beiswenger, Lt. Col., USAFR, for their input and encouragement. I'll be forever grateful to J. K. Humber Jr., D.C.; Mark Baker, D.C.; Don N. Parkerson Jr., D.C.; Wayne Neal, D.C.; Judi Gerstung, D.C.; and Linda Force, D.C.; for providing case histories and moral support while also keeping me in good health during the stressful times.

My heartfelt appreciation also goes to my talented daughter Marie, for her generous gift of time and energy in creating and maintaining my Web page www.healthcare-alternatives.com. I will always be touched by her loving dedication to helping me reach more people with the vital messages in *The Estrogen Alternative, Preventing and Reversing Arthritis Naturally,* and *Today's Health Alternative,* through the many hours of computer design work she has contributed.

And my love and thanks to my husband, Jack, for sharing his refreshing and clear communication skills. He furnished the missing "flow" to the work. His gift for words, analytical ability, and prudent judgment provided a consistent sounding board for my endless questions. He also helped me clarify my personal objectives and stay focused on them. He taught me necessary computer skills and usually stayed calm in the face of my recurring crises with so-called user-friendly software. His counsel held everything together.

And I can't thank Bill Martin, my brother-in-law, fervently enough for his suggestions and constructive criticism upon carefully reviewing an early draft. His objective eye zeroed in on better readability and accuracy, while his professional advice in the area of the sciences stimulated all of us to do more research.

Later came the difficult task of final revision and organization of the manuscript. For this and much more I am indebted to Connie Smith. Thanks to her painstaking regard for detail and priorities, our critical deadlines were all met. She brought to the book the accuracy and meticulous editing skills needed to do justice to a vital subject. Connie's personal research played an important role in unraveling and interpreting the differing viewpoints of various authorities. Her astute sense of judgment concerning complex issues was continually employed, as was her intelligent guidance. Her inspiration and strength motivated me to engage in honest reflection right to the end of our mission.

I'm truly grateful for the support and confidence of John Hart, M.D., FACOG. He received specialty training in obstetrics and gynecology at the University of Virginia (1981). This book is dedicated to doctors like him who have gone that extra mile to help women seek answers and safer ways of addressing their female disorders and related problems resulting from hormone imbalance. He is a true ally in the fight for freedom of choice in health matters.

Last, I must acknowledge the late Dr. John R. Lee and Dr. Raymond F. Peat. Their published findings are beginning to enlighten a countless number of people, helping women at long last to find more satisfying answers to age-old problems. My personal thanks to them are reflected in many references throughout this book. I am also deeply grateful for their personal tutelage in scientific and medical terminology in preparation for this book's publication. I am honored that they agreed to become active participants in this work.

And with both heart and mind I give thanks to the Lord for guiding me onto the paths of the above talented souls. I am grateful for His endowing us all with curiosity and concern about an issue so crucial not only to our physical health, but also to our mental and spiritual well-being.

ॐ

*Dedicated to the doctors who are not limited by prejudice or greed,
and who reason and act beyond the prevailing orthodox medical practice
in order to pursue greater truth for the benefit of humanity; and to
the multitudes of patients who suffer needlessly from having met only
silence from the medical and pharmaceutical industries concerning
the natural healing opportunities that have helped so many.*

A Bombshell That Changed HRT Medical History

A shock wave hit the country on July 10, 2002, when the "long-overdue" news regarding the dangers of synthetic hormone replacement was brought to public awareness. It was broadcast on TV and radio stations as well as all the major newspapers and Internet sites. From the *Wall Street Journal* to holistic health magazines, they all reported, one after another, that a major study—known as the Women's Health Initiative (WHI)—had shown an earlier increase in the risk of breast cancer, coronary heart disease, stroke, and blood clots for women using the conventional hormone replacement therapy (HRT) as compared to those taking a placebo. The findings came from a research project sponsored by the National Institutes of Health, a study that followed 16,000 women who were prescribed the estrogen/progestin combination drug Prempro. According to the results published in the *Journal of the American Medical Association (JAMA)*, there were a total of 2,082 cases of breast cancer in this group of women.

According to the *New York Times*, the WHI study involved 40 clinical sites across the country with thousands of women participating, each of whom was given the combination HRT or a placebo. They offered the following interpretation of the risks involved: Half the women took the drug for a year and the other half did not. Women in the first half had 8 more occurrences of aggressive breast cancer, 7 more heart attacks, 8 more strokes, and 18 more occurrences of blood clots.[1] Headlines from the following news sources flooded the media in the days and months immediately following the July 2002 announcement.

USA Today (Health & Science), "U.S. Halts Study on Hormone
   Therapy," July 9, 2002.
CBS.com, "Red Flag on Hormone Replacement," July 10, 2002.
CBS.com, "Limits of Hormone Therapy," July 11, 2002.
CBS.com, "MDs to HRT Patients: Don't Panic!," July 16, 2002.
CNN.com, "The Pros and Cons of Halting Research," July 17, 2002.
New York Times, "Survey Halted, Drug Makers Seek to Protect
   Hormone Sales," July 17, 2002.
Newsday, "Hormone Decision is all about Risk," July 17, 2002.
Newsweek, "The End of the Age of Estrogen," July 22, 2002.
Newsweek, "What's a Woman to Do?," July 22, 2002.
Time, "Should Anyone Take Hormones?," July 22, 2002.
New York Times, "Facing the Hormone Dilemma," July 22, 2002.
Wall Street Journal, "Alternative to Hormone Replacement Therapy,"
   July 24, 2002.
U.S. News and World Report, "Making Sense of Menopause,"
   November 18, 2002.

All this news came as a shock to many in the medical community, because medical practitioners have sworn by these synthetic hormones since they were first introduced approximately fifty years ago. Warnings about such dangers first surfaced when it was found these hormones were associated with the development of endometrial cancer. In 1947 Dr. Saul Gusberg of Columbia University "called the ready use of estrogen 'promiscuous' and warned that what was going on was a human experiment." He had observed too many estrogen users coming in for D&Cs for abnormal bleeding caused by endometrial overstimulation, as well as documented cancerous and pre-cancerous changes of the uterus.[2]

For some of us, none of this was *new* news. In fact this *old* news has continued to surface and resurface throughout the years. The dangers of traditional hormone therapy were reported in the first edition of this book seven years prior to this recent study. The media's unfortunate misinterpretation led many to believe that before the 2002 WHI study, no one had any idea of the possible dangers of the use of HRT in any and all of its many forms. We wrote then: "Millions of menopausal women are taking such potentially lethal combinations daily. And sadly, the recommendation to do so is justified by the statistics that *heart disease* is the number one killer of post-menopausal women—the persuasive rationale for taking HRT." Now that this rationale has been proved wrong, perhaps it's time for us to delve into the studies showing what has been, and what will always be, a far superior alternative to synthetic HRT.

The *World Health News* couldn't have stated it better: "The simplicity and safety of the solution is almost shocking. One might ask why every suffering woman is not using botanical progesterone,"[3] and why is there such a lack of education concerning the dual relationship between estrogen and its essential but *neglected* partner called progesterone? The tragic results of breast cancer, stroke, heart disease, and other side effects caused us as authors to reflect on the words of our first edition in 1992: "Perhaps someday the prescribing of synthetic hormones to women will be labeled *malpractice*, and the prescribing of any form of estrogen unopposed by natural progesterone will be a *violation of insurance codes*."

Because women have been given the wrong hormones for so long, we often hear stories such as this one from the *New York Times:* "Cheryl Kipfer (56) from Omaha is really confused as to what to do. She learned that she had bone loss, and her doctor recommended that she continue with HRT every day. 'I am afraid,' Ms. Kipfer said, 'afraid of fractured bones if I stop taking the hormones, afraid of breast cancer if I continue. If I was taking it for hot flashes, I would come right off,' she said. But what about osteoporosis?"[4] It's sad when women such as Cheryl are not informed by their medical doctors about how supplementing with progesterone (transdermally or sublingually) will help to rebalance their hormone levels. And how progesterone is the hormone that is even proactive in building build bone mineral density (BMD),[5, 6] which can help women prevent and even reverse osteoporosis.

Reading about Cheryl's frustration caused me to flash back to a conversation I had with a discerning senior citizen who called me to say "thank you for writing that book. . . . I've been on estrogen most of my life because the doctor said it was good for my bones and heart. Since then I have had three heart attacks and suffer from severe osteoporosis." She told me that the research in my book made so much sense that she became confident enough to put to use what she read. She now feels better and stronger at her age than she has for decades. Thank goodness she heard of this natural alternative before the doctor put her on Fosamax.

Drugs such as this, as well as Evista (SERM—selective estrogen receptor modulators), Tamoxifen, Arimidex, Lipitor, and Raloxifen, will increase one's chances of Alzheimer's disease, neuronal cell death, memory loss, and other diseases associated with dementia.[7–10] Today there may be new names for such designer drugs, but they all have their list of harmful and often long-term side effects. If you are thinking of taking such medications, I encourage you to read further in this book where we document the dangers reported by those researchers *who are not in the business of profiting from the sale of drugs.* We all need to be alert to these facts especially when reading articles and reports that are often quoted in popular journals and on the Internet that use research sponsored by drug companies, which are slanted to make us think it is still okay to use synthetic hormones.

We have tried to be extremely cautious about sources and sensitive to who has sponsored studies that we have used for our investigation in the writing of this book. In contrast and seldom mentioned, Wyeth-Ayerst, the giant drug company, financed the book *Feminine Forever* (1968). Understandably so, it was quite enthusiastic about the drug Premarin and became a bestseller. It is not a coincidence that in 2001, Wyeth received more than two billion dollars in sales from Premarin.

Further evidence of the spread of such biased information comes from Dr. Nadin F. Marks, associate professor at the University of Wisconsin at Madison, where he explains that the pharmaceutical industry sponsors scores of promotional articles written for gynecological and obstetrical journals and textbooks in which the doctors are convinced that "a woman's life could be destroyed if she didn't have estrogen in her body."[11] Do these words still sound convincing to us? How much longer will these deceptions continue to be imposed upon us through such powerfully clever organizations? When will we realize the impact that this well-organized propaganda has on our health? How many more trials are going to be organized using vulnerable women who are in need of healthy solutions rather than perilous ones? What does it take to stop this madness?

Many drug marketing campaigns have a simple goal—to establish in every woman's mind the belief that prescribed estrogen alone, or an estrogen/progestin combination, is not only safe but also is essential for them in every way. This kind of irresponsible ad blitz has caused many vulnerable women to learn about cancer the hard way. Billions of dollars in grant money has been used to continue this reckless prescription to cancer and other fatal diseases. Of great concern now are the millions of American women who are still on this runaway freight train. Education regarding the alternatives available is essential for women to understand why they need to get off this track as soon as possible; that they not buy into the self-serving promises that "the benefits will outweigh the risks"; and, most of all, that they learn about safely balancing hormone levels through the use of natural progesterone, as well as the additional safe alternatives discussed in the appendices and throughout this book.

Unfortunately, we can realistically predict that with all the vested interests at stake (grants from the pharmaceutical industry and the "medical specialists" working to produce a "better" synthetic HRT), another estrogen or combo drug will soon show up under a new label. And it will likely have similar lethal or debilitating side effects. And sadly, the new substances will once again be hailed as a miraculous "breakthrough" and will surface with different names and different promises (see appendix B).

Even as this fourth edition is going to press, some within the medical community have concluded that a monthly menses was really overdoing it on the part of our creator. This group of doctors and researchers are telling teenagers and cycling women that it's only necessary to have a period three to four times a year. Hence, the new buzz word *menstrual suppression*. And thus the latest and greatest synthetic hormone, Seasonale, is being marketed as the answer to all that messy monthly hassle and discomfort.

At this writing it is evident that the shocking news has already been forgotten. The results of clinical studies, not to mention the tragic testimonials of women involved in the WHI trials, don't seem to matter very much to the pharmaceutical and medical establishments. Once again the cover-up shows itself loud and clear as we hear commercials for the "improved, low dose" of Prempro. It is being advertised in a new campaign that promises relief, but that still carries the same risks and warnings regarding the dangers of this drug. A drug that was only recently removed due to its serious and potentially fatal effects. If it has the same warnings and contraindications, how can simply lowering the dose make it safe? Such ads are used to encourage susceptible women to rush to their gynecologist requesting the latest version of HRT. We can be sure that once again there will be more experimental trials using other women in order to feed this multibillion-dollar menopausal industry. Before that happens, we encourage you to read the fine print on the "new and improved synthetic drugs."

Through independent studies included in this fourth edition, we hope that readers will become empowered with facts concerning real causes and effective cures for breast cancer and other female disorders. Instead of being duped by magazine and TV advertisements sponsored by high-profile companies that discourage us from seeking a healthy life through prevention, the reader will have a clearer understanding about what's behind the fundraising "runs" and "walks." Perhaps we need to think twice about pink ribbon days (see Breast Cancer Awareness in appendix D), or the invasive chemotherapy procedures given to cancer patients that often result in heart attacks (as occurred with one of my own relatives).

As we become better educated about safer alternatives and become more aware of the social, economical, and environmental influences which prolong harmful health habits, we will be able to understand more clearly the distinction between the *politics* and the *evidence*. Our mission as authors is to give you the facts that will assist you in weaning yourself away from synthetic hormones as well as antidepressants and other drugs. Perhaps it is now time for all women to take matters into their own hands when it comes to the issue of hormone balance rather than just taking *what the doctor prescribes*.

Introduction

We can drift along with general opinion and tradition, or we can throw ourselves upon the guidance of the soul and steer courageously toward truth.

Helen Keller [1]

In our lives we often face situations that are new, perhaps even overwhelming. We find we have to make educated choices without sufficient education being available to us. As women, we may be barred from the knowledge critical to managing our own unique health problems from puberty through old age. Natural hormone replacement therapy, for example, is seldom provided as an option, and few of us know about it. Instead, the medical world continues to stick with its same conventional therapies, exposing us to the hostile and long-term side effects of synthetic hormones.

This story begins years ago before much was known about the physiology of the menstrual cycle. For many women the monthly cycle came and went with little or no discomfort. But for a significant number it was, as it is now, a time of physical and emotional affliction, often quite severe, and there was little that could be done about it.

Gradually, however, help began to arrive. The role of hormones in the menstrual cycle came to be understood better. Doctors began prescribing synthetic hormones as an antidote to the distress of premenstrual syndrome (PMS) and later in life's progression, menopause. Women were given the hope that these chemically-altered hormones would rid them of the unpleasant menstrual or menopausal symptoms that many of them experienced. But unfortunately, far too often, such hormones just made the symptoms worse.

Today, we have a fresh opportunity to halt the onslaught of hot flashes, night sweats, bloating, tension, fatigue, cramping, mercurial moods, and depression that may accompany an imbalance in our essential hormones. That opportunity is NHRT: natural hormone replacement therapy, as opposed to the usual synthetic HRT. I invite you to learn how and why plant-derived progesterone can help prevent the symptoms of PMS and menopause, including osteoporosis, fibrocystic breast disease, cardiovascular disorders, and painful endometriosis; how it can help with many pregnancy-related problems; and how it may help reverse diseases ranging from vaginal atrophy to heart disease and even cancer.[2, 3]

Part of our challenge is to find qualified, open-minded, good medical doctors to work with us. One of those high on my list is the late Dr. Robert S. Mendelsohn. His insight and spirit captured the hearts of many, and his philosophy echoes over and over again in a wealth of articles and books about health.

Besides drawing from the wisdom of Dr. Mendelsohn, I'm delighted to introduce to the reader several other eminent minds. One you will be hearing about in the course of this book is Julian Whitaker, M.D. Often, while browsing in health food stores, I've heard people talking about the latest breakthroughs in natural healing publicized in his newsletter. Many of these customers were at one time exhausted and disheartened by adverse reactions to the various drugs that had been prescribed to them. Natural options such as those presented by Dr. Whitaker help to ease the decisions we must sometimes make concerning our health.

After reading the following paragraph from his newsletter *Health & Healing*, I knew immediately he would be added to my cadre of out-of-town medical advisors. He says, "In medical school . . . I was taught that the only tools that work to help people are drugs and surgery. In the twenty years since then, I have learned that a lot of what I was taught is just plain wrong. There are treatments for our most serious diseases that are not only safer than surgery and most drugs, but also *more powerful*." He continues, "The medical profession tends to promote what is good for the profession, not what is necessarily good for the patient. The doctor's joke, 'Better hurry up and operate before the patient gets well!' is truer than you think."[4]

I shudder to think of the patient who wants to make haste and "just get it over with" before looking into existing alternatives. I was such a patient many years ago. Now, shaped by life's experiences, I have learned to be much more inquisitive.

One day, reading one of Dr. Whitaker's newsletters, I enthusiastically jumped out of my chair and ran to tell my husband, Jack, about the abundance of information it gave on natural hormone replacement therapy. After having looked for so many years, I couldn't believe that such knowledge was suddenly available. I was so delighted I could hardly get the words out of my mouth. From this moment I was on the path that finally resolved my long-standing misery—the path that would eventually lead to the publication of this book.

I soon became immersed in the findings of natural hormone research. I came across some incredible accounts, both personal and clinical, involving botanical progesterone.

The chronology of events begins in the year 1938 with the first adaptation of plant hormones to conform to human progesterone. In time, this discovery by research chemist Dr. Russell E. Marker[5] was followed by the work of other pioneers. Three decades later came Dr. Katharina Dalton's studies on the use of progesterone in prenatal care, recorded in the *British Journal of Psychiatry* (1968).[6] Ten years after that (1978), the *Journal of the American Medical Association* made further extraordinary revelations regarding natural hormone replacement;[7] and in 1989 the research of Joel T. Hargrove, M.D., and his colleagues on micronizing (finely grinding) progesterone for better absorption appeared in the *Journal of Obstetrics and Gynecology*.[8] A couple of years later (1991), a landmark review by Jerilynn C. Prior, M.D., on progesterone and the prevention of osteoporosis was published in the *Canadian Journal of OB/Gyn & Women's Health Care*.[9]

And for some of the most thorough and comprehensive work of the present day, we are indebted to the late John R. Lee, M.D., a leader in the field of natural progesterone. Raymond F. Peat, Ph.D. (an early mentor of Dr. Lee), Alan R. Gaby, M.D., Jonathan V. Wright, M.D., Betty Kamen, Ph.D., C. Norman Shealy, M.D., Ph.D., and Jane Heimlich are some of the many others who have pursued the truth and have been willing to share it with all women.

The chapters to follow will emphasize the accumulated knowledge of these noted authorities on subjects that range from combating stress and lowering cholesterol to fertility, easier pregnancy, and successful breastfeeding. The last chapter of the book, as well as appendix F, is devoted to helping women locate a doctor interested in correcting the complex deficiencies that occur before, during, and after menopause.

My book was inspired by physicians who realize the importance of natural foods, vitamins, minerals, herbs, homeopathy, chiropractic, and, most specifically, botanical hormone replacement therapy. I hold in great esteem those who put themselves on the firing line, up against many of their colleagues, for the sake of what is best for their patients' health.

The health care practitioners who will be featured in this book recognize the injustice the medical community has promoted in the name of "consumer welfare." Their compassionate efforts to reeducate the public have encouraged me to seek out, try, and then share these ideas. Although I wish I'd come across this information when I was younger, I feel blessed that it came my way at all. Now, past menopause, I actually feel more energetic than ever before. I have regained my health and vitality since discovering the natural way.

The revelations in these chapters should be read by all women and by those who care about them. We must start early to prevent chronic disease. Fatigue, headaches, heart disease, osteoporosis, and cancer, for example, can have various causes. Among these are a decline in hormones, unwholesome diet, food additives, environmental toxins, and nerve interference. Let's say, for our purposes, that the cause is indeed a hormone deficiency. If we take prescription drugs to cover up what is really a decline or lack of natural progesterone, more often than not our condition becomes worse.

Yet, the subject of hormone replacement is complicated because no two women's bodily needs are the same. For instance, past trauma or stress may cause some women to experience premenopausal symptoms in their thirties. Even the woman who sails through menopause without feeling any changes whatsoever is still at risk for cancer, heart disease, and osteoporosis. But regardless of how much estrogen we have, progesterone is our real concern because of the fact that very little is made anywhere in the body once ovulation ceases. As progesterone declines below one's estrogen level a hormone imbalance, with its many complications, is established.

Needless to say, it's important to know as much as possible about natural versus synthetic hormones and the side effects of the latter. First of all, you should know that *natural* progesterone is seldom prescribed by medical doctors. Yet it was first crystallized from plant sources in 1938 and is readily available today. Most doctors don't know about it and don't even consider it when making recommendations to their patients. Why not? Probably because it is not a prescription drug. Although it may not be carried by your local pharmacist, it is available in natural compounding pharmacies (which are listed in appendix G) and health stores. However, most physicians haven't educated themselves or their patients about the benefits of such treatment.

John R. Lee, M.D., sheds some light on the reason why it's so hard to get information on natural progesterone from our traditional health care providers:

> Pharmaceutical sales success and profit are . . . also dependent on the patentability of the compounds to be sold. Since natural compounds (i.e., the hormone molecule as made by the ovary) cannot be patented, it

is in the interest of the pharmaceutical industry to create compounds which are not identical to the natural hormone and are nowhere found in nature.[10]

Some medical doctors have told their patients that Provera, a synthesized compound, is progesterone. It is not![11] In fact, Dr. Lee informs us that it mimics only some of the activity of progesterone and is not identical. He says that altered and synthesized hormones such as Provera "may also provoke biologic responses which are undesirable or toxic. This is seen, for example, in the extensive lists of warnings, precautions, and side effects which accompany the descriptions of the synthetic hormones as found in the PDR (*Physicians' Desk Reference*)."[12] See appendix B.

Synthetic material does wonders in the making of cars, clothes, and Tupperware—but how desirable can it be for our biological needs? Before I started using natural hormones on a regular basis, I asked the pharmacists at the Women's International Pharmacy some questions. The research material they sent convinced me that natural progesterone is effective and is a plant-based substance containing no animal by-products. They explained that the botanical hormone diosgenin is a sterol, or saponin—an oil manufactured by many plants, including the wild yam, and easy to extract.

In the body, we make (synthesize) progesterone from pregnenolone, which is synthesized from cholesterol. In the lab, the chemist makes (synthesizes) progesterone from diosgenin. This *diosgenin* from the wild yam—like the stigmasterol from soybeans—is actually a precursor to a number of hormones. Thus, with only slight modification it can be made to duplicate the progesterone molecule the body produces so that it can be fully utilized as needed.[13]

The ensuing chapters will present a wealth of studies concerning the many applications of this natural hormone. We'll see how women who have suffered for most of their lives with various female problems have not only derived relief from their disorders but often achieved reversal of life-threatening illnesses such as osteoporosis and cancer.

We have no time to lose. I challenge women everywhere to use the information gathered here to evaluate for themselves all the pros and cons of hormonal treatment. We need to know the varied and multiple benefits of the natural form of progesterone over the synthetic, and to be thoroughly informed about the serious risks of pharmaceutical hormone products. As you will see in appendix G, even in the realm of natural hormone replacement therapy, there are wide variations in bioavailability and effectiveness in the multitude of new botanical products that are flooding the marketplace.

Unfortunately, previous generations have not had much choice in these matters. I can't help thinking of my own mother. Although she was a nurse, she didn't have this knowledge. I watched her slowly weaken from osteoporosis and disorders of the heart and kidneys. She became frail and bent over. Osteoporosis made her hip pain so severe that she was hardly able to lie on one side or even sit.

Because of my own experience with hormone imbalance, I have come to consider health problems as teachers, progressively opening my eyes to the power of the medicine found in nature. There is no need to be dependent on synthetic hormones or other drugs, which often cause sickness and premature aging. Age should not be a matter of how many years we have been living but rather a matter of the integrity of the tissues of the body. One's "age" is also shaped by a positive mental outlook—by seeking what is good and acting upon what is sound, not only for the body but for the mind and spirit.

This leads me to reflect upon the philosophy of a truly great woman who suffered from severe limitations. Helen Keller, rather than dwelling on her misfortune, actively sought ways in which she could be of some service to her fellow human beings as a contributing member of society. Her own constraints and her strong religious faith led Helen to understand and express in her writings a conflict we often face:

> We can drift along with general opinion and tradition, or we can throw ourselves upon the guidance of the soul within and steer courageously toward truth. . . . We have a choice in every event and every limitation and . . . to choose is to create.[14]

This book doesn't pretend to have all the answers, but it does provide a thought-provoking look at the choices now available. During the relatively short span of a few years that it took to compile and write it, the procession of ever-changing information has marched on. To the best of my ability, I have presented an accurate picture of natural hormones based on what we know today. Of course, some parts of this picture might change tomorrow.

But one thing we do know for certain is that what the medical profession *has* been doing in the way of hormone replacement is not working. We know there is a better way, and we've opened a dialogue that is bound to lead us there—as long as we continue to ask the right questions with open minds. Naturally, those at high risk or with a history of serious health problems should do their homework and ask even more questions. Here we've tried to initiate this process.

Seldom in the past have our medical options been made very clear to us; yet, these decisions can have such a profound influence on our lives. Since my venture into natural healing I have personally felt an exhilaration, never experienced before, about the choices that are now available among the more gentle forms of health care. As we realize and experience their harmony with nature, we will also discover a gift of life.

PART I

Natural Hormone
Replacement
from
God's Garden

ONE

Sick and Tired of Being Tired and Sick

Study sickness while you are well.
Thomas Fuller [1]

Something was wrong. I was in my forties, and the symptoms of menopause had already appeared. Hot flashes, bloating, irregularity, trouble sleeping, night sweats, emotional tension—I realized that I needed some kind of help to cope! The hormonal changes that every woman experiences at midlife were playing havoc with my body. So I went to see my gynecologist. He responded with the standard, widely accepted medical treatment: a program of hormone replacement therapy (HRT) using synthetic hormones. Specifically, this meant a prescription for Premarin (a conjugated estrogen) and Provera (medroxyprogesterone acetate, a progestin). These are manufactured substitutes for two hormones that play a central role in every woman's sexual and reproductive life—hormones whose supply and balance are gradually altered as a woman passes through and beyond the normal childbearing years.

I had thought to myself, "Here I am in menopause. Finally, I'll have freedom from my monthly periods." But instead I was told that I needed to take these hormone supplements and continue drug-induced monthly cycles for the rest of my life. For twenty-five days each month I was to take one tablet of Premarin, and from the sixteenth through the twenty-fifth day of each month I was to take the progestin tablet. Then I was to stop taking both drugs for five days.

Even though I couldn't help feeling that my body was being artificially regulated, my first reaction to the drugs was generally positive. My menstrual cycle stabilized, the symptoms diminished, and I began to feel confident about my doctor's advice. By the second day my body was adjusting well. I became calmer and slowly began to feel better in many ways. "Why didn't I do this sooner?" I thought. "Such a simple solution to all of these problems!" I *wanted* to believe that routine HRT was the answer.

Before long, though, my honeymoon with synthetic hormones came to an end. In the second month I started to worry. There were some unpleasant new side effects, including weight gain, bloating, painful breasts, and tension. I wondered whether this was not the answer after all—at least, not the whole answer. Perhaps a change was in order. Maybe the dosage of the Premarin or Provera needed to be decreased or one or both of them discontinued, or maybe the whole approach was wrong. Disappointed now with my doctor's treatment, I consulted an endocrinologist, then an internist, and later still another gynecologist. All offered different suggestions, but none of their drugs helped my symptoms without bringing on some other abnormal discomfort. This trial-and-error period continued for several years.

Speaking with other women going through similar experiences, I heard a common complaint. They had gone down this same road with doctors who had prescribed variations of the same treatment, and as we all tend to do, followed their doctors' advice and just "hung in there." Women would come home from an appointment in tears of frustration because the doctor had made no change in their treatment regardless of the unpleasant reactions. The typical advice they got, as did I, was "You need to be patient. Just keep taking the pills a little longer until the body adapts." Generally a physician will urge a woman to continue her treatment, either varying the dosage or keeping it the same, on the premise that her body will eventually adjust to synthetic hormones. I can tell you that such advice will drive some women to their psychiatrists or closest medical centers in an attempt to deal with the drugs' multiple side effects.

I wanted my doctors to be right. So I did what they prescribed, over and over again. At first I'd be encouraged, because the drugs were making a few changes that I thought were good. But as time went on and it was clear that my body was reacting poorly, I began to feel additional symptoms: sharp uterine pain and inflammation and infection of the cervix, which was often quite painful. My bloating became more severe, along with digestive disorders such as colitis.

I feared another D&C (dilation and curettage), which some physicians routinely administer to women on HRT, and I dreaded the painful cauterization of cervical tissue that I'd been told was necessary to deal with the cervical inflammation. Yet I'd learned that the scar tissue resulting from some of the treatments I'd already had was probably causing even more harm to surrounding tissue! I grew more anxious still when a second endometrial biopsy (removal of a piece of the uterine lining by means of a plastic catheter) had to be performed in order to check for any deterioration of my uterus. Frustrated, I did not know what to do. I had to make up my mind before my next doctor's appointment, when he'd indicated he would probably recommend a hysterectomy.

As I continued to ask questions, I began to understand that the doctors I had been seeing all along didn't necessarily have all the answers. They didn't seem to comprehend completely the complexities of menopausal problems, the PMS problems of younger women, or the side effects of the synthetic hormones they were prescribing. Not only were their answers contradictory to each other, I sensed a lack of conviction on their part that this was indeed the right way to go. I thought to myself, *Is it any wonder women become confused, afraid, and discouraged during what can already be a stressful time?*

I decided I would have to take things into my own hands—maybe spend more time at the health store instead of the drugstore, and at least learn enough to direct my own treatment. I had lots of unanswered questions about why these hormone supplements were not working. What were synthetic hormones all about? Where did they come from and how did they work? What were the side effects—both immediate and long-term? Were alternative treatments available? What specific nutrients and exercises would help? And of course, the question that hung over it all: Whose advice should I believe, and what should I do?

Thus began my journey of discovery into the world of estrogen and progesterone and the roles these hormones play in women's health—a journey that not only led me to the answers to my many questions but in the process prepared me to recognize the variety of available alternatives. The answer has restored peace and health to my life.

THE SEARCH BEGINS

My goal became to find a complete and sound alternative treatment for my menopausal problems. After consultation with my doctor I immediately stopped using the synthetic progesterone substitute because it was causing dreadful feelings of stress throughout my body. I accepted his advice on the estrogen supplement, though, and continued to take it.

But I also began looking into other measures I had heard about, such as nutrition, herbs, and homeopathic remedies recommended specifically for menopause. I changed my diet to include more raw vegetables, fresh fruits, whole grains, seeds, and complex carbohydrates and less meat. These changes helped reduce some of my discomfort. I also added to my diet some known antioxidants, including vitamins A, C, and E, plus selenium as well as vitamin B complex and zinc. I learned that zinc plays an important role in enzyme activity, especially in relation to the lymphocytes, and is needed for the absorption of vitamin A.[2] I had also become aware that many studies have shown that antioxidants help protect the body from toxins.

As long as I kept up my chiropractic treatments to enhance nerve flow and transmission, I was much less susceptible to gynecological infections and other disorders. I had learned that even though the right diet is important, the nervous system is the major regulator for all hormonal performance. I believe that spinal misalignments and subsequent nerve interference should always be addressed because of the close interconnection between the spinal nerves and the endocrine system.[3]

But those were the early years. Once the full force of menopause came upon me, some of the old symptoms resurfaced—though they were less pronounced than before. So either something major was still missing, or what I was taking (or doing) needed to be changed. I was ready to try anything just to feel normal. I talked to many other women in the same predicament, and eventually one of them gave me a new idea. She was a former nurse and knew about the Estraderm patch, a "time-release" patch that is placed on the surface of the skin so that estrogen is absorbed in small doses over time. I wondered why my doctor hadn't mentioned this.

I asked my doctor to substitute this method for my oral Premarin, and he agreed. This small adhesive pad did, in fact, seem to work better for me initially. Certain symptoms, such as the joint pains I'd been experiencing, temporarily went away. I felt more energetic at first, but I knew we hadn't found the solution yet.

I had read that estrogen should never be taken alone, so I sought out a female gynecologist and asked her about combining it with progesterone to cancel out the carcinogenic effect of the estrogen. When I told her I'd had a very bad reaction to Provera, she prescribed another of the synthetic substitutes for progesterone. Only later did I learn of the incredible difference between synthetic progesterone and natural (bioidentical) progesterone.

Before long I again lapsed into some of the same symptoms, and again it was from the effects of the synthetic hormones: nervousness, bloating, uterine cramping, and some sleepless nights. So I went to another doctor, and he decided to reduce the dose of estrogen to the lowest level available in patch form. As the months went by it became apparent that this wasn't working either. I knew something still wasn't right and was disappointed with all the experimenting. The vaginal dryness that had troubled me before I began HRT returned with all its associated pain and discomfort. I had also developed strange pains on the side of my breast, near the lymph nodes.

My doctor switched me to yet another synthetic progesterone substitute in the lowest dosage available. There followed more adjustments: less estrogen, then more, then back to Provera, then less of it, and so on. But nothing seemed to help. I kept trying in vain to find the right balance between the two drugs, thinking that the doctor knew best. I did not understand why my body was reacting as it did to these substances, or why they seemed to be doing more harm than good as time progressed.

I decided one day to stop the treatments completely. This decision came after I got out my magnifying glass and read the fine print that presented the risks and warnings on the leaflets accompanying the drugs. Some possible adverse reactions to synthetic hormones are liver disease, malignancy of the breast or genital organs, fluid retention, cystitis-like syndrome, headaches, nervousness, dizziness, edema, mental depression, insomnia, fatigue, and backache. The warnings on the package go on to point out that the drugs can cause or aggravate conditions such as epilepsy, migraine, asthma, and cardiac or renal dysfunction.[4] And all of the other estrogens and progestins normally prescribed have similar lists of side effects.

No wonder I was feeling bad. I began to resent the fact that the knowledge I desperately needed on such important health matters is not made readily available to women. At times I wondered how I would ever get through postmenopause if I couldn't get a grip on these menopausal years. Frankly, I was now afraid to take estrogen and the progesterone substitutes, which I understood at the time to be the only available source of progesterone.

But admittedly, I was getting some benefit from these drugs. When I stopped taking them, the old symptoms flared up. I even noticed that my chiropractic adjustments held better when I was on HRT. I also experienced an interesting phenomenon during these years of off-again, on-again hormone replacement: every time I stopped taking my hormones, I felt joint aches and knee pains. The more I monitored my hormone therapy by such signs and symptoms, the more suspicious I became that hormones (or the lack thereof) might very well be contributing to this reaction. I have since learned that other women have also come to associate muscle and joint pains with menopause.

On one hand, not taking the drugs was an obvious way to avoid the adverse reactions they could cause; on the other hand, giving them up meant losing their temporary benefits. A constant battle raged within my mind and body. I went back on the Estraderm patch, but in the meantime started reading everything I could find on the subject of hormones to try to find a new direction.

My hopes were turned into real fear when I read this statement in a report by Dr. Brian Henderson: "The patch produces higher levels of the most potent form of estrogen (estradiol) than does Premarin, giving a woman almost as much hormone as she would have made herself." Dr. Henderson continued, "The effect of that should be to make one's breast cancer risk go up substantially more on the patch than on Premarin."[5] It took that warning of a worst-case scenario for me to end my nearly ten years of experimenting with synthetic hormone replacement. I never found any combination or dosage of synthetic hormones that gave me enough benefits to compensate for the side effects that always accompanied their use. I felt blessed that I had not yet contracted cancer, but I remained terribly confused. Where could I turn next?

The beginning of the solution came to me when Dr. Julian Whitaker's *Health & Healing* newsletter arrived. What he had to say sent my hopes soaring. The information and phone numbers he included provided me answers to some of the questions I had asked doctors for so many years: "What specifically does *progesterone* do? How can we get natural hormones? Do we always need a prescription?" Could it be that what I was about to explore would actually resolve what had seemed a never-ending quest? Was it possible that my fears and anxieties could be a thing of the past? I truly hoped so.

My mailbox soon began to fill up with research reports and abstracts that I had requested. They told me that there was a natural, plant-based source of progesterone that had none of the side effects of the synthetic substitutes. Eager and willing, I kept rereading the encouraging words of Dr. John R. Lee from a statement in the periodical *Medical Hypotheses:* "Progesterone is inexpensive, being available from many plant sources. . . . Furthermore, it is remarkably free from side-effects."[6]

More information arrived in an educational brochure distributed by the Women's Health Connection in Madison, Wisconsin:

> The process of producing natural progesterone, which is made from yams and soybeans, was discovered by Russell Marker, a Pennsylvania State College chemistry professor. While experimenting with sapogenins, a group of plant steroids, in the jungles of Mexico in the 1930s, Marker realized that progesterone could be transformed by chemical process

from the sapogenin, diosgenin, which is found naturally in yams.

Unlike medroxyprogesterone [the chemical name for Provera], natural micronized progesterone is an exact chemical duplicate of the progesterone that is produced by the human body.

Another immediate difference between medroxyprogesterone and natural progesterone is that the synthetic hormone can actually lower a patient's blood level of progesterone. Some women who take medroxyprogesterone to combat PMS or oppose estrogen in menopause, report headaches, mood swings and fluid retention.

The more information I acquired, the more questions I had. How, why, and where does natural progesterone work in the body? The answers later came to fill a whole chapter of this book. But I am getting ahead of myself. I was so relieved to find that such a natural hormone existed that I immediately ordered a jar of cream made from these naturally occurring plant sterols. No prescription was needed. When it arrived, I quickly read the directions and applied the cream to my skin. It is a fat-soluble compound that is absorbed into the skin and taken up by the fatty layer beneath. From there it is transferred into the bloodstream to circulate throughout the body.

In the days and months that followed, I experienced a peace of mind that I had not felt in many years. Enjoying my new sense of well-being was like living in a new body—no sharp uterine pains, no bloating, no tension. Best of all, my energy level was high, and I was able to sleep at night. I continued using the progesterone every day, secure in the knowledge that it was safe. It brought innumerable health benefits without artificially continuing my menstrual periods for the rest of my life.

I quickly learned that with *natural* hormone replacement therapy (NHRT), it was important for me to use the product daily for three weeks out of every month. I added this to my regimen of vitamins, minerals, other nutritional supplements, chiropractic care, and exercise. I found that all of these components were vital for optimal health and in supporting my natural HRT program. The plant-derived progesterone had greatly reduced the irritating conditions I've already described, such as fluid retention, colitis, joint pain, and sleep disorders. As my discomforts slowly diminished, I realized that this remarkable "phytohormone" had eliminated much of what used to be stress and had given me new stamina and energy.

I gradually became more active yet calmer when dealing with family and business issues. The benefits for me were obvious very quickly. Like most women I have talked to, I found that applying the contents of approximately one two-ounce jar of progesterone cream each month to various areas of the skin is quite sufficient to remedy the majority of problems. Further details on when and how to use the cream will be offered throughout the book; for other modes of hormone use, see appendix A.

Indeed, I have learned that progesterone can be found not only in the cream form but also in a capsule form (micronized for better absorption). I had my internist call in a prescription for a specific dosage of this to one of the numerous pharmacies that specialize in formulating natural products. At prescription strength, it is covered by most insurance companies, which makes NHRT quite affordable. The suppliers are located in various cities throughout the country (see appendix G). You can also order sublingual drops (applied under the tongue) or a micronized spray (applied to the mucous membranes of the cheeks) rather than the cream form. Some studies have found that the sublingual method provides approximately three times the concentration found in some of the nonprescription creams.[7]

I added this prescription for micronized capsules to my natural hormone program for two simple reasons: (1) I knew exactly how many milligrams I was taking, and (2) it was covered by insurance. At the time, I didn't want to bother with the blood or saliva testing because of the inconvenience and the expense. My choice served me well for several years, and I had never felt better.

As I read and learned more, however, I realized that although the prescription indicated exactly how many milligrams I was ingesting, this was not necessarily the amount of progesterone that was being absorbed by my body. Questions arose for me, such as, "After progesterone is altered in the liver, how much of the real progesterone are you getting? Is your liver functioning at a hundred percent efficiency?" I didn't have the answers, so I thought it prudent to begin dissolving my pills sublingually.*

At the same time I am quite happy with the results of using the transdermal progesterone cream on a routine basis. I have found that it also has many other uses. For instance, I sometimes massage it where I have back, hip, or knee pains. Doctors now report that rubbing progesterone cream or oil directly onto the joint or painful area helps their patients.[8]

It's important for all of us to ask lots of questions prior to choosing the type of product (creams, pills, or drops) to use. We need to evaluate these according to strength, purity, and quality of the delivery system and relate these to the degree of our symptoms and estrogen dominance. I have

---

* Since individual needs can vary greatly, depending on the health of one's liver and adrenals, some women may want to obtain an adrenal stress and hormone level evaluation.

concluded that it's well worth the time and effort required to move toward the goal of satisfying one's unique requirements.

I've learned a great deal about progesterone, especially since coming upon one of the most informative books of all on the subject: *Natural Progesterone: The Multiple Roles of a Remarkable Hormone*. Its author, John R. Lee, M.D., instructs us not only about progesterone's molecular structure and the interplay of our natural hormones but also about the many advantages of using the cream. "How long should a woman stay on this natural progesterone cream?" Dr. Lee is often asked. He replies, "I want them to stay on it till they are ninety-six and then we'll reevaluate!"[9]

Later, after putting into practice what I knew at last to be essential to my overall health, I learned of the wide-ranging implications of natural hormone replacement therapy for other health problems. Principal among these are cancer, osteoporosis, and heart disease. It is well known that the use of synthetic hormones increases a woman's risk of breast and endometrial cancer; the use of natural progesterone changes those odds. As for osteoporosis, only recently has the importance of this type of hormone therapy become known for treating bone loss. I will show you evidence that natural progesterone therapy can halt and even reverse the effects of osteoporosis. Sections of this book cover each of these subjects, as well as the connection of progesterone to cardiovascular problems.[10]

For decades the medical community promoted estrogen for its health benefits for the heart only to find that it could actually cause long-term side effects such as heart disorders, blood clots, stroke, and even cancer.[11-14] The first edition of this book was published in 1997. It explained then, as it does today, that natural progesterone offers protection in its antispasmodic effect in the body. In fact this natural hormone functions as a vasodilator to prevent or regulate coronary artery spasms, whereas progestins such as Provera often contribute to cardiovascular disorders.[15-18] On this subject it was interesting to read a *Health Dispatch Newsletter* from Dr. David Williams (August 4, 2003) reporting that estrogen can elevate homocysteine levels and contribute to clogging of the arteries by depleting vitamins B_6, B_{12}, and folic acid.

Throughout this book we see, however, that the use of natural progesterone is the hormone that should have been heralded for its variety of physiological benefits. Studies demonstrate that natural progesterone, the all-too-often overlooked hormone, is effective in opposing estrogen's stimulatory effect as found in cancer and other such "cellular over-growth" diseases—both benign and malignant.[19, 20] Raising progesterone levels has also been shown to be effective for a variety of physiological disorders from osteoporosis and postpartum depression to premenstrual epilepsy. Research continues to show us that rebalancing of hormone levels by focusing on progesterone deficiency is crucial in achieving wellness.[21–28]

As we unearth solutions that guide us toward optimal health, we often discover that the answers are found not in just one area of the natural sciences but in many. Raw foods, natural nutritional supplements, and exercise are among the many healthy ways we can encourage the body's innate healing power. By addressing hormonal, neurological, and nutritional deficiencies, we can better attain a greater mental clarity and a more serene confidence in God's power. Through these channels we can turn our negative stress and anxiety into positive opportunities for growth, learning, and service to others.

VICTORY AND RESPONSIBILITY

The thought of the legions of women who have met conflict and contention with their physicians in the search for better health prompts me to recall the struggle of Helen Keller, as depicted in a recent book about her life, *Light in My Darkness*. I could not help but be affected by what her editor described as Helen's "unwavering faith in God's plan, as she fought and then found through her religion that every human life is of sacred importance and dignity."[29]

Faced with misfortune, we either succumb to our impediments and prejudices, or overcome them. And as Helen aptly expresses it, "Life is either a daring adventure or it is nothing."[30] As we forge ahead with the knowledge we have at hand, we are better prepared for tomorrow's challenges—a bit wiser concerning our choices and more mindful of how to protect ourselves and our dignity.

As for myself, the moment I learned what is good and natural for homeostasis—our internal balance—is a moment of truth I will never forget. I knew then (and my experience confirmed) what I must also convey to others who are suffering from the grim side effects of synthetic hormones and other related medication.

Trust your own intuition. If at first your doctor says, "Oh, you're too young to worry about menopause and hormone replacement therapy," you can ask for tests such as those for LH (luteinizing hormone) and FSH (follicle-stimulating hormone), which measure hormone messages between your pituitary and ovaries. Do this before you are given a diuretic or pills for pain, insomnia, "nerves," or high blood pressure. However, note that although FSH does go up at menopause, Sandra Coney in *The Menopause Industry: How the Medical Establishment Exploits Women*, says there is disagreement among doctors as to the level that confirms the reaching of menopause. Furthermore, she says, "hormones can fluctuate wildly during the menopausal transition (40–50 years old) and even for some months after the last period; . . . therefore, biochemical tests cannot accurately predict whether a woman is menopausal [and] are really not much use."[31]

According to Dr. John R. Lee, Harvard University's Dr. Peter Ellison "has shown that you can get a more accurate measure of the functional level of estrogen and progesterone by measuring it in saliva" rather than in the blood. "It's logical," he says, "and less expensive."[32] To find out where you can order a saliva hormone level test kit to use in the privacy of your own home, see chapter 7. Certain laboratories also perform a more comprehensive version of this test, if ordered by your doctor.

Without any testing, the doctor may just prescribe stopgap medication, with the reassuring words, "This will calm you down so you can get through the day. It will also help you sleep."

Does this sound familiar? And keep in mind that, with so many other patients needing attention, once you have left the office you may be "out of sight, out of mind." In the end, *you alone* are responsible for yourself. No one else is likely to be willing to invest as much time or effort as you are in your own welfare.

I invite you to learn how and why plant-derived progesterone can help prevent the symptoms of PMS, menopause, osteoporosis,[33] fibrocystic breast disease,[34] and painful endometriosis[35] and may reverse disorders ranging from blood clotting to vaginal atrophy[36] and even some forms of cancer.[37] And should progesterone alone not prove effective, I encourage you to examine your diet and research other natural alternatives such as maca, which is one of a variety of support systems we discuss in chapter 6.

I hope that for others who, like me, have experienced PMS or childbirth difficulties or the complicated trek through the premenopausal, perimenopausal, and postmenopausal passage, this book will provide some well-deserved solutions.

TWO

The Myth of Estrogen Deficiency Versus the Reality of Progesterone Deficiency

*The medical mindset of estrogen prescribed alone represents
a victory of advertising over science.*
John R. Lee, M.D.[1]

Most women don't want to run to their doctors for every ache or minor illness that comes their way. They'd rather just wait it out and let the body heal itself. Or maybe, like me, they're simply afraid to go—anxious about being misdiagnosed or having to bring home yet another package of potent prescription drugs, with their usual side effects. Or they're concerned about having to endure a deluge of tests, perhaps to be told that there is nothing wrong and to be presented with a huge bill.

As we age, our bodies can come to seem less friendly, putting us through many tests and challenges. I've seen this particularly in my older relatives and friends as they've begun to suffer from joint pain and arthritis in their fragile bodies. And it's hard to forget my own mother and elderly aunts, maneuvering cautiously and living as best they could with their pain. Nor are they alone among the countless women who have become dependent on family, friends, or nursing homes. Because most have never been exposed to natural hormone replacement therapy (NHRT), they are especially prone to increasing osteoporotic symptoms and heart problems, which force upon them sedentary lifestyles.

The great news is that we can avoid or lessen the severity of these conditions. Our challenge is to overcome our lack of education about what happens in a woman's body at puberty, during the menstrual cycle, and finally just before, during, and after menopause. The average woman is in the dark about the underlying causes of many of the problems she'll encounter at these times. As a result, she may accept treatment or therapy that is not really in her best interest. Unless we all take charge of our own bodies, we will continue to experience the same traumatic consequences.

In the pages to come, we'll discuss all this in detail. But first I would like to review some relevant basics about a woman's hormonal system, define some terms we'll be using, and look at some standard medical therapies.

THE RIGHT BALANCE OF HORMONES

Both progesterone and estrogen are vital to the life and well-being of every woman. These hormones are produced primarily in the ovaries, beginning at puberty and continuing, in the case of estrogen, for the rest of her life. The two hormones exist in a delicate balance, and variations in that balance can have a dramatic effect on one's health. Additionally, the amount of these hormones that the body produces from month to month and year to year can vary, depending on a whole host of factors such as stress, nutrition, and exercise.

Finally, at the onset of menopause there is a radical change in the ovaries: the production of estrogen decreases significantly and the production of progesterone virtually stops. This causes a major shift in the fine balance between the two hormones that the body has attempted to maintain to that point. This imbalance leads, inevitably, to the unpleasant menopausal symptoms many women experience.

This might be a good place to point out that the chemical building block for many of the body's hormones is cholesterol. Not enough emphasis is placed on the importance of our good cholesterol. Cholesterol is the first step in a complex process. It is converted into pregnenolone, which is the precursor of both progesterone and dehydroepiandrosterone (DHEA). From one or the other of these hormones, in turn, come androstenedione, testosterone, and the estrogens. So progesterone, estrogen, testosterone, and DHEA are all made from cholesterol.[2]

Estrogen is thought of as *the* female sex hormone. It is responsible for triggering all of the changes that take place in a girl's body at puberty and for sustaining them in later life, and it plays a vital role in the menstrual cycle. Unlike progesterone, which is a single hormone, estrogen is actually the general name for a group of perhaps twenty different female hormones of very similar structure and function. The most important of these are *estrone, estradiol,* and *estriol.*

In this book we will generally follow the layperson's convention of speaking of estrogen as if it were a single hormone. But bear in mind when we do so that we are really speaking of the actions of one or more of the particular estrogens. In the final chapter we will discuss how exposure to and accumulation of the variety of estrogens, whether naturally derived (phytoestrogens), prescribed (HRT), or environmental (xenoestrogens), are heavily taxing our hormone balance. And as Dr. Norman Shealy points out, "estrone, estrodial, plant estrogens . . . and the petrochemical estrogens are potentially carcinogenic, particularly for the breast, uterus, ovaries, and probably the male's prostate."[3]

Both progesterone and estrogen in their ovarian production (endogenous) have many functions in the mature woman's body, but the most important for our initial consideration is probably their role in the control of the menstrual cycle. Here the two opposing hormones work in careful balance to control the woman's reproductive functions, time the cycle, and sustain any eventual pregnancy. On cue from follicle-stimulating hormone (FSH), which triggers an egg to mature, estrogen starts the endometrial buildup and controls the first part of the cycle. Without an adequate level of estrogen, the cycle will not start. Normally estrogen production gradually builds to a peak just before ovulation, then drops for the remainder of the cycle, dropping again at the end.

On the other hand, the ovaries dramatically increase their output of progesterone at the time of ovulation (release of the egg), about twelve or thirteen days into the cycle. They are prompted to do so by luteinizing hormone (LH) from the pituitary gland. The level of progesterone rises rapidly to a peak in three or four days, surpassing the level of estrogen, and remains elevated in order to develop and maintain the endometrium (uterine lining) in the event of conception. Progesterone dominates and controls the cycle during this latter half.

Progesterone is essential to the survival of the fetus and its continuing development until birth. Its name, in fact, is derived from this principal function: "pro-gestation." It has many other roles in a woman's body, though, and exerts a much broader impact on her health and vitality than might be supposed.

If conception does not occur, within ten or twelve days the levels of both progesterone and estrogen drop quickly, menses takes place, and the cycle starts over again. The dramatic drop of progesterone is the trigger that causes the body to shed the endometrium. In addition, it has been discovered that the presence of sufficient progesterone prior to ovulation (that is, for at least a week prior to its normal surge) prevents the release of an egg by either ovary. Knowledge of this phenomenon led to the development of birth control pills, which employ synthetic progesterone-like compounds that simulate this specific function of progesterone.

At menopause the body may reduce its production of estrogen but it almost completely halts the production of progesterone. The amount of estrogen in the body drops below what is necessary to start another menstrual cycle—so no cycle can start. However, estrogen is still present. The level of progesterone, on the other hand, drops to near zero in the ovaries. For all practical purposes, the female body becomes deficient in progesterone. This, then, is the condition of a woman's body after menopause—the presence of some estrogen accompanied by a virtual absence of progesterone.

Dr. Jerrilyn Prior explored the fluctuation of estrogen levels and found that prior to menopause they do not decline, but become more variable.[4] This is also documented by the study conducted by S. R. Cummings et al. who found a continuous adequate production of our own "endogenous" estradiol even after menopause in more than two-thirds of the women studied.[5] This data confirms our premise that we do not need estrogen replacement therapy but that progesterone is the hormone of choice—and only in its natural form.

In optimal circumstances before menopause, any negative physiological effects of estrogen are suppressed by the opposing effects of progesterone. In the menopausal woman, though, the imbalance of these hormones causes the deleterious effects of estrogen to surface. They include tendencies to increased body fat, salt and fluid retention, depression and headaches, and increased blood clotting—root causes of the well-known complaints of many menopausal women. As we shall see later, this same imbalance between progesterone and estrogen is frequently a cause of PMS in premenopausal women.

It's obvious, then, that a large number of women could benefit from the use of supplemental progesterone. It is very effective in treating or preventing the above conditions as well as menstrual irregularity, cramping, miscarriages, infertility, incontinence, endometriosis, hot flashes, night sweats, vaginal dryness, cardiovascular disorders, and more—because it restores the balance between estrogen and progesterone.[6-8]

Until recently the market was waiting for an abundant and inexpensive source of supply. A source was actually identified more than fifty years ago when scientists found progesterone-like substances occurring naturally in numerous plants. One of these was a substance found in the wild yam called diosgenin.* More important, researchers soon discovered that this natural substance could be easily converted to a compound that is bioidentical to the human progesterone. Today this hormone is formulated into a reliable, inexpensive, transdermal cream.[9] So the supply is now at hand.

The Standard Treatment

Unfortunately, natural substances themselves are not patentable and don't yield the large profit margins of proprietary drugs. So the pharmaceutical industry immediately went to work inventing synthetic (and profitable) prescriptive progesterone-like products derived from this same source of natural progesterone. Soon a whole new class of substances, called progestins, was created by the industry. These progestins are widely used today in birth control pills and are too often the drugs of choice in the medical field for treating PMS and menopausal symptoms. One of them, Provera, was the drug originally prescribed for my own use. No attention was given to the possible use of the safer and natural forms of progesterone.

Just a note about names at this point, because there is a fair amount of confusion about what to call these synthetic substances. Some of the literature, and perhaps some doctors, may refer to progestins by the name "progestogens," "progestations," "progestens," or, in Europe, "gestagens." For the sake of clarity we will use the name "progestin" in this book. Just be aware if you see any of the other names that they are referring to exactly the same group of synthetic substances.

Many doctors mistakenly persist in referring to these substances as "progesterone," but that is a serious error. There is only one progesterone—the natural substance. The progestins so widely prescribed are synthetic substances that are chemically different from progesterone. This chemical difference causes all of the progestins to have significant side effects, whereas progesterone has no known side effects. That's important enough to repeat: the progestins all have possible serious side effects. (For more information on synthetic compounds listed by their chemical or brand names please see appendix B.) This information should not be taken lightly. Natural progesterone, on the other hand, produces no known adverse reactions and instead produces numerous benefits.

---

* Diosgenin is one of a hundred phytogenins (in *Dioscorea* and other plants) that have a hormone-mimicking character.

THE PERILS OF BEING A PATIENT

Many of us have strong concerns about taking artificial substances anyway. Deep down we know that most of the synthetic hormones and drugs we use won't correct the actual cause of our symptoms but will only temporarily relieve them and camouflage the problem. Yet, we often don't know where to turn. We listen to the doctor as he firmly advises us to continue with the prescribed medication. He gives us a fleeting sense of hope that we are going to put an end to this misery by saying, "You haven't given the medicine enough time," or, "Give it three to six weeks (or months) more."

You may have already experienced some side effects or felt worse since beginning the drug. You wonder, "What do I do now? How can I cope?" In my own case, I tried to find a way to deal with this dilemma and my resentment of a system that was not getting to the cause of my problems. To use the words of author Peter S. Rhodes, I tried "internal considering."[10]

Putting myself in the shoes of the medical doctors who were doing their best to treat me at the time, I said to myself: "Doctors are busy people with full waiting rooms and many interruptions for emergencies. When they go home, they're tired, and it's all they can do to try to keep up with all the latest findings." They must continually deal with new information and the stream of articles in scientific journals. Of course, that heavy schedule also includes business seminars given by drug companies and conferences with their representatives.

Soon, my "internal considering" began to fade. I had tried to give my doctors the benefit of the doubt, but I was well aware of what is certainly no secret: that doctors are heavily influenced by the pharmaceutical companies' sales force and by promotions for various drugs. I realized that the advice they would be giving me could be prejudiced.

Then and there, I decided to substitute action for consideration. The frustration I'd encountered forced me to face my own ambivalence. If I wanted unbiased answers to my questions, the time had come for me to do my own trail-blazing and to take responsibility for my own health. It was time to go to work. The following is what I found.

A VERY PROFITABLE BUSINESS

The puberty-to-postmenopause population provides the drug companies a booming business. This multibillion-dollar bonanza for the U.S. pharmaceutical industry, however, is taking its toll on more than half a million women, especially those going through the midlife crisis. And whether we are talking about human or synthetic estrogen, it is estrogen in all its many forms that we need to oppose before it gets out of hand. It's no wonder more and more books are being written about the medical establishment's exploitation of women and our need to protect ourselves from becoming "hormonal guinea pigs."[11] What is sad is that misinformation about estrogen is being given to vulnerable women who are desperately looking for relief.

The commercially adulterated substances that are used today to create estrogen and progestin products, notwithstanding their poor utilization by the body, are misrepresented to the consumer as the "fountain of youth." In contrast, however, the plant-based progesterone that the body is able to utilize is virtually ignored, having little place in the profit-driven world of drug promotion. However, botanical progesterone is a phytohormone that is considered bioidentical to human progesterone. This is explained by Norman Shealy, M.D., Ph.D., who says, "The wild yam *(Dioscorea)* . . . produces diosgenin, a vegetable steroid. The simple addition of hydrochloric acid and warm water converts diosgenin to natural progesterone."[12] He tells us that when it is produced in this way it becomes an exact chemical duplicate of human progesterone.[13] Needless to say, since it is bioidentical, it has the same physiological effects as our own ovarian-produced progesterone.

No matter what "authorities" say, "estrogen is a potentially dangerous drug with significant side effects," warns Dr. Lawrence Riggs of the Mayo Clinic.[14] Nevertheless, the pharmaceutical industry has cultivated a great market among menopausal women by publicizing estrogen as "essential to a woman's good health and her womanhood."[15] However, as sales increase, so have breast and endometrial cancer.

PROMOTING ESTROGEN: A POWER STRUGGLE

Estrogen is considered one of our most potent prescription drugs. In *The Menopause Industry: How the Medical Establishment Exploits Women*, Sandra Coney recounts this sordid tale: "Warnings about the dangers of estrogen had been made sporadically for nearly 30 years. In particular, it was known that estrone, the form of estrogen in Premarin, could be associated with the development of endometrial cancer. As early as 1947," she discloses, Dr. Saul Gusberg of Columbia University "called the ready use of estrogen 'promiscuous' and warned that what was going on was a human experiment." He had observed too many estrogen users coming in for dilation and curettage (D&C) for abnormal bleeding caused by endometrial overstimulation, as well as documented precancerous and cancerous changes of the uterus.[16]

With time and with more investigation of the serious problems that were occurring, the FDA finally insisted that all prescriptions be accompanied by warnings about the risk of cancer, blood clots, gallbladder disease, and other complications. When this estrogen scare reached the public, sales began to decline. Without a moment to lose, however, the American Pharmaceutical Manufacturers' Association and the public relations firm for Ayerst Pharmaceutical, Hill and Knowlton, wasted no time in producing sales strategies and an intense promotional campaign. This included articles sent out to magazines *(Reader's Digest, McCall's, Ladies' Home Journal, Redbook)* and 4,500 suburban newspapers in order to "preserve the identity of estrogen replacement therapy as effective, safe treatment for symptoms of the menopause."[17]

Those with monied interests were so opposed to the FDA's plan for packaging the warning inserts that they took legal action, for "patient information would reduce sales of estrogen drugs and, therefore, reduce profits." Other organizations that joined in opposition were the American College of Obstetrics and Gynecology, the American College of Internal Medicine, and the American Cancer Society. They claimed that "giving patients information violated the physician's right to control how much information to disclose to patients and threatened medicine's professional autonomy." Eventually the U.S. National Women's Health Network introduced a brief to the court in favor of the FDA,[18] and the FDA won out.

Nevertheless, synthetic HRT remains a booming business. But because of the risks involved with the drugs, a variety of profitable tests, procedures, and drugs is called for along the way—from blood tests, biopsies, and mammograms to hysterectomies, D&Cs, pain relievers, blood pressure medication, diuretics, and frequent doctor visits. And there are as many as 175 different possible treatment combinations to experiment with when bad reactions occur![19]

Many of us don't recognize when we may have been given the wrong type of hormone. We are completely dependent upon what our medical doctors advise with respect to trying new formulations that have just come on the market. Yet, year after year, as we fail to get results from medicines developed through costly technology, we can't help but perceive the undercurrents of greed associated with products that are promoted at the sacrifice of public health. Slowly but surely, we are beginning to think twice about what's in store for us and are asking more questions that challenge the physician's monopoly of information.

What the medical establishment calls breakthroughs are often justified in the name of "consumer protection." However, we need to be mindful and learn as much as we can about what is best for our welfare. I think we should seriously consider the words of John Lee, M.D., more than a decade ago concerning this frustrating situation:

> The emerging realization that estrogen should never be given unopposed, i.e., without progesterone, due to its risk of developing endometrial carcinoma makes natural progesterone a valuable addition in those cases where menopausal symptoms require treatment. . . . It is amazing to me that, given the extensive supporting medical references presently existing, estrogen without concomitant progesterone is still commonly prescribed.[20]

Previously I have discussed the different forms of estrogen. In this section I must reemphasize that two forms of synthetic estrogen, estradiol and estrone, are often prescribed in spite of being potentially tumor-forming. "It is believed but not proven that estrone is even more carcinogenic than estradiol,"[21] says Dr. Lita Lee. This is not good news, because orally administered estradiol is mainly converted to estrone in the small bowel.[22]

The next time your doctor prescribes these chemical compounds, you might want to ask this question: Why is Premarin, which consists of estrone and estradiol,[23] being prescribed when these hormones have been implicated as potential causes of cancer? This predicament has become quite serious as we are now finding that with what our own bodies produce (endogenous form) and that which we acquire from the environment (exogenous form), most women already have too much estrogen. In fact, the *New England Journal of Medicine* points out that the majority of older women exhibit ample estradiol levels many years after menopause[24] and sometimes even have higher levels of estrogen than younger women. This information sheds a different light on the commonly held belief that when a woman turns fifty (or thereabouts), she automatically needs a prescription for estrogen. Unfortunately, that seems to be the working premise and the reason for Premarin's domination of the drug market.

A study reported by Graham A. Colditz, M.D., in *Cancer Causes and Control* showed a 59 percent increase in breast cancer risk for women who had used synthetic HRT for more than five years, and an additional 35 percent risk for those fifty-five years of age and older.[25] In conjunction with Harvard Medical School, Dr. Colditz extended his study of 121,700 nurses for a total of sixteen years. A later report published in the *New England Journal of Medicine* (June 15, 1995) concluded with similar figures and noted "a clear, significant increase in risk" associated with standard, long-term synthetic hormone replacement therapy.[26] And in July of 2002, yet another major study proved that use of Prempro (estrogen/progestin combo) in conventional HRT showed an increased risk in women of breast cancer, coronary heart disease, stroke, and blood clots.

I have personally witnessed many of my own friends and colleagues, after twenty or thirty years on various estrogenic substances, undergoing mastectomies of one breast, second mastectomies two years later, and within about four more years dying. They were denied a decent quality of life in what should have been their golden years. We must all become better informed and learn from education—not desperation and misinformation—to avoid a possibly tragic outcome in our own lives and the lives of family, friends, and coworkers.

As every body is different, including needs and deficiencies, we will discuss in this chapter and in chapter 5 how a variety of herbs have proved helpful in relieving hot flashes and other symptoms of hormonal imbalance. I have personally found some herbs such as don quai, chasteberry, and licorice (considered adaptogens) to be helpful. Of course, because of our stressful lifestyles, it's always important to have such herbs accompanied by natural transdermal progesterone. As we learn from Dr. Lee, "Lack of progesterone interferes with adrenal corticosteroids by which one normally responds to stress. . . ."[27]

Interesting to also learn from author Norman Shealy, M.D., Ph.D.: "natural progesterone is the only known replacement hormone which does not suppress or turn off the body's own production of that hormone."[28]

BOTANICAL PROGESTERONE THERAPY

The need for natural progesterone is confirmed and reiterated in numerous research papers. Progesterone has been utilized for more than thirty years with no reported increase in cancer incidence.[29] In fact, a "Women's Health Report" in *McCall's* tells of research indicating that "progesterone deficiency—which women with PMS have—actually increases the risk of developing breast cancer."[30] This article records an astute observation that the stress that occurs during PMS often triggers ailments that do not seem at all related to one's hormones.

Who would guess that colds, flu, asthma, allergies, epilepsy, migraine headaches, and various endocrine disorders might be connected with a severe progesterone deficiency? Phil Alberts, M.D., who heads a PMS treatment center in Portland, Oregon, explains that problems such as these, seemingly unrelated to PMS or menopause, tend to manifest themselves at times when a woman's immune system is depressed due to hormone imbalance.[31] Progesterone is the real missing ingredient for increasing vitality, enhancing sexual libido, and reducing sleep disturbances.[32]

Upon finishing my personal research, I was overcome with strong feelings about the injustices inflicted upon the thousands of women who need this information and desperately deserve to be helped. However, turning my thoughts to a more positive sort of reflection, I began to think of all the medical doctors who are looking for better and more natural ways to help women avoid PMS and menopausal symptoms.

The physicians mentioned throughout this book are among the many who are now making available information on the benefits of natural HRT. More and more, you may come across published accounts by such individuals. For example, Niels H. Lauersen, M.D., says, "In my practice, hundreds of women who were severely handicapped by PMS have been completely symptom-free with progesterone."[33] We can place further reliance on the reinforcement of progesterone when we read in books such as those written by medical doctors Hohn Lee, Norman Shealy, and others that progesterone also seems to assume a preventive role in PMS and other conditions.[34, 35]

No wonder we feel gratitude for those who have introduced us to this natural treatment. We need to hear about this safe solution over and over again, otherwise we will continue to be enticed into trying synthetic hormones that only steer us further from homeostasis, the hormonal and metabolic balance we want to achieve.

THE PROTECTION AND POTENTIAL OF PROGESTERONE

One of the first things women ask is whether there are any adverse side effects with natural progesterone. All of my investigation says there have been no negative results—only positive. In fact, Dr. Niels Lauersen tells us: "Progesterone is not believed to be cancer causing. No human cancer has been reported during progesterone treatment; quite the reverse, progesterone has been used in treating specific uterine cancers."[36]

Dr. John Lee mentions that when the proper progesterone dose is determined, "because of the great safety of natural progesterone, considerable latitude is allowed."[37] Occasionally, a slight feeling of drowsiness may indicate that you're using more than your body needs. And don't be alarmed if you should happen to read about side effects in products containing natural progesterone or USP progesterone. A pharmacist assures us that since the Food and Drug Administration (FDA) makes no distinction between natural and synthetic progesterone, federal law requires that all known reactions be listed, even if in reality they apply only to the synthetic formulas (progestins).

Not only does natural progesterone have no serious side effects, it is a precursor of other hormones including adrenal corticosteroids, estrogen, and testosterone. Dr. Lee informs us that it participates in the ultimate formation of all the other steroidal hormones.[38] Progesterone is beneficial in treating or preventing

- irregular menstrual flow; cramping
- bloating; depression; irritability
- migraine headaches; insomnia; epilepsy
- miscarriages; infertility; incontinence; endometriosis
- hot flashes; night sweats; vaginal dryness
- hypoglycemia; chronic fatigue syndrome; yeast infections
- heart palpitations and other cardiovascular disorders
- osteoporosis (reversible by increasing bone mass)[39–42]

With progesterone, blood pressure often returns to normal,[43] body fat is burned up for energy, and cell membrane function is safeguarded.[44] Progesterone not only has an anti-inflammatory effect but also helps balance cellular fluid, which protects against hypertension.[45]

It's important to be especially careful if you have been convinced that you need to take estrogen for the purpose of preventing heart disease. Epidemiologic investigations and many other studies show that estrogen has no coronary benefit and that its use increases not only the risk of cardiovascular disease but also the risk of stroke or even bleeding from a brain artery. Doctors have been giving estrogen on the basis of a study "limited to postmenopausal women free of any history of cardiovascular disease or cancer." Statistics can be easily manipulated, with mainstream medicine's focus on estrogen and its eagerness to prescribe estrogen hormone replacement therapy. As Dr. Lee says, the media have perpetuated the estrogen myth, even though the hype was built on flimsy evidence.[46]

It should be noted that the severity of endocrine or reproductive system disorders can be affected not only by hormonal imbalance but also by poor diet[47–49] or by nerve interference within the neuromusculoskeletal system.[50] Many doctors do not adequately address these factors or the probable underlying progesterone deficiency, which is often accompanied by an overabundance of estrogen. Instead, they rely on treatment with antidepressant drugs, aspirin, ibuprofen, other analgesics, or sleeping pills. Fortunately, a much more effective remedy is available in the form of natural progesterone cream, which offers these further benefits:

- protects against breast fibrocyst formation
- keeps the uterine lining healthy, helping to prevent fibroids, etc.
- assists thyroid hormone action
- normalizes the blood-clotting mechanism
- restores libido (sex drive)
- acts as a natural antidepressant[51-53]

Adverse symptoms can begin when a woman is in her thirties or even at the onset of menses in her teen or preteen years. So it is important to be thinking about natural alternatives in the years prior to menopause. Prevention is essential for any health condition, and the sooner we look into natural sources, the sooner we can start to think, look, and feel as young as we are. After studying what natural progesterone does for the bones (see chapter 4), the heart, and the body as a whole, we can better understand the need for it as part of a natural hormone-balancing program.

Now You Don't Have to Refuse Hormone Supplements

I so often hear women repeating the same thoughts I once had: "I won't take hormones. I don't believe in taking pills." That's because many people don't make the distinction between natural ingredients and most of the drugs that are continually portrayed on TV. Yes, NHRT (natural hormone replacement therapy using bioidentical progesterone) is in a different class, as it represents a natural replacement that the body needs; and yes, we do need to continue to resist commercial inducements to take pills, and to try to ignore the medical hype.

Concerning the need for NHRT, Dr. Betty Kamen states in her book *Hormone Replacement Therapy: Yes or No?* that even if you don't have menopausal symptoms and have a good diet and exercise regularly, the use of natural progesterone is still recommended to fortify one's body against the stress of daily living. And to be realistic, she points out, no diet is perfect anyway; and we all cheat on top of that.[54] No matter how diligent we are in maintaining a proper diet, there are always days when we want to escape from the stresses of life, saying, "Everything will be OK. Here, have a treat—something sweet. It will make you feel better!"

Cravings for ice cream, doughnuts, or other simple carbohydrates can be pretty powerful. When stress takes over your senses, no one has perfect control, and if you do, you are the exception. It's easy to forget in that moment that the sugar will only stress one's system more. Alan Gaby, M.D., explains how sugar depletes the body of "magnesium, folic acid, vitamin B6, zinc, copper, manganese, and other nutrients that play a role in maintaining healthy bones."[55] But, while using natural progesterone does not justify such lapses, we can take some comfort in the knowledge that it helps support the adrenals, our stress glands, and helps protect against hypoglycemia.

Dr. Kamen confirms my own experience as to the need for natural progesterone when she says, "Perfect lifestyles/diet may be impossible for perfectly good reasons. Don't feel guilty. Feel better! Natural progesterone could make the difference."[56]

Natural HRT has made me feel like myself again. And I truly believe it will begin to reverse whatever damage the synthetic HRT may have done to my body. Fortunately, I did take antioxidants back then (and still do) to fight any free radical damage, and I added other vitamin and mineral supplements to my daily diet to help counter what might have been toxic to my system.

It is interesting to note that progesterone, a precursor of other hormones, is so nearly perfect for our body chemistry that even its promoters can't exaggerate its importance. Without it I can testify that I felt stressed, run-down, and dependent on medical help; with it, I feel energetic, calm and, most important, free. Menopause does not have to be treated as an illness. It can be better viewed as a challenge! Once a woman establishes proper hormonal, nutritional, and neurological balance through natural methods, she'll find she's taken a great step toward increased vitality.

It's Safe, It's Sound, It's Easy

For some practical guidance, we can now hear from the professionals in order to understand which form of progesterone is the most appropriate for our use. In appendix A we describe the ways of hormone application, but first it's important to provide a little history on how these guidelines were established.

The most popular way to apply natural progesterone is with transdermal cream. Dr. John Lee reports that he has been using transdermal natural progesterone with postmenopausal women since 1982 and has seen remarkable success.[57] "Progesterone," he says, "like all gonadal steroids, is a relatively small and fat-soluble compound which is efficiently and safely absorbed transdermally. Not to use it in cases of progesterone deficiency is imprudent, to say the least."[58] He cautions, however, that any product containing mineral oil may "prevent the progesterone from being absorbed into the skin."[59] Furthermore, according to Dr. Raymond Peat, certain components of mineral oil (found in many cosmetics) are toxic, and any that does get into the system does not metabolize.[60]

The cream is now available in many brands and formulations and at varying strengths. Researchers have measured the levels of hormone in women who were using various wild yam creams that do not contain USP (U.S. Pharmacopeia) progesterone. While many of these creams worked well, some were found not to have much effect. However, according to Aeron LifeCycles Clinical Laboratory in San Leandro, California, (800) 631-7900, most of the creams that contained USP progesterone did produce hormonal changes in most women.[61] (See chapter 4.)

Christiane Northrup, M.D., in her book *Women's Bodies, Women's Wisdom*, also recommends natural progesterone over synthetic because it is compatible with the body and does not have the side effects (bloating, depression, etc.) produced by progestins.[62] Dr. Peat agrees that transdermally applied progesterone is effective for most symptoms as well as for long-range maintenance.[63] Dr. Lee points out that in the beginning stages of treatment some of the application may be retained in the subcutaneous fat layer sometimes delaying the initial physical response. However, the longer a woman uses the cream, the greater the benefits.[64]

Alleviation of symptoms as a clinical response provides a good yardstick for comparison. As with many forms of health care, starting with the least invasive product (in this case the mildest) gives you a baseline for evaluating your response. You can always switch to a stronger product or add to your initial treatment program.

THE ESTROGEN DEBATE CONTINUES

It seems most women of a certain age are either on estrogen, pondering whether to start it, or contemplating getting off it. Some have been made to believe that it is the cure-all for PMS and menopause, heralded to end all our female problems. Chapter 3 demonstrates clearly how this type of promotion has led to relentless suffering and needless disease. Here we will discuss another form of estrogen called *estriol*, which has been rumored to be a safer and weaker form of estrogen, and its usage in other countries.[65]

As seen in many studies, the more potent estrogens, estradiol (brand names: Estrace, Estraderm) and estrone (brand names: Premarin, Ogen, etc.), can cause the lining of the uterus to thicken and increase a woman's risk of endometrial and breast cancer (further discussed in chapter 4). Estriol, on the other hand, has a weaker stimulatory effect on the uterus[66] but, unfortunately, has still been found to cause hyperplasia (tendency to stimulate cell over-growth). Important to note here: vitamin E supplements provide a safe means by which you can increase the ratio of estriol to estradiol and estrone.[67] Other research confirms this, showing increased effectiveness with decreased toxicity to the tissues when utilizing a base of natural vitamin E (*tocopherol*, but not the cheaper *Tocopherol acetate* some manufacturers use).[68]

For these reasons we are not suggesting the utilization of any of these forms of estrogen in this edition. There are just too many other natural alternatives available that we have found to be safer. And needless to say, what might be completely effective for one woman may not be a cure-all for another. If you find that hot flashes and other discomforts are still bothering you even after using natural progesterone (as directed and for a minimum of three months), you might try adding maca root and/or other progestagenic or adaptagenic herbs, which we will talk about in greater detail in chapter 6.

But, regardless of what other supplements one chooses to use, we find that progesterone should always be the foundation and cornerstone in our hormone-balancing regime. Speaking of which, one knowledgeable pharma-cist at Women's International Pharmacy says that another reason the trans-dermal cream form of progesterone may be more effective is if a person's liver is not functioning fully due to dietary deficiency or drug overstimulation. A sluggish liver could also be further comprised by alcohol or disease (such as hepatitis). This pharmacist tells us that transdermally applied progesterone is most efficient because it acts systemically before it acts locally. The benefit of this direct effect is that it cuts down on some of the work the liver has to do.

I have found the use of transdermal progesterone cream to be adequate for my needs. During periods of excessive stress, I slightly increase the amount, as I've learned that it's a precursor of the adrenal hormones.[69, 70] I've also had good results with pregnenolone, which is itself a precursor of progesterone, DHEA, and other important hormones.[71–73] Pregnenolone is available in powder, capsule, or cream form and is beneficial not only for hormone replacement but also for relieving arthritic pain. When I combine these safe and natural supplements with my daily nutritional program, it seems to take care of all my postmenopausal problems.

In the journal *Fertility and Sterility* (April 1995) we find evidence that nat-ural progesterone applied directly to the breast does offer protection against estrogen's stimulatory effect on breast cells.[74] Other skin sites that are ideal for applying transdermal progesterone are discussed in appendix A. Also, please refer to the section on breast cancer in chapter 5.

Excess Estrogen Equals Excess Weight

Contrary to popular opinion, researchers make it clear that menopause does not mean an absolute end to estrogen production. There are other areas of the body that assist the ovaries in the postmenopausal production of estrogen. This occurs because the adrenal glands produce a hormone that is converted in estrogen in the fat tissue. This process, says author Sharon Gleason, "will maintain low levels of estrogens to minimize symptoms."[75]

Dr. John Lee states that a sign of *estrogen dominance* is weight gain caused by both water retention and fat deposition at hips and thighs. This is an interesting point, because I have found that many women wonder why they are gaining weight even though they are exercising and on a strict diet. One of my neighbors thought she had gained weight because she had given up smoking. At the same time, however, her doctor had put her on estrogen therapy for her menopausal problems, informing her (albeit incorrectly) that this hormone would be good for bone growth and make her feel a lot better. After talking to her I couldn't help but think that the generally accepted accumulation of a "middle-age spread" could very well stem from the cumulative effect of environmental, prescribed, and endogenous estrogens along with the rapid drop in progesterone level that can begin during perimenopause.

Another case is highlighted in *The Menopause Industry*, by Sandra Coney. This woman, prescribed Premarin for her joint problems and pelvic inflammation, began to put on weight "at an alarming rate" and was then switched to different forms of estrogen, including Estraderm patches and implants. The unfortunate result was a thirty-five-pound weight gain, fluid retention, and breast discomfort.[76]

In contrast, botanical progesterone is a natural diuretic. It burns fat (often caused by high doses of synthetic estrogen already in the body) for energy and lowers cholesterol levels[77]—once again helping to avoid another unwanted side effect of conventional HRT.

Other Side Effects of Estrogen Dominance

Dr. John Lee reminds us that if a woman decides to take estrogen for any length of time, it sould always be accompanied by the use of natural progesterone. He says that estrogen "allows influx of water and sodium into [the] cells, thus affecting aldosterone production leading to water retention and hypertension. Estrogen," he continues, "[also] causes intracellular hypoxia [oxygen deficiency], opposes the action of [the] thyroid, promotes histamine release, promotes blood clotting thus increasing the risk of stroke and embolism, thickens bile . . . promotes gall bladder disease [and] causes copper retention and zinc loss."[78]

Is it any wonder that so many women feel miserable when using synthetic estrogens? And is it any wonder that Dr. Lee says, "Something is wrong with the ongoing, medically endorsed estrogen theory"? Prescribed alone, estrogen can lead to breast or uterine cancer as well as heart attack and stroke[79–82] even five years prior to menopause.[83] Other consequences of estrogen dominance, he says, include "heightened activity of the hypothalamus [and] hyperactivity of adjacent limbic nuclei leading to mood swings, fatigue, feelings of being cold, and inappropriate responses to other stressors."[84]

Just before menstruation, as Dr. Lee says, too much estrogen in the body often causes edema, or swelling and bloating. Dr. Ray Peat agrees: "Under the influence of estrogen, your body retains extra water."[85] This, he says, is one reason we often crave extra salt.

Some authorities recommend cutting down on salt the week before one's period in an effort to reduce bloating and breast tenderness. However, Dr. Peat points out the often-overlooked fact that sodium "is essential for [maintaining] adequate blood volume, and that it is almost always unphysiological and irrational to restrict sodium intake." He explains that "reduced blood volume tends to reduce the delivery of oxygen and nutrients to all tissues, leading to many problems."[86] (For more on the wise use of sodium, please see page 174.) Perhaps it's time for women to question their doctors before they are ushered into the commonly prescribed HRT that can raise their estrogen to unsafe levels and bring with it a variety of risky side effects, which have proved over and over to be instrumental in the development of cancer.[87–90]

FIBROCYSTIC BREASTS

Estrogen dominance in the body causes fibrocystic breasts. However, Dr. Lee assures us, "Restoring hormone balance with natural progesterone usually results in prompt clearing of the problem. . . . When natural progesterone is used . . . during the two weeks before menses, fibrocystic breasts revert to normal within 2–3 months."[91] One patient, who came to him fearful of breast cancer, reported having undergone repeated needle drainage and biopsies. But as one might expect, after a course of progesterone and an improved diet, not only had her cysts disappeared, but many other symptoms were also relieved.[92]

Dr. Lee's instructions for use of the progesterone cream are quoted in the popular book *Alternative Medicine*. "Using this progesterone transdermally," he says, "from day fifteen of the monthly cycle to day twenty-five will usually cause breast cysts to disappear."[93]

Concerning fibrocystic breasts, Dr. Nina Sessler says:

> Avoiding caffeine and other methyl xanthine derivatives such as black tea, most colas, and chocolate, as well as many nonprescription and prescription medicines which contain methyl xanthines, has been shown to help a great deal with the discomfort. Many physicians recommend vitamin E (400–800 I.U.) and . . . vitamin C can also help reduce the inflammation that often accompanies FBC [fibrocystic breasts].[94]

On the other hand, noted breast surgeon and author Susan M. Love, M.D., states that most studies of caffeine and benign breast disease have been either inconclusive, unscientific, or contradictory and that the popular perception of a connection may or may not be a reality. She points out that individual physiological differences could account for caffeine's affecting one person but not another.[95]

Some years ago, Dr. Linda Force had surgery on her breast to remove a fibrocyst. Following the surgery her breast swelled to twice the normal size and was very painful. The surgeon had not removed all of the cyst because it would have created too much deformity. Dr. Force says, "As time went on, I controlled the problem by watching my diet and avoiding caffeinated beverages. But when I was thirty-five and developed PMS, the breast discomfort intensified. This is when I went to Dr. William Douglass, who dispenses rectal progesterone therapy over a three-month period. For those months only, I was fine. After that, my discomfort was not as bad as it had been previously, and I learned to tolerate it. But every month when my period would start, my breasts would swell and become very sore."

Fifteen years after the first surgery to remove her fibrocysts, Dr. Force was still suffering from the cysts, which were getting more and more painful as time went by. Her medical doctors were advising her to undergo surgery again if they didn't clear up. That's when I provided her with literature about transdermal progesterone cream. It explained how the decline of progesterone can create estrogen dominance which in turn can cause any number of disorders such as fibrocysts, weight gain, endometriosis, depression, and more. I mentioned to her that many women who suffer from fibrocystic breasts rub the cream directly on their breasts and that it has done wonders in reversing their condition. I assured her that it is botanically derived and converted in the lab to a molecule that is bioidentical to human progesterone. Rebalancing hormone levels with this supplementation would address her *hormone deficiency disorder*.

As a doctor, she quickly understood the dangers and side effects of unopposed estrogen. The fact is that when estrogen is administered to women with fibrocystic breasts, their condition becomes worse. However, it is easily treated with progesterone therapy.[96]

Beginning her treatment immediately, she conscientiously applied the cream to the sites of the lumps in her breast and to her abdomen twice daily, once in the morning and once at night. As the weeks went by, she saw subtle improvements during her periods—more regularity and less clotting. After three months, her fibrocysts had disappeared and she was free of the pressure and pain she'd previously had. Her relief at having avoided the prescribed surgery and drugs was evident. And as a true health care provider, she soon made this important information about natural progesterone cream available to all her patients and staff.

UTERINE FIBROIDS AND OVARIAN CYSTS

Dr. John Lee refers to fibroids that develop in the uterus as

> another example of estrogen dominance secondary to anovulatory cycles and consequent progesterone deficiency. They generally occur in the 8–10 years before menopause. If sufficient natural progesterone is supplemented from day 12 to day 26 of the menstrual cycle, further growth of fibroids is usually prevented (and often the fibroids regress).[97]

Ovarian cysts are often found in women taking birth control pills, which suppress the natural release of the developing egg. It is then often retained as a cyst rather than resorbed. We never hear from our doctors or from health news on TV that this artificial birth control suppresses ovulation, which prevents the monthly release of ovarian progesterone. Nowhere is it acknowledged that our endogenous progesterone plays a crucial role in promoting and maintaining a balance of the female hormones that protect against bone loss and other female disorders. Nowhere is it made clear how this chemical suppression leads to ovarian "burn-out." Nowhere do they correlate the epidemic numbers of women arriving at the infertility clinics with their use of birth control pills for three or more years. Nowhere do they tell women that their natural monthly cycles do not recover as easily as before they were blocked by the effects of birth control pills.[98]

However, we are enlightened by some doctors, such as John Lee, whose approach is to administer just the progesterone directly. He says that "natural progesterone, given from day 5 to day 26 of the menstrual month for two to three cycles, will almost routinely" cause disappearance of these cysts by suppressing normal FSH (follicle-stimulating hormone), LH (luteinizing hormone), and estrogen production and giving the ovary time to heal.[99]

Another common problem is the accumulation of small cysts that develop underneath the surface of the ovaries—a condition known as polycystic ovaries. It is linked to surplus body fat, in about 50 percent of cases, as well as a high level of androgen and circulating insulin, with many associated health risks including diabetes, hypertension, and heart disease. The signs of this problem include lack of normal ovulatory cycles, hirsutism (excess facial hair), or extra weight (often carried around the waist). Dr. Christiane Northrup tells us, "When a woman's normal hormonal cycle is blocked by chronic androgen overproduction, neither she nor her ovaries will experience the natural cyclic changes associated with normal ovarian function. Her hormonal levels remain static. Thus, a woman's ovaries contain many small cysts from underdeveloped eggs."[100]

Some of Dr. Northrup's suggestions for the treatment of polycystic ovaries include an organic whole-foods diet, avoidance of partially hydrogenated fats and oils (see also chapter 6), a well-balanced nutritional supplement, exposure to daylight, and emotional grounding—along with the use of natural progesterone to counter the estrogen overload that is known to contribute to these ovarian cysts, as well as other reproductive disorders.[101]

Studies have been reported in the *Journal of the National Cancer Institute* as far back as 1951 in which progesterone even produced evidence of regression of cervical tumors.[102] It's reassuring to know that progesterone can protect us in so many ways; but we must all be alert to the fact that the long-range harmful effects of estrogen dominance in the body are not widely recognized.

ENDOMETRIOSIS

Majid Ali, M.D., calls endometriosis, which he says afflicts five million American women, "a painful, often disabling disorder that can lead to infertility." It is sometimes treated, mistakenly, with synthetic birth control pills. He blames estrogen "overdrive" for the "growth outside the uterus of misplaced cells that normally line the uterine cavity."[103] Linda G. Rector-Page,

N.D., Ph.D., adds that this tissue often attaches to other organs, and there is a backup of some of the heavy menstrual flow.[104] Dr. Ali maintains that treatment with synthetic estrogens, so widespread among doctors, is a grave error.

With estrogen so commonly prescribed, Dr. John Lee confirms that within a year after taking estrogen a pap smear will often indicate cervical dysplasia, "soon followed by a hysterectomy. I consider this medical malpractice," he says, "but it happens to hundreds of women every day."[105]

Women on Menopause, by Anne Dickson and Nikki Henriques, reveals that unopposed estrogen was first linked in 1970 to "abnormal cell growth in the endometrium," resulting also in the possibility of endometrial cancer.[106] Today, women need to be aware of the many other serious side effects when estrogen is administered alone and their progesterone levels are down: nausea, anorexia, vomiting, headaches, and fluid retention leading to weight gain. It is important, say the authors of this book, for women who have other physical disorders to avoid supplementation with only estrogen, for it can exacerbate high blood pressure, diabetes, migraine, and epilepsy.

It is important to note here that the repetitive, monthly use of bleached tampons (which often begins in the early teens) may very well be a contributor to one's total estrogen exposure. Prolonged use is now thought to initiate cellular overgrowth within the reproductive tract, which may manifest in the form of endometriosis, cervical hyperplasia (excess cell growth of the cervix), or uterine fibrocystic conditions. According to the *Women's Book of Healing Herbs,* "Many herbalists believe that the rise in endometriosis is linked to a rise in environmental pollution, specifically to highly toxic substances like dioxin (used in some pesticides). . . ."[107] This is a chemical that is produced in the tampon bleaching process and is known to mimic estrogen.[108]

Herbalist Rosemary Gladstar, director of the Sage Mountain Herbal Education Center and author of *Herbal Healing for Women,* echoes the growing realization that endometriosis is a "hyperestrogenic disease."[109] So making lifestyle changes that will reduce our estrogen exposure is critical in our efforts to avoid or even reverse such prevalent medical conditions as endometriosis.

This is a condition that is not without its complications. Sandy MacFarland was only nineteen when her gynecologist suggested she have a hysterectomy for her endometriosis. According to the Endometriosis Association, this condition, which affects girls and women from the ages of eleven to fifty, is "the leading cause of hysterectomy."[110] Fortunately, Sandy's father was a nutritionist, and he decided to try to correct what he thought might be a hormone imbalance with natural progesterone. This decision not only saved Sandy's uterus but also normalized her once-irregular periods.

Most people, however, are not as lucky, as we'll see in another woman's all-too-typical experience. When I met one of my former tennis partners I hadn't seen in almost ten years, she told me she'd had a total hysterectomy because of endometriosis. She'd been on Premarin for more than six years prior to the hysterectomy and has continued to take it many years after the surgery. Now, however, she was experiencing endometrial tissue buildup in her colon. She was depressed because the hysterectomy hadn't really solved her problems. The doctor, as a last resort, had just written her a prescription for Prozac (another top-selling drug) to be used along with the estrogen therapy. Unfortunately, too often these routine approaches do nothing but cut out, cover up, exacerbate, or create new conditions in a misguided attempt to heal the original problem.

Some women are also being diagnosed with a variation of endometriosis know as "adenomyosis," which is "internal endometriosis." This occurs when the uterine wall grows thick and spongy as it becomes saturated with blood.

It's worth noting that in 1995 the *Journal of the American Medical Association* published the results of a trial called "The Postmenopausal Estrogen/Progestin Intervention (PEPI)," in which one of the adverse reactions of Premarin was a "significantly increased risk of adenomatous or atypical hyperplasia"[111] as a result of estrogen dominance. Many factors contribute to such an overload, and the resulting diseases take on varying forms. Documentation tells us how to combat such abnormalities. The *New England Journal of Medicine* makes it clear that "excessive estrogen is associated with most of the risk factors that have been linked to endometrial carcinoma."[112] Another study shows that any decline in the rate of growth of endometrial tumor cells depends on the concentration of progesterone in the tissue.[113] It's encouraging to know that the application of transdermal natural progesterone can help to assure adequate tissue saturation.

HYSTERECTOMIES: FORCED MENOPAUSE

Hysterectomies are recommended for numerous reasons, often unwarranted. They are frequently suggested when women complain of adverse reactions to their prescribed estrogen or progestins. A doctor may recommend a hysterectomy instead of offering natural therapies that facilitate the body's own healing process. Gail Sheehy, in her book *The Silent Passage*, tells us that doctors will justify to their patients a more radical surgical approach by explaining that they won't have to take the hormones that have been causing such irritating side effects. The surgery will free them from the worry of having to protect their uterus with hormones.

Gail Sheehy asked one doctor if he took the ovaries out as a routine procedure. The doctor nonchalantly told her, "In a postmenopausal woman, the ovaries are of no use anyway." In dismayed retrospect, Sheehy asks, "Wasn't this extreme?" This doctor was disregarding the fact that the ovaries continue to manufacture a small amount of testosterone, which, as Sheehy points out, "strongly influences a woman's sexual desire and energy."[114] This is not, however, an endorsement of the use of supplemental testosterone for women who have had hysterectomies, or even for women with an intact uterus. In healthy women, natural progesterone will normally increase libido and without any of the adverse effects of testosterone.

We might want to think several times before considering a hysterectomy. Every organ has an integral role to play throughout one's entire life. In her book Sheehy tells us that "between 33 and 46 percent of the women whose ovaries had also been removed complained of reduced sexual responsiveness."[115] Dr. Howard Judd of UCLA, an expert on the postmenopausal ovary, emphasizes that "the concept that the ovary burns out is not true."[116]

Sheehy relates that most women who have undergone hysterectomies are in the age group of twenty-five to forty-four. When the cervix and uterus are removed, some women feel the effects of menopause within two years of the surgery. However, an oophorectomy (where the ovaries are removed) will generally bring on the state of menopause immediately. It's sad that such surgically induced menopause will often befall women when they are quite young.[117]

The Wall Street Journal reports, based on a study in *Obstetrics & Gynecology,* that "each year 600,000 women in the U.S. have hysterectomies, but more than 400,000 of them probably didn't have to," and that more than 50 percent of those surgeries were actually inappropriate. The *WSJ* went on to say, "The loss of the uterus can also cause bladder-control problems" and may trigger early menopause for young women.[118] Furthermore, it's a matter of fact that these reproductive surgeries, and medical therapies such as radiation and chemotherapy "have never been evaluated by systemic studies and are used simply because doctors have always believed that they work" says Dr. Kevin Patterson.[119] In a book entitled *Sex, Lies, and Menopause: The Shocking Truth about Hormone Replacement Therapy* studies show that such treatments are not as much prescribed because evidence proves it to be so, but is prescribed because this is how doctors have always done it! How long will the quality of our health be dependent upon hanging onto the coat tails of Tradition! Because of this we see a "sorry margin of success."[120–122]

In these times of such medical mistreatment we all need to speak out about the studies that alert us to the truth of the matter, not the studies that give more fuel to the prescriptive drugs that are causing severe health problems, often needing more drugs to cover up their side effects. We need to bring evidence to the forefront in more studies and books on this subject. (See appendices D, E, F, and G for some of the best studies and books we have found.)

Menopause usually begins around the ages of forty-five to fifty, and the last period is experienced in the early fifties.[123] However, ovarian dysfunction can begin at thirty. Undue trauma, or more than normal physical or mental stress, can bring on menopause years sooner. If a woman smokes, has a poor diet, is on medication, or has undergone surgery, chemotherapy, or radiation, she will also experience a dramatic loss of progesterone, which accelerates the aging process. And the degree of menopausal symptoms can also vary enormously in accord with each individual's genetic differences.[124]

STROKE AND BLOOD CLOTS

My personal experience with blood clots began two months after the laboriously long and difficult delivery of my son. As I was adjusting to my newborn baby, who had colic throughout the night, the meaning of stress became clear beyond doubt. Dr. Lee has mentioned that when stress is heightened, a woman is predisposed to anovulatory cycles (menstrual periods with no ovulation). Additionally, he says, "Lack of progesterone interferes with adrenal corticosteroids by which one normally responds to stress."[125] Also during the immediate postpartum phase, progesterone levels are near zero until ovulation resumes. This in turn will create a state of relative estrogen dominance with all its associated symptoms and risks.

I had no way of understanding then the underlying and multiple reasons for my stress and immense weakness, or why my body could not adapt to the demands of taking care of an infant during the night and a two-year-old during the day, while cooking for family and friends who had come to join us at this time of celebration.

As the days proceeded, I rapidly lost motor control on my left side. Within two months after the birth, my left side had become paralyzed as the result of a blood clot that had lodged in a blood vessel wall on the right side of my brain. This embolism left me helpless and traumatized for several months. The neurosurgeon, my OB/GYN, and other specialists were completely mystified as to the cause of my condition.

This postnatal paralysis all took place years ago. Now, however, after sifting through much research, I can't help but speculate that progesterone deficiency was perhaps one of the causes for my stress and that natural progesterone might have rescued me from the trauma I had endured. I recall, too, that Dr. Peat writes that during stressful times in a woman's life, supplementation with the hormone progesterone is urgently needed to correct imbalances in the endocrine system.[126] Have these doctors and researchers solved the mystery that was so puzzling to my specialists decades ago?

Recently, the memory of my personal crisis really hit home when I heard on the news that two days after giving birth, a woman had died from a blood clot in her brain. This story caused an instant flashback to my own experience. I realized what could have happened to me and may very well be happening to others, all because of a lack of information about the tragic consequences of high estrogen/low progesterone levels. In fact, progesterone may help many at-risk women to avoid strokes and other stress-related disorders.[127]

Again I reflect on my own vulnerable state of needing help after my doctors were not able to understand why a blood clot could have formed on my brain when only thirty-two years of age. However, when all the news about stroke and heart problems flooded the newspapers in the summer of 2002, I couldn't help but put the puzzle together. The answer to my own personal problem came to me loud and clear when reading about how the National Institute of Health put an immediate halt on their major study on conventional hormone therapy due to strokes, blood clots, and increasingly high risks of heart disease and breast cancer.[128]

Chapter 5 speaks about the myriad other ways that estrogen mimickers enter our bodies. This occurs through the saturating impact of environmental toxins, which have proven to have a dramatic effect in raising estrogen levels. This is due to the fact that these excitotoxins from our environment are processed in the body as pseudoestrogens affecting not only women, but also men, by stimulating cell overgrowth including cancer cells. Authors such as Ted Mangum, M.D., confirm that "we do not live in the pristine world of our ancestors but instead in a world saturated with toxins, many of which have potent and troublesome estrogenic activity."[129]

THE HORMONAL DUET: POINT AND COUNTERPOINT

Needless to say, the above experience took place during my childbearing years. Comparing the premenopausal stages of life with the menopausal and even postmenopausal stages, we view hormone replacement in different ways.

Our needs differ depending on many factors: our symptoms, age, diet, amount of exercise, level of stress, and other lifestyle habits.

We also need to remember that the menopausal or postmenopausal woman does have some estrogen—it's the progesterone that is no longer produced anywhere in her body to any noticeable degree. It makes one wonder why medical doctors have been prescribing estrogen replacement for so many years—often to the exclusion of progesterone. Yet, researchers are proving over and over that progesterone is an important hormone, and as Norman Shealy, M.D., Ph.D., states in his book, it is a "major regulator of estrogen, testosterone, and cortisol . . . [It] is the most versatile hormone in the human body."[130]

Estrogen and progesterone interact with each other, and each of them sensitizes receptor sites for the other. Dr. Peat points to recent research showing that progesterone protects by toning down the estrogen receptors. Why take supposedly antiestrogenic drugs, such as Evista (see page 115) which is associated with serious risks,[131] when we know that progesterone does the work naturally? It energizes enzymes and the liver's detoxifying system that modify estrogen so it can be excreted from the body. Additionally, it acts as a neurosteroid, has a positive effect on the immune system, and promotes efficient respiration. And of significance in these days of confusing media representations about estrogen's role in heart disease and the conflicting ideas and inconsistent advice given to us by our physicians who specialize in this area is this reassuring statement by Dr. Peat about progesterone: "In the circulatory system, it regulates heart action and vascular tone, preventing venous pooling of the blood and orthostatic hypotension, [and] helping to keep the pulse pressure in the low range indicating efficient circulation."[132]

Dr. Betty Kamen writes, "Estrogen regulates the neurotransmitters of the brain—substances which control the function of our nervous system," including the thinking processes and motor activity. An excess of estrogen relative to progesterone can result in cortical hyperstimulation. Since this process permits the brain cells to communicate with each other,[133] it may be of value to begin natural progesterone supplementation when severe PMS or menopausal mood swings, agitation, depression, and anxiety arise.

Additionally, according to Dr. Peat, estrogen in excess can act as an "excitotoxin" to the brain, eventually causing an energy drain (cellular exhaustion) by stimulating the brain beyond the nervous system's capacity to respond. He says that even an average estrogen level can be a serious problem when there is insufficient progesterone to balance it and that "it is best to have five to ten times as much progesterone as estrogen."[134]

ESTROGEN/PROGESTERONE ASSESSMENT

Use the following list to assess whether you have an estrogen imbalance or dominance problem. The progesterone column shows how progesterone can balance the effects of estrogen overload.

Symptoms of Estrogen Overload	Benefits of Progesterone Supplementation
Weight gain	Utilizes fat for energy
Insomnia; Hot flashes; Night sweats	Calming effect
Breast, uterine, and ovarian cancer	Stops cells from multiplying
Fibrocystic breasts	Protects against fibrocysts in breast
Endometriosis; Cervical hyperplasia	Reverses cellular growth syndromes
Depression	Natural antidepressant
Fluid retention (bloating)	Natural diuretic
Thyroid imbalance	Assists in normalizing thyroid action
Blood clots; Heart problems	Normalizes blood clotting
Elevated blood pressure	Regulates blood pressure
Migraine headaches	Restores oxygen to cells
Infertility	Promotes conception
Risk of miscarriage	Prevents premature contractions
Irregular menstrual flow; PMS	Relieves cramping: antispasmodic
Cramping	Normalizes periods
Acne; Psoriasis; Keratoses, etc.	Heals skin irritations
Inflammation	Precursor to cortisone
Slows bone loss	Stimulates bone growth
Loss of libido	Restores energy
Vaginal atrophy and infection	Fights infection; Relieves dryness

PART II

Opening Up a New World of Hope and Healing

THREE

The Seasons of a
Woman's Life

To be surprised, to wonder,
is to begin to understand.
José Ortega y Gasset [1]

There is no reason for an active woman to endure the symptoms of hormone imbalance when safe, natural relief is readily available. We all have enough on our hands trying to solve the host of life's other challenges without adding more. If we don't take the time to provide for our needs, even menial tasks and minor problems can take us over the edge. An incident as simple as having to answer a child's question or give someone directions becomes unbearable. Discomfort, dizziness, or fatigue brought on by menstruation or menopause weakens one's energy and enthusiasm. How easy it is to lose stamina, confidence, and the ability to help oneself, one's family, and others. But simple preventive measures can empower today's woman to rise to any occasion and meet the daily demands of business and family.

The women of this generation need to take heed of what nature has not provided for those of past generations. They did not have full knowledge about hormone therapy, nor did they have the alternative choices we have today. You might have been blessed with one of those "super moms" with genetic vitality and strength. However, many women suffered from heart disease, osteoporosis, or cancer because the slowly diminishing supply of their own natural estrogen and progesterone created an imbalance between these two hormones, and eventual disease.

Now, with the incredible number of artificial hormones that have been introduced (see appendix B), women may encounter unexpected and unpleasant side effects such as bloating, weight gain, emotional tension, and insomnia. And as the years pass, they may have to deal with endometriosis, thyroid disorders, fibrocysts, heart disease, osteoporosis, and cancer. Often labeled chronic complainers, some become dependent on psychiatric care to cope with their pain and to deal with the emotional problems brought on by these health conditions. Let's take a look at some of the beginning signs of hormone deficiency and the symptoms of this cruel onslaught.

YOU'RE NOT CRAZY; IT'S JUST YOUR HORMONES

Long ago, in another generation, women experiencing symptoms of PMS or menopause were often accused of insanity, and even institutionalized. As early as 1931, several years after both PMS and menopause had been classified as forms of emotional and psychological disturbance, literature on the subject actually admitted that there were physical problems associated with the "change of life."

Today, women are not routinely institutionalized for exhibiting symptoms of hormonal stress, but at the mercy of impulsive moods, hypertension, irritability, depression, and crying spells, we are often diagnosed as having a "nervous breakdown." Many types of medication are prescribed, from sedatives to muscle relaxants. In Great Britain, says Sterling Morgan, "[natural] progesterone treatment for PMS is so accepted that in three different murder trials, women were sentenced to take progesterone. Their defense was that they had committed violent crimes because they were pre-menstrual!"[2]

Dr. Katharina Dalton, in her book *Once a Month*, tells of her experience with patients who exhibited psychological and physical symptoms ranging from what she calls "cyclical" criminal acts (including child abuse and murder) and suicidal inclinations to asthma attacks and excessive weight gain—all related to premenstrual syndrome.

When she traced the history of these tendencies, she found coincidentally that in every case they had begun at puberty with each woman's first menstrual period. Many of these women had been on medication deemed appropriate at the time for their particular manifestation of symptoms, but it was not until they switched to supplemental progesterone that relief came almost immediately. Some, even those who had been in prison, no longer had to be institutionalized.[3]

As for menopause, historically far too little has been done to help women through what is for some a severe illness—especially when one considers osteoporosis, a very crippling disease and the result of untreated hormone imbalance. And medical science still wants to set PMS aside as a mystery, rather than a reality to be dealt with. As Dr. Stuart Berger states in his book *What Your Doctor Didn't Learn in Medical School*, PMS "has managed to remain something of a medical enigma."[4]

The PMS and menopause conundrum does, however, continue to be discussed and written about in medical publications. There appears to be a consensus that perhaps 40 to 60 percent of women under the age of fifty are affected to some extent by PMS.[5] For women in the childbearing age range, it is somewhat less common, with perhaps 20 to 40 percent afflicted. But fully a fourth of these, 5 to 10 percent, have such severe PMS that it significantly disrupts their lives.[6]

It is interesting to note Dr. Katharina Dalton's comment that "target cells containing progesterone receptors are widespread in the body, although most are found in the brain, particularly in the limbic area [near the brain stem], which is the area of emotion, rage and violence."[7, 8] The body's other receptor sites for progesterone are in the eyes, nose, throat, lungs, breasts, liver, adrenals, uterus, and vagina.[9, 10] "All these," says Dr. Dalton, "are areas in which symptoms of PMS may occur such as headaches, asthma, laryngitis, pharyngitis, rhinitis, sinusitis . . . mastitis, alcohol intolerance and congestive dysmenorrhoea." In fact, as many as 150 symptoms throughout the body have been recorded that relate to PMS.[11]

Carol Petersen, R.Ph., of Women's International Pharmacy, says that around menopause or when symptoms escalate, the estrogen dominance that is at the root of all this is often intensified by the introduction of synthetic progestins such as Provera, for they block the brain receptors from receiving natural progesterone. Dr. John R. Lee describes how such an imbalance can wreak havoc even without drug intervention, simply as a result of a woman's deficiency of natural, balancing progesterone:

> Low premenopausal progesterone, as a consequence of anovulatory cycles, can induce increased estrogen levels and lead to symptomatically significant estrogen dominance prior to menopause. The most common age for breast or uterine cancer is five years before menopause. And there is more. The hypothalamic biofeedback mechanism activated by this lack of progesterone as a woman approaches menopause, leads to elevation of GnRH [gonadotropin-releasing hormone] and pituitary release of FSH and LH. Potential consequences of this are increased estrogen production, loss of corticosteroid production, and intracellular edema.

Heightened activity of the hypothalamus, a component of the limbic brain, can induce hyperactivity of adjacent limbic nuclei leading to mood swings, fatigue, feelings of being cold, and inappropriate responses to other stressors . . . . Hypo-thyroidism is suspected despite normal thyroid hormone levels.[12]

To sum up this section, note the words of John T. Hart, M.D., from the third edition foreword of this book: "Depression is treated as a Prozac deficiency, water retention with a diuretic, weight gain with appetite suppressants—whereas the solution can be as simple as counteracting estrogen overload with what she is no longer able to produce on her own—namely, progesterone."

What Causes Severe Premenstrual Cramps?

Speaking from my personal experience—life could have been so sweet if I'd had a glance into the future! But then again, it might not have been as enlightening or purposeful. The struggle to reach our goals is often as rewarding as their final attainment. Even uncovering small pieces of information that eventually lead up to the big picture can be fulfilling.

One such piece came to me in the mail in a medical report from which I learned that cramping starts when the adrenal gland has been drained of its cortisone reserve. Another article came from the *Cancer Forum*, published by the Foundation for Advancement in Cancer Therapy, presenting Dr. Lee's findings that progesterone is a precursor of cortisone, which is made by the adrenal glands.[13] It also functions as a natural antispasmodic.

In reading about this, I could easily remember suffering from severe cramps as a teenager. The pain would be so intense that wherever I was—at work or school—I would often faint. I would end up in the clinic for the rest of the day with a hot water bottle, hot tea, and aspirin every two hours. As women of menstrual age continue to have these problems, it's appalling that education on natural solutions is not available from most of our doctors. Instead, unnecessary suffering continues, and medical doctors continue to prescribe the common synthetic drugs.

Yet, many women have found progesterone to be a pain-relieving hormone. Cramping at the onset of a period can be painful and disruptive, but progesterone helps alleviate the discomfort by assisting the adrenal glands to create cortisone. According to Betty Kamen, Ph.D., some physicians now advise the "application of one-half teaspoon of the cream to the abdomen every 30 minutes until cramping subsides."[14]

Anecdotal testimony comes from Dr. Linda Force, who tells me that prior to using the progesterone cream, she had a problem with clotting during her periods. But administering the cream has given her a normal, even flow and kept her periods regular. She now applies it every morning and evening, right up to the time her period begins. When her period stops, she starts all over again.

Be aware, however, that many doctors fail to associate our symptoms with PMS or menopause. They do not typically recognize and acknowledge our difficulties as being related to progesterone deficiency, but rather attempt to treat only our symptoms.[15] An example of this can be seen with many post-menopausal women who are not aware of the significance of the decline in their progesterone levels. They are finding that even though they eat low-fat foods, their cholesterol levels have become elevated. Since they are often put on *unopposed* conjugated synthetic estrogen, their LDL (less desirable) cholesterol has consistently risen. This is the result of estrogen dominance. Instead of neutralizing this dangerous hormone with natural progesterone, the doctor will often prescribe one of the many drugs that lower cholesterol. Meanwhile, the estrogen in their bodies remains unopposed and continues to be threatening.

It is vital to keep our thoughts focused on the natural alternatives to these drugs. In appendix F and appendix G of this book you will learn how to have natural progesterone prescribed by your doctor, or where you can obtain natural progesterone in a variety of forms without a prescription.

It's comforting to realize that experts have found a combination of all-natural ingredients that will work to create a proper balance between a woman's own estrogen and progesterone. Replacement of the body's own natural progesterone addresses any deficiency, and the result is relief from many worrisome symptoms.

PREMENSTRUAL EPILEPSY AND DEPRESSION

Dr. Ray Peat has detailed studies showing that when epilepsy occurs prior to menstruation, it is often relieved by progesterone therapy. This therapy has also been used with success in suicidal depression, Reynaud's phenomenon, Meniere's disease (inner ear), kidney disorders, and abnormal liver metabolism.[16]

This has been validated by Dr. Dalton, who says, "One of the most satisfying experiences is to diagnose and treat a woman with premenstrual epilepsy. She can be treated with progesterone and freed from all anticonvulsant tablets with their many and unpleasant side effects."[17] She tells of patients who have responded completely to progesterone treatment and have even been able to have their driver's licenses restored.[18] Dr. Betty Kamen, in her book *Hormone Replacement Therapy: Yes or No?*, concurs that progesterone has an effect on epileptic seizures because of its barbiturate-like action on brain metabolites.[19]

The following item, which appeared on the Internet, seems to corroborate those statements. It came in from a woman who had suffered in the past with epilepsy. She wrote: "Many years ago, at my absolute worst, I was having 30–50 seizures a day. Since I went on 200 mg. of natural progesterone (capsule form) a day, I have been nearly seizure-free. I know the vitamins and nutrients that I'm on are also helping."

Dr. Dalton's experience and study make clear that many of the uncomfortable symptoms normally associated with a woman's monthly cycle occur just prior to and during the first few days of menstruation, and occasionally at ovulation. It is not uncommon to experience pain, depression, and headaches continuing through the first day or two of each menses. However, all these ill effects, often aggravated by stress and its consequential depletion of progesterone, can be bypassed. Once the progesterone is replaced in our bodies naturally, many of our problems clear up. We *can* avoid the sufferings of hormone deficiency, and whether in our teens or in the postmenopausal period, we can learn from the studies that continue to surface,[20] and be thankful for the efforts of Dr. Katharina Dalton.

PROGESTERONE, STRESS, AND THE ADRENAL GLANDS

It is becoming more frequent for women to hear or read negative statements about progesterone in health-care magazine articles and even by doctors who have posted statements on their Web sites. However, their comments often seem to be inconsistent when it comes to their knowledge of progesterone and the full scope of its physiological effects. They will give a positive list of natural progesterone's many benefits one time, and *then* will use phrases like "beware," "use progesterone with caution," or "disrupts the adrenal function." They say things off the cuff without taking the time and effort to back up their comments with adequate documentation and studies.

As researchers, authors, and postmenopausal women who have been using natural transdermal progesterone for well over a decade, we can testify to its benefits in improving energy, bone mass, and overall health. The true need to separate facts from fiction is to go to the source and learn from the pioneers on the subject. For instance, one researcher on the subject, Raymond Peat, reports that progesterone will even "energize the adrenals and thyroid.[21] And Norman Shealy, M.D., Ph.D., states that progesterone is a "major regulator of estrogen, testosterone, and cortisol... [It] is the most versatile hormone in the human body."[22] Another authority, the late John R. Lee, M.D., tells us "because of the great safety of natural progesterone, considerable latitude is allowed."[23] Many doctors also agree that in an effort to stabilize our adrenal glands, we not only have to be on a diet that focuses on normalizing our pH balance, but we need to be aware how supportive it is to provide these glands with their natural building block—progesterone.

Our suggestion to our readers regarding those who take a negative and uninformed stand is to also "Beware" and "Use Caution" when reading their alarming messages on the Internet and elsewhere. We now have every opportunity to ground ourselves in the fundamentals of natural hormone rebalancing, so we will be prepared to face the skeptic about progesterone's use on the adrenal glands.

Even though circulating progesterone is produced in the ovaries, Dr. John Lee says that progesterone is also manufactured by the adrenals (our "stress glands"), where it is converted into the corticosteroid hormones. This progesterone is immediately and continuously used to supply the multitude of adrenal functions.

Niels H. Lauersen, M.D., says that "when natural progesterone drops, the normal conversion by the adrenal glands cannot take place, salt may build up, fluid may be retained, and hypoglycemia may ensue. Synthetic progestins generally make PMS symptoms worse, so if a woman is about to be treated with progesterone, she should be sure that it is natural progesterone."[24] According to Dr. Lee, this will balance out the estrogen dominance that is contributing to these symptoms.

Dr. Robert Lindsay, an osteoporosis expert, confirms that the synthetic hormones cause an increase in stress. He says, "If [they're] given ten milligrams of Provera in combination with . . . Premarin, many women feel premenstrual and crabby and irritable. They call up and say, 'Why did you give me that stuff?'"[25] Natural progesterone, however, not only protects against hypertension by reducing the build-up of intracellular sodium, as reported in 1990 by the *Journal of Epidemiology*, but also has an antistress effect on the pituitary.[26] This does not appear to be true with synthetic hormones, which increase cellular sodium and may lead to increased hypertension.[27]

Sterling Morgan writes that progestins can "cause temporary hypoglycemia by blocking adrenal production of glucocorticoids, which regulate blood sugar."[28] It's understandable that women so often decide to discontinue synthetic hormones. "Such problems," the author says, "are practically unknown with the natural kind [of progesterone] since it is totally compatible with the human body."[29] And Dr. Peat explains how progesterone aids in many allergic diseases, including the autoimmune and "collagen" diseases. It does so by helping to maintain blood sugar levels and by stabilizing lysosomes—cellular components that are involved in the inflammation process.[30]

Dr. Lee says that women in their thirties (some even earlier, and long before actual menopause) will on occasion not ovulate during their menstrual cycles. From my understanding, this can occur after a vigorous athletic training schedule, trauma, injury, harsh dieting, use of some methods of hormonal contraception, or severe emotional stress. Dr. Lee elaborates:

> Without ovulation, no corpus luteum results and no progesterone is made. Several problems can result from this. One is the month-long presence of unopposed estrogen with all its attendant side effects leading to the syndrome known as PMS. Another is the present, generally unrecognized, problem of progesterone's role in osteoporosis. Contemporary medicine is still unaware that progesterone stimulates osteoblast-mediated new bone formation. . . . A third is the interrelationship between progesterone loss and stress. Stress influences limbic brain function including the functioning of the hypothalamus.[31]

Dr. Lee makes clear that *stress can cause missed ovulation.* A decline in progesterone disrupts the production of adrenal corticosteroids. Stress is thereby heightened, causing a woman to be vulnerable to anovulatory cycles.[32]

We often hear about the physical stress caused by excessive exercise. Studies show that stress endured by long-distance marathon runners causes a loss of 4.2 percent of their bone mass in one year. This is due to stress factors that inhibit ovulation, and thus progesterone production.[33, 34] Dr. Peat explains that toxins build up at this time and can also contribute to a progesterone deficiency. Needless to say, the entire body can be affected by this hormone imbalance.[35]

Raising DHEA Levels with Phytohormones

Stress can also deplete another of our vital hormones produced by the adrenals: dehydroepiandrosterone (DHEA). This is the most abundant hormone in the human body, and yet until recently it has received the least attention from medical science! C. Norman Shealy, M.D., a neurosurgeon, has been doing research and giving seminars on the importance of DHEA in men and women. He says that the normal range in men is 180 to 1250 ng/dl (nanograms per deciliter) and in women 130 to 980 ng/dl. Dr. Shealy has found that the patients who fall in the low normal range and below tend to have adrenal exhaustion. These individuals cope poorly with stress, and many have physical and mental disabilities (often serious diseases).[36] According to Dr. Alan Gaby, as well as others, low levels of DHEA have been associated with premature aging, breast cancer, osteoporosis, rheumatoid arthritis, heart disease, obesity, diabetes, poor immunity, and even lupus and Alzheimer's disease.[37, 38]

Preliminary studies suggest that DHEA and progesterone have a heretofore unsuspected link, and that the use of natural progesterone cream—or progesterone's precursor, pregnenolone—may safely help DHEA levels to stabilize. Dr. Shealy and other researchers believe that in most cases this approach is far better than taking synthetic DHEA supplements, as it allows the body's wisdom to determine just how much of the hormone to make.[39] In extreme cases, sometimes DHEA is given for temporary relief, along with progesterone for balance. But a young person taking DHEA simply for increasing energy might damage her adrenals by signaling them not to produce any more of the hormone. And as Dr. Dean Raffelock explains, "large doses of DHEA which the body can't use are shunted into estradiol, which is exactly what we don't want."[40]

A Convincing Argument

Parallel research indicates that *Dioscorea*, the wild yam plant, contains natural precursors to DHEA. The *Journal of Clinical Endocrinology and Metabolism* states that higher levels of DHEA have been associated with a more active immune system and a decrease in diseases of the major organ systems.[41] Joe Glickman Jr., M.D., refers to various studies showing that people with low DHEA levels are more prone to hardening of the arteries, strokes, and cancer. In a twelve-year study of more than 240 men, those who had higher DHEA levels had a lower death rate from all these diseases.[42–46] Dr. Glickman even predicts that DHEA "may prove of significant benefit in treating AIDS."[47]

Raising DHEA levels may also reduce gastric cancer, as well as have a general anticarcinogenic effect on the breast, lung, colon, thyroid, skin, and liver.[48–52] Moreover, the *Journal of Neuroscience Research* reports that DHEA "greatly increases the number of nerve cells and their ability to establish connections to other nerve cells," suggesting that DHEA levels may help prevent Alzheimer's and other age-related senility diseases.[53]

The important factor to remember here, says Dr. Glickman, is that in its synthetic (prescription) form, DHEA could have damaging side effects to the liver.[54] Using a natural plant source seems to be the key to the many benefits of this hormone—especially in prevention of diseases brought on largely by the wear and tear of chronic stress to the system. Dr. Neecie Moore informs us that we can beneficially raise our DHEA levels (just as we can our progesterone levels) with the precursor found in the wild yam. She illustrates with the story of one doctor who raised his DHEA levels 91 percent in sixty days with *Dioscorea*.[55] (See chapter 5 for more about raising one's DHEA with progesterone.)

The more I have learned about natural progesterone, the more intrigued I have become with it. In case you are debating whether or not to take natural progesterone and are wondering whether it is really necessary, Dr. Ray Peat gives some more reasons: "When progesterone is deficient, there tends to be hypoglycemia," he says. Furthermore, natural progesterone has a stabilizing action in the muscle tissue and many other areas of the body, "such as the uterus, blood vessel walls, the heart, the intestines and the bladder. Less visibly, progesterone stabilizes and normalizes nervous, secretory, and growth processes. Biochemically, it plays a major role in providing the material out of which all the other steroid hormones (such as cortisone, testosterone, estrogen and salt-regulating aldosterone) can be made as needed."[56] In short, he says, progesterone plays a multitude of roles in normalizing body functions.

MENOPAUSE: THE RIGHT AND WRONG WAYS TO EASE THE TRANSITION

Now let's explore further some of the evidence as it relates to menopause—keeping in mind that most doctors deal with this critical period in a woman's life with a well-known prescription drug, the use of which has recently become more and more controversial. The synthetic estrogen known as Premarin is given to more than twenty-two million women per year and is one of the ten most prescribed drugs.[57] The prescribing of Provera (medroxy-progesterone), touted as being for "prevention," tried to keep pace. And, as we previously discussed, Prempro (the combination form of the two hormones) was used in the 2002 WHI trials that had to be stopped because of its role in causing an early increase in breast cancer, blood clots, and other possibly fatal reactions. However, even that hasn't been enough to stop the drug companies from introducing a modified, lower dose version of Prempro to the market place in 2004. How sad, when the truth of the matter is that both Premarin and Provera are synthetic hormones that are very difficult for the body to metabolize and thus are capable of causing extreme reactions.

In spite of the many dangers, physicians will frequently prescribe a synthetic form of progesterone (progestin) because they erroneously say it prevents breast and ovarian cancer in women on estrogen. Unfortunately, they do this without warning us about the potential for triggering coronary vasospasms, stroke, and cancer.[58–63] Although the trial in the summer of 2002 was halted due to these harmful and sometimes fatal outcomes, nevertheless prescriptions for Premarin/progestin are still being handed out to women of all ages. That's right, the trials were suddenly stopped, but the prescriptions did not.

In good conscience, why would physicians continue this practice? Why do companies spend millions of dollars on double blind studies and then not adhere to the facts from the trials that clearly demonstrate these harmful effects on women? And why do double-blind studies continue to use vulnerable women for their business purposes if it is not going to serve the general public as a whole? At one time they used animals for experimental purposes, but now they are using women, women who are desperate for help.

Todd Mangum, M.D., tells us that Premarin is "foreign to humans and problematic for us to metabolize. Because of this, the use of Premarin often increases an undesirable form of estrogen known to be carcinogenic . . . even though it might be called natural, it is still far from bioidentical for women."[64] Unfortunately, what women really need and what they are sold are extremely divergent. It's based on corporate profits rather than patient benefits. Perhaps we should take a look into the past and see if there could possibly be any sane justification for this approach. Let's start from the very beginning and see if there's some rationale as to why women have suffered so needlessly and for so long.

History Behind Conventional HRT

Since 1942 Premarin has been heralded as the "fountain of youth" pill. In 1952 it was rumored that it would "enhance verbal memory" in the elderly. In 1959 *JAMA* publicized how it could protect women from becoming osteoporotic and that there was no need to fear cancer when using Premarin. In 1962 *JAMA* once again reassured menopausal women that Premarin's estrogen would reduce reproductive cancer. Robert Wilson's 1968 book, *Feminine Forever*, sponsored by the drug manufacturer Wyeth-Ayerst, recommended estrogen as the cure for menopause. In 1970, approximately 14 million prescriptions were written for Premarin. In 1973, men were used in trials where they were given Premarin "to prevent heart attacks and strokes." The trials came to a halt again when it turned out that the men were "having more heart attacks and blood clots."[65] In 1975, documentation in the *New England Journal of Medicine* showed estrogen use increased the risk of endometrial cancer in menopausal women.[66] In 1976, a study showing a link between estrogen and breast cancer was published in the *New England Journal of Medicine*. In 1982, experts report in *Cancer Research* that HRT was the leading factor in reproductive cancers. In 1985, the Framingham Heart Study showed that cardiovascular events rose in women taking estrogen more than with those not using conventional hormones. In 1989, a Swedish study found that when "women switched to combination HRT, their breast cancer risk more than doubled."[67]

From 1990 to 1995, Premarin was the top-selling drug in the United States. In 1995, Prempro (the combination Premarin and progestin) pill was approved by the FDA.[68] In 1989, and again in 1994, studies found links to other forms of cancer.[69] In 1995, we were again told that estrogen increased the risk of breast cancer[70-72] and ovarian cancer.[73] In the same year *JAMA* published a national study showing an increased risk of coronary heart disease when the synthetic combo was prescribed.[74] More warnings came in 1996 when the same synthetic hormones were linked to endometrial cancer.[75]

In considering the harmful effects of these chemically altered hormones, let's first reflect on a statistic reported in *Science News* (March 8, 1997): "Heart disease kills three out of every four post-menopausal women."[76] One clue as to why emerges from a study (Hermsmeyer et al.) done at the Oregon Regional Primate Research Center. Estrogen was given daily to eighteen rhesus monkeys who were in simulated menopause because their ovaries had been removed. One third of them were also given natural progesterone, and another third received synthetic medroxyprogesterone acetate (Provera or MPA), "the most widely prescribed progesterone for postmenopausal U.S. women."[77]

At the four-week interval, the monkeys received chemical injections to simulate a heart attack. This triggered "unrelenting constriction in the coronary artery, cutting off blood flow"[78] in those receiving the estrogen/MPA combination or no hormones at all. Immediate treatment was necessary to prevent them from dying.[79] In this study the animals treated with estrogen alone or in combination with natural progesterone experienced a quick recovery of blood flow without any kind of emergency care. The scientists involved, whose findings were reported in the March 1997 *Nature Medicine* and the March 1, 1997 *Journal of the American College of Cardiology,* stated that they were very surprised to find that the commonly prescribed synthetic progesterone was such a dangerous drug.[80]

The dilemma in the orthodox medical approach is the real discovery of this investigation. On one hand, doctors were no longer to prescribe estrogen alone,[81] yet as a result of the Oregon study the conventional solution of combining it with Provera was also no longer tenable. One has to wonder how long it will take this information to come to light. Millions of menopausal women are taking such potentially lethal combinations daily. This approach is justified by the statistic that "heart disease" is the number one killer of postmenopausal women—the persuasive rationale for taking HRT.

The natural progesterone as utilized in this study is impressively effective and seems such an obvious solution. One reason natural progesterone offers such protection is its antispasmodic effect in the body, functioning as a vasodilator to prevent or regulate coronary artery spasms, which may, conversely, be induced by the administration of Provera.[82]

In 1998, the "first major placebo-controlled trial of HRT showed that hormones do not help women who have already had a heart attack and, in fact, caused more heart attacks, strokes, and other cardiovascular events."[83] Women put their faith in the rhetoric offered by their physicians (based on pharmaceutical promotions) that it was good for their heart and other female problems. The *Journal of American Medical Association,* in the 1998 HERS study, disproved this theory after a clinical trial was conducted involving 2,763 women. The participants were given daily doses of oral estrogen and progestin. After this four-year investigation, it was discovered that these synthetic hormones "did not reduce the overall rate of coronary heart disease (CHD)" but did increase the rate of thromboembolism (blood clots), as well as gallbladder disease.[84, 85]

In 2000 the Women's Health Initiative told women that if they wished they could drop out of the study. In 2001 Premarin prescriptions rose to more than 11 million. In 2002 this news from Washington shocked the world: Government scientists brought one of the largest HRT studies to an immediate halt when the National Institutes of Health found that these synthetic hormones "significantly increased the women's risk of breast cancer, strokes, and heart attacks . . . [The] use of estrogen and progestin increased otherwise healthy women's risk of a stroke by 41 percent, a heart attack by 29 percent, and breast cancer by 24 percent."[86]

There's no excuse for this ongoing mistreatment. Study after study demonstrates that women are being duped and used as guinea pigs. They continue to be deceived by "health" schemes promoted by glamorous celebrities who are paid handsomely to endorse the establishment propaganda.

Advertisements sponsored by powerful organizations have a vested interest in marketing synthetic HRT and promoting yearly mammograms. This is very unfortunate considering the fact that non-invasive screening tools and safer forms of HRT are available. (See appendix D for more information.) They continually maintain their stronghold by switching product names, ingredients, and dosages. Thus they manipulate the naïve and symptomatic. Well-compensated drug company strategists in the area of "women's health" can be depended upon to continue to find new ways to meet their goals, often at the expense of women who are desperately seeking help.

A *New York Times* article revealed one of their new advertising schemes. It includes the hiring of celebrities such as Lauren Bacall, Kathleen Turner, and Rob Lowe to talk about specific diseases. They "casually plug a product without mentioning that, oh by the way, they've received payment in return for their pitch . . . state the health problem . . . instill a little motivating fear . . . suggest an action to take . . . then name the miracle remedy that you need to ask your doctor about."[87] These endorsements featuring alluring movie stars have become an effective marketing tool for the drug companies. A clever and profitable ploy? Yes! But is this the way we want to get our medical advice? How much longer are vulnerable and uninformed women going to be used for corporate profits?

Women Who Speak Out

In a personal account, Gail Sheehy tells us in her book *The Silent Passage: Menopause* what happened when she added synthetic Provera to her regimen:

> I felt by afternoon as if I had a terrible hangover. This chemically induced state was not being subdued by aspirin or a walk in the park. It only worsened as the day wore on, bringing with it a racing heart, irritability, waves of sadness, and difficulty concentrating. And to top it off, the hot flashes came back! . . . . By night I couldn't go to sleep without a glass of wine, and even then was awakened by a racing heartbeat and sweating.[88]

It's frightening to learn that most of our traditional medical doctors prescribe progesterone's counterfeit, Provera, despite the fact that, Sheehy points out, "it has never been approved for treatment of menopause by the U.S. Food and Drug Administration."[89] She continues:

Notwithstanding, the FDA's Advisory Committee on Fertility and Maternal Health Drugs stated in '91 that this combination of hormones "may be used indefinitely by a woman with a uterus." Asked what proportion of the female population over age fifty would be suitable candidates for long term consumption of estrogen alone or combined with synthetic progesterone, the committee replied, "virtually all." A blank check.[90]

Some of these synthetic hormones have been on the market for approximately fifty years. However, year after year since then, women have come home with their prescriptions and continued to have the same miserable reactions and apprehensions about taking them. Many never even fill their prescriptions, and some who do will not have them refilled, especially after reading the manufacturers' warnings (see appendix B). We are afraid and often don't know where to turn. Gail Sheehy expresses what many women have experienced:

> I didn't require a ten-year clinical trial and double-blind study to guess what was going on. Taking synthetic progesterone with the estrogen for half of each month was like pushing down the gas pedal and putting on the brakes at the same time, and it had left my body confused and worn out.[91]

Before we go into some of the conditions that accompany menopause, keep in mind the numerous physiological benefits of natural progesterone—versus the associated problems that are known to be aggravated by use of synthetic progestins, such as cardiac insufficiency, epilepsy, migraine headaches, depression, high cholesterol levels, and kidney disorders.[92] When you ask your doctor for natural progesterone in lieu of the synthetic substance, he may say that the artificial hormones have been proved to mimic our natural hormones perfectly. If so, refer your doctor to an article in the *New England Journal of Medicine* that appeared in 1993.[93] Remember that this information, urgently needed by women, was discovered by scientists who held themselves above the politics of medicine. Dr. Betty Kamen's words aptly summarize this news:

> Progesterone is the primary building block for all the other steroid hormones. This alone distinguishes natural progesterone from synthetic progestins. . . . The one similarity between the synthetic and natural forms of progesterone is that . . . each can trigger uterine bleeding similar to menstrual flow, if needed.[94]

This ability to trigger a monthly menses became one of the major factors in the development of birth control pills. Mistakenly, it was believed that if a woman had a "period" each month, her ovaries would remain healthy.

As we highlight the many benefits that develop with natural progesterone supplementation, I must relate to you a surprising turn of events described to me by a friend. I had told her Dr. Linda Force's story of how the application of progesterone had cleared up her fibrocystic breast disorder. My friend then decided to use the natural progesterone cream on the lump on her breast, which at one time she'd had to have drained. This fibroid of hers would come and go, and at this point she was not overly concerned because she thought that with proper diet and exercise it would eventually go away.

However, after thinking about progesterone therapy for a while and learning that it was natural and had no side effects, she decided to use the cream as a preventive measure and apply it directly to the lumpy area on her breast. When we met the following month, she was elated with the results of the progesterone cream. She told me that after the first few days of using it, she began to experience other unexpected benefits. Not only did the lump go away but *so did her hot flashes*. This was a surprise to her, because everything she had read indicated that supplemental estrogen was the only remedy for hot flashes.

Of course, if she'd had the opportunity to read any of Dr. John Lee's writings, my friend would have understood that a high percentage of women with hot flashes respond to the progesterone alone. He sees no need for additional estrogen (preferably estriol) unless the hot flashes do not subside within about six months of the beginning of progesterone treatment; and it should then be a very individual and informed decision. Every body is different and will experience benefits in its own unique way. My friend also mentioned that her insomnia was no longer a problem. As long as she used the progesterone cream, she was able to sleep through the night without the usual interruptions that are brought on by hormone imbalance.

Another friend, Dianna Widerstrom, shares her experience: "Two weeks before my period, my breasts would swell so badly that they would be painful to the touch or whenever I lay on my stomach. (I had been diagnosed as having fibrocystic breasts six years ago.) When I finally started my period, I would pass blood clots the size of a silver dollar. At this time I also experienced a tremendous amount of water retention. During all this stress to my body I would also become very irritable.

"As I was relating my problems to a dear friend, she told me about progesterone cream. I began using the cream, and after the first month I saw several changes in my body—the breast lumps had reduced tremendously; the clotting wasn't as bad, nor was the water retention. After three months, the lumps were completely gone and the blood flow had become even. All these things have had a positive effect on my personality, which hasn't gone unnoticed or unappreciated by my husband.

"After several more months I decided to take a month off the cream. What a mistake! I'll never do that again! My breasts became lumpy and very sore. I was passing blood clots again (though not as large as before); my periods no longer had a nice even flow, and I retained a lot of water. This all proved to me that my body needs and works well with progesterone. (I've also discovered that dandelion root extract works well to reduce water retention.)

"I am a salon owner and have decided to sell the cream in my studio. Several of my clients use it and have seen major changes in their bodies, and thus their lives. Unfortunately, we are not always able to obtain these natural ingredients from our doctors."

Hot Flashes, Breast Swelling, and Infections

Estrogen is produced by the ovaries and is also stored and manufactured after menopause in body fat. When it is needed, it is released and then metabolized by the liver.[95] As we get older, the body tells us when our hormones are declining. According to the experts, the two major signs of low estrogen are hot flashes and genital atrophy. Although Dr. Lita Lee says, "I have never seen a menopausal woman (whether natural or surgical) who did not successfully ameliorate hot flashes with progesterone treatment,"[96] I have personally talked with several menopausal women who experienced an *increase* in breast swelling, water retention, insomnia, or headaches during the *initial* stages of progesterone treatment.

I asked Dr. John Lee why this might be. He explained that before these women started their progesterone therapy, they were estrogen-dominant. Estrogen dominance tunes down the estrogen receptors. The body is trying to protect itself from too much estrogen. Progesterone, however, temporarily increases the sensitivity of the receptors. Thus, for a short duration one might experience estrogen-like side effects, such as breast swelling and bloating, which in time (after a two- or three-month period of progesterone application) usually subside.

He illustrated that a similar thing happens with a woman who is in her perimenopausal phase. She is still making, as he put it, "a ton of estrogen" and is menstruating regularly; but she has no progesterone to bring about orderly periods, so they are sometimes heavy and sometimes light. The body is now making more estrogen than it really needs, because the receptors are not very attentive to it. When you then add progesterone, you restore estrogen dominance for a while as the receptors resume normal sensitivity. At this time there may be a period of adjustment when some women experience various uncomfortable symptoms; all that estrogen they are making may suddenly flare up as swollen breasts, weight gain, water retention, and headaches.

These estrogen side effects last only for the first month or two, if they're even noticed at all. By the third month, the body's progesterone level is sufficiently high to oppose this action. Dr. Lee's suggestion to women with these problems, therefore, is that if you will just persevere for two to three months, your progesterone level will rise enough to do its beneficial work and the temporary side effects should disappear.

VAGINAL ATROPHY

Another common problem associated with menopause is vaginal atrophy, which can be extremely painful with intercourse. Many women have found that a mixture of pure progesterone oil, and/or unrefined coconut oil or extra virgin olive oil can be applied to the vaginal lining to be helpful. Along with this, a capsule of vitamin E tocopheral and vitamin A inserted into the vagina itself will be even more effective. This combination will make the vaginal wall more elastic, and less susceptible to infection. As you continue these applications, the function of the mucus-secreting cells will provide a beneficial effect.

Elaine Hollingsworth's *Take Control of Your Health and Escape the Sickness Industry* speaks about other herbs, such as chastetree and motherwort to help restore the vaginal lining.[97] Dr. Carlton Fredericks suggests that the use of vitamin A and E cream for atrophic vaginitis is much safer than the synthetic estrogen creams (Cynonal or Premarin) so frequently prescribed by medical doctors. He says, "Both have side effects and may also irritate you."[98] Another natural alternative comes from Dr. Jonathan Wright, who tells us that the use of 100 mgs of Panax ginseng has been shown to be effective in thickening vaginal mucosa, with the effect of a disappearance of vaginal dystrophy.[99] For more information on this subject see appendices A and F.

As for the progesterone cream, many women feel great when they first start using it. Then, after three months, some women may find that their symptoms seem to return. An answer to this dilemma comes from David Smallbone, M.D., who practices homeopathy and nutrition and has been advocating progesterone to his patients for many years. He maintains that when symptoms start up again, it's because "the body is beginning to convert the progesterone into other hormones, so that progesterone activity appears to take a dip." At this point, he advises "a very slight increase" in the dosage for another three months[100] to bring the system back into balance. This kind of fine-tuning is necessarily an individual and ongoing process.

Dean Raffelock, D.C., who is a clinical nutritionist in Portland, Oregon, gives another reason some people seem to develop uncomfortable symptoms when they first start using progesterone. This occurs in a small group of women who, even though they have been found to be highly estrogenic and low in progesterone, are usually found to have serious liver dysfunction. If the liver is not healthy, it won't be able to break down the steroid hormones.[101]

To support the liver, it's important for us to eat foods containing sulfur, such as broccoli, cauliflower, brussels sprouts, beans, molasses,[102] cabbage, kale, garlic, onions, eggs, and fish.[103] Supplements that contain sulfur can also be helpful in the process of detoxification, including glucosamine sulfate (GLS) and methyl-sulfonyl-methane (MSM). If you take MSM, Dr. Raffelock advises that you make sure that you are also getting about 1 mg of the mineral molybdenum daily.[104]

Also important are B complex vitamins. As an example, Dr. Raffelock explains that the active form of B_6 (pyrodoxyl 5-phosphate), in concert with magnesium, ensures the adequate functioning of the liver's various metabolic pathways and assists in breaking down the sex steroids for their necessary elimination. We can help to detoxify the liver every day, not only through good diet but with homeopathic liver remedies[105] and herbal supplements such as dandelion and milk thistle, which are beneficial to the liver by means of their alkalinizing effect on pH levels.[106] Such an overall approach will allow for better utilization of progesterone and help prevent the buildup of excess estrogen, with all its concomitant complications.

Even if your doctor thinks your symptoms indicate a need for estrogen treatment, remember that natural progesterone should be the first treatment for at least two or three months. Applied topically, it is very effective for many women.

Along with progesterone, Dr. Lee also talks about estriol for vaginal dryness and "atrophic mucosa" (shrinking membranes) after menopause. The condition will in turn "predispose women to vaginal, urethral, and urinary bladder infections. . . . To treat the infectious agent," he says, ". . . with antibiotics is only temporarily successful because the underlying real cause . . . is loss of *host resistance* secondary to hormone deficiency."

Dr. Lee says that in his clinical practice, estriol treatments have "resulted in the reemergence of friendly lactobacilli [bacteria] and the near elimination of [undesirable] colon bacteria, as well as the restoration of normal vaginal mucosa and a resumption of normal low pH (which inhibits the growth of many pathogens)."[107] Where estrogen had been contraindicated to his patients, Dr. Lee was surprised to find that the natural progesterone therapy also cleared up the vaginal dryness and mucosal atrophy after three to four months of use. His experience and that of many other doctors is confirmation of our need to find the right individual balance of hormones in their *natural* form.

HOW DO DRUGS AFFECT OUR HEALTH AND HORMONE LEVELS?

Dependency on medication is a disease in itself, as it leads to an addiction to many drugs. The average American may think at first, "I'm not dependent on medicine!" However, reality strikes when we take a look inside the medicine cabinet. For example, consider those antibiotics prescribed so frequently and without consideration of their long-term effect. Because antibiotic therapy results in the destruction of useful bacteria, it creates an ideal environment for the overgrowth of more harmful bacteria or fungi (yeasts).[108] Consequently, other infections take over and virulent, drug-resistant strains of many disease-causing organisms evolve. Dr. Julian Whitaker says, "13,300 hospital patients in 1992 died from infections that could not be controlled by antibiotics."[109]

We might well turn our attention from *anti*biotics to *pro*biotics—a word used in the informative book *Alternative Medicine*. Providing our own friendly bacteria with proper nutrition will eventually create and assure an excellent state of homeostasis. According to this book, some of the probiotics include *Lactobacillus acidophilus, Lactobacillus bulgaricus, Bifidobacterium bifidum,* and *Bifidobacterium longum.*[110] While antibiotics such as penicillin kill our good bacteria, and steroids such as cortisone and birth control pills may also harm the flora of the bowel, these beneficial bacteria can thrive on live yogurt and diets that are rich in complex carbohydrates (organic raw vegetables, whole grains, legumes) and low in sugar and fats.[111]

Many women suffer from an overgrowth of *Candida albicans*, a fungus common to all of us and harmless when kept in check by friendly bacteria. Often difficult to control, this condition is more widespread than we generally recognize. Its symptoms may include chronic vaginal irritation, thrush, an itchy skin rash, headaches, extreme fatigue, and problems of the gastrointestinal or urinary tract or the neuromuscular or respiratory system.[112, 113]

Frequently brought on by antibiotic therapy, candidiasis may also be related to the use of contraceptive and other corticosteroid drugs as well as to dietary factors (e.g., excessive sugar) and to progesterone deficiency. The amount of sugar in many women's diets not only feeds the yeast but upsets our hormone and mineral balance. Dr. Lee brings the point home:

> One can of Coke contains nine teaspoons of sugar. Dumping nine teaspoons of sugar into your body is a setup for wildly fluctuating blood sugar levels, weight gain, insulin resistance, and adrenal fatigue—a perfect setup for hormone imbalance! Just as bad are the diet sodas with aspartame [NutraSweet], a synthetic chemical containing substances called excitotoxins, which are known to cause brain damage and may contribute to hyperactivity, learning disabilities, and Alzheimer's.[114]

To treat yeast infection and the associated uncomfortable discharge, doctors often prescribe one of several fungicidal creams, such as Monistat-7 or similar over-the-counter drugs. Thinking of my own experience with these products stirs up an unpleasant memory of vaginal tissue burning and irritation. But having this additional side effect to compound my other menopausal troubles would not have been necessary, had I known then about *natural* hormone treatment.[115]

NATURAL HORMONES RAISE "GOOD" CHOLESTEROL AND LOWER THE "BAD"

Another area of concern relates to our cholesterol levels as we age. Have you had yours checked lately? If you are menopausal, have you noticed that it's been higher than it used to be and that all those "cholesterol-free" products don't seem to be having any effect on lowering the "bad" cholesterol?

Diet and exercise are certainly important, but there's another factor that has been greatly overlooked in controlling cholesterol. Gail Sheehy also suggests a relationship between hormones, cholesterol, and cardiac disease:

> The most significant predictor of heart disease is the HDL level. Bad cholesterol levels normally increase in women for some ten to fifteen years following the cessation of periods. Again, dangerous changes in cholesterol count or blood pressure do not announce themselves with obvious symptoms, not until there is a medical catastrophe. "If your HDL level is low, and your LDL level is relatively higher—even if you're

walking around with a total cholesterol count of 100—you're going to be in trouble," says Dr. Estelle Ramey.[116]

As you may recall from our discussion in chapter 2, clinical experience emphasizes the need for stabilizing estrogen with progesterone to counter the risks of lowering our supply of HDL cholesterol, which can occur in the presence of chronically high estrogen levels. Conventional estrogen treatment, by itself, can cause many harmful side effects and further accelerate this problem. The 2000 edition of *Facts & Comparisons* states "Some progestins* may elevate LDL levels and decrease HDL." (See warnings in appendix D.) The question is, then why take cholesterol-lowering drugs when we have a safer and more natural alternative in supplemental progesterone from plant sources?

The Natural Pharmacy, compiled by some of the world's leading experts in nutrition, states that "steroidal saponins (such as diosgenin) account for some of wild yam's activity," and have "also been shown to lower blood triglycerides and to raise HDL cholesterol (the 'good' cholesterol)."[117]

Lowered HDL levels are known to be a significant indicator of the potential for heart disease. And, as reported in the *Phoenix Tribune* on February 5, 1998, the American Heart Association calls heart attacks and strokes "the No. 1 killer of women in America" over and above all forms of cancers.[118]

Since the onset of cardiovascular disease is usually symptomless and gradual, it is of utmost importance to raise our HDL levels throughout our perimenopausal and menopausal years without dependency on synthetic heart medications. As we mention elsewhere in this book (see appendix A), wild yam may not confer the same benefits as when its diosgenin is converted to USP progesterone; however, it appears to have a role in the non-drug approach to women's health care.

LUTEAL PHASE DEFICIENCY

A common complaint of many younger women today is, "My periods have completely stopped" or, "My periods are abnormally frequent or irregular." Medically, these symptoms are referred to as "luteal phase defect" and are caused because the corpus luteum is not producing its optimal output of ovarian progesterone (18–25 mg) from ovulation to day 26 (the second half of the menstrual cycle). Explained simply, estrogen is the dominant hormone during the first part of the cycle (the follicular phase). But if it continues to predominate in the second part of the cycle (the luteal phase), this

---

* Synthetic progesterones

indicates low progesterone production and could bring about any of these menstrual abnormalities, referred to as hypermenorrhea, polymenorrhea, or amenorrhea.[119]

Failure to correct such a deficiency can have a major impact if and when a woman finds out she is pregnant. At this time clinically low progesterone, as found with luteal phase deficiency, can trigger miscarriages. This problem will be discussed further on in this chapter.

NEW THOUGHTS ABOUT CONCEPTION/CONTRACEPTION

But what about those still in their reproductive years? According to Dr. Samuel Epstein, in *The Politics of Cancer*, "Worldwide use of birth control pills, in spite of conclusive evidence of carcinogenicity of estrogens in experimental animals, constitutes the largest uncontrolled experiment in human carcinogenesis ever undertaken."[120]

The average person is confused. Statistics show that approximately "ten million women in the United States"[121] and as many as fifty million worldwide are using oral contraceptive agents.[122] And the average layperson is confused as to whether it is progesterone or estrogen that is prescribed for contraception. According to *Goodman and Gilman's The Pharmacological Basis of Therapeutics*, "Progestational agents . . . in combination with estrogens are used widely as oral contraceptives." Ethinylestradiol, mestranol, and many other combinations are listed.[123] However, Dr. John Lee tells us that the commonly prescribed synthetic contraceptive ethinylestradiol is considered dangerous "because of high oral absorption and slow metabolism and excretion [which are] true of all synthetic estrogens."[124]

The long-term side effects are often tragic. Since progestational agents were introduced in the 1950s, the number of synthetic forms of the drugs has increased abundantly, and many are used clinically as contraceptive agents. Norethynodrel was one of the very first progestin compounds to be used. Among other highly potent progestins are chlormadinone acetate and cyproterone acetate.[125] The U.S. Food and Drug Administration issued a warning concerning medroxyprogesterone, one of the most commonly prescribed and one that seems to cause the most agitation and discomfort. Evidently the agency had not approved it for contraceptive use because of "potential serious side effects."[126] Nevertheless, it continues to be used.[127]

Scientists have studied the action of progesterone receptors in animals. They've demonstrated, as Dr. Katharina Dalton attests, that "progesterone receptors will only transfer molecules of progesterone to the cell nucleus, but not molecules of the artificial progestogens. . . . [Yet] these substitutes for progesterone are used in the contraceptive pills and in other gynecological conditions."[128]

Dr. Ray Peat cautions that the use of estrogens, birth control pills, and even IUDs can cause progesterone deficiency.[129] One study shows, in fact, that the intrauterine device blocks ovarian production of progesterone[130] by a mechanism called *luteolysis*—a process in which the IUD's chronic uterine irritation causes degeneration of the corpus luteum (the source of ovarian progesterone).[131] Such artificial means of contraception can cause severe cramping, infertility, weight gain, and other seemingly unrelated problems, with breast cancer included among the long-term reactions to the Pill.[132] A 1966 study by Spellacy and Carlson demonstrated the danger of prolonged pancreatic stimulation by oral contraceptives. This increased the level of free fatty acids and the tendency toward diabetes.[133]

Be cautious of studies that say there is no need to worry about cancer risks when taking birth control pills. Learn from women like Barbara Joseph, M.D., herself a survivor of breast cancer, who has found the reverse to be true. She documents a definite correlation between "the pill" and breast cancer in younger women.[134] Oral contraceptives were first prescribed in the mid-1960s. A long enough time has passed since then to witness the large number of women who have been stricken with breast cancer from these synthetic drugs.[135]

The *Journal of the National Cancer Institute* published long-term studies of women who were prescribed birth control pills with a lower concentration of estrogen. The conclusion was that "women who start taking oral contraceptives before age 18 and continue to take them for more than 10 years increase their breast-cancer risk threefold."[136]

Dr. Ray Peat cautions that the unexpected can occur when the body is exposed to the dangers of chemically altered hormones. As Dr. John Lee tells us, "Some of these drugs [have] resulted in permanent loss of ovary function. . . . [And] vaginitis occurs more often among women taking contraceptive pills. . . . Contraceptive pills prevent the normal hormone-generated mucus from being produced to protect them. Birth control pills work, after all, by suppressing normal hormones."[137]

Oral contraceptives have also been clearly linked with the development of blood clots.[138] Clotting may occur in the veins of the legs—a condition known as deep venous thrombosis. Since blood clots in the leg (calf, thigh, etc.) can easily travel to the lungs (pulmonary embolism), these are quite serious. *The Complete Book of Menopause* states that "pulmonary embolism can be fatal and [is] the basis of the major concern about deep venous thrombosis."[139] We see time and again the importance of introducing natural progesterone to oppose the dangerous effects of too much estrogen. In place of the artificial and harmful progestins, Dr. Alan Gaby compares the different results produced by the use of natural progesterone and its synthetic version. He says:

> Whereas progesterone aids in conception and helps maintain pregnancy, progestogens inhibit ovulation and are therefore used for birth control. . . . Many women who have had severe side effects from birth control pills or from other hormone regimens containing progestogens improve when they receive natural progesterone.[140]

Some medical doctors and many women wonder why we have not been using natural progesterone as a contraceptive, since it has never exhibited any serious or long-term side effects. For while progesterone, given from the time of ovulation, maintains pregnancy—given before, in some situations and at the right strength, it may be able to prevent it. (Apparently it is all in the timing—which can be tricky—taking into account individual cycle variations and responses.) This urgently deserves further study. However, at this stage there is a certain amount of disagreement as to the application of natural progesterone to contraception, and just how much guarantees "safety." *Therefore, the discussion that follows is not to be considered a recommendation*, but merely a starting point for more investigation.

When asked about progesterone having contraceptive action in premenopausal women, Dr. John Lee replies that he uses progesterone in cream form mainly to establish normal physiological levels. There are varying potencies of creams on the market; some are probably so mild as to have no contraceptive effect, while others may have the potential to prevent ovulation in some women.

When a woman would like to have a baby, Dr. Lee advises the patient to wait until day twelve or fourteen to start progesterone. This avoids any inadvertent interference with ovulation. If she is not interested in conceiving and is deficient enough in progesterone to warrant a few extra days of treatment each month, he sometimes moves that up to day eight or ten.

Dr. Lee tells us, "If sufficient [natural] progesterone is provided prior to ovulation, neither ovary produces an egg. This inhibition of ovulation is the original mechanism of action of progestin contraception. . . . Similarly, the high estriol and progesterone levels throughout pregnancy successfully inhibit ovarian activity for nine months. Therefore adding natural progesterone from day 10 to day 26 of the cycle suppresses LH and its luteinizing effects."[141]

The reason for taking higher levels of progesterone before ovulation is that at the time of ovulation, when the follicle converts to the corpus luteum and starts producing progesterone at a mammoth rate, the other ovary senses the excess progesterone and immediately halts its own ovulation process. In normal circumstances, both ovaries are stimulated in the first half of the month by the follicle-stimulating hormone, and both start making an egg. When one of them ovulates and starts producing progesterone, that's a signal for the other one to stop. If both ovaries ovulated, we'd have fraternal twins quite often because sperm may enter both fallopian tubes. But fraternal twins occur only once out of every three hundred births—meaning that the rest of the time, one ovary ovulates enough ahead of the other ovary to shut it down. That's the basis of birth control pills. While higher doses do stop ovulation, it is now known that the major contraceptive mechanism of synthetic progestins is that even at low doses they occupy progesterone receptors in the endometrium and prevent implantation of the fertilized ovum (egg).

Lita Lee, Ph.D., is one who also believes that natural progesterone is "nature's contraceptive and can . . . prevent pregnancy without harmful side effects."[142] Nonetheless, I must share with you a conversation I had with Wallace Simons, R.Ph., President of Women's International Pharmacy, concerning birth control (or to use his terminology, "ovulation control"). Referring to Dr. Katharina Dalton's claim that using natural progesterone from day eight through the end of her cycle will make a woman contraceptively safe, he stressed, "*Don't count on it.* I can think of three cases where it did not work, and they have three beautiful babies to show for it." (Dr. Lee informs us that Dr. Dalton recommends much larger doses than most doctors.)

Wallace Simons added, "We have women who are using synthetic progestogen pills for birth control and they absolutely will not give up this protection, yet want to use the natural progesterone for their PMS problems and especially to ward off the side effects of birth control pills. At first we said, 'Sorry, you must get off the progestogens first.'" But the pharmacy had so many requests for this combination that they finally began to recommend the natural progesterone along with the synthetic after the tenth pill of the pill pack during the second half of the menstrual cycle, and it worked just beautifully.

So even though the subjects' receptor cells have been at least partially blocked by the synthetics, the body somehow utilizes the natural progesterone to offset any discomfort. I asked Simons if there was any way one could use just the natural progesterone for ovulation control. He replied, "No, and I have a two-year-old granddaughter to prove that. We cannot tell you it's a birth control."

In essence, then, the authorities seem to agree on the principle; it's the application that can be risky. For greater safety it might be wise to combine natural progesterone for ovulation control with a barrier method of birth control. As for surgical contraception, too few women are aware of Dr. Dalton's warning: "Sterilization should be avoided; it can lower the blood level of progesterone and increase PMS."[143] Not only is this true of tubal ligation, "previously thought to be a convenient permanent solution,"[144] but vasectomy has been linked with long-term hormone imbalance and cancer in men.[145] However, many men are opting for this surgical procedure and then balancing their hormone levels with the use of transdermal progesterone and DHEA.

FERTILITY AND INFERTILITY

Increasingly in the area of fertility therapy, holistically-oriented medical doctors are concentrating on prescribing more natural substances for women. It would be wise to try to locate one in your area who will work with you and understand your needs when it comes to natural hormone replacement therapy.* A case in point: natural progesterone for conception. Although under ideal conditions it sometimes works as a contraceptive, progesterone is also used in some fertility clinics.[146]

In the July 1997 issue of the *Vegetarian Times* we learned that "10 million Americans are affected by infertility."[147] The stress, depression, and financial drain that results from a continual focus on fertility treatments, however, may now be an ordeal of the past. Let's hope so, considering that the price tag on many of the high-tech testing procedures ranges in the area of $10,000.[148] We know of people whose personal experience at fertility clinics involved expenditures totaling as high as $50,000 to $60,000 per attempt. Couples need to be informed that there are better solutions than the standard use of drugs, surgery, and expensive diagnostic procedures. These approaches can often be painful and dangerous and do not even ensure a healthy pregnancy or child.

As Dr. Lee makes clear, "Progesterone is the most important hormone in fertility and pregnancy."[149] Yet we don't hear about progesterone very often from conventionally-trained doctors, even though seventy years ago it was discovered that progesterone, which is produced in the corpus lutea of the

---

* Information for your physician can be found in appendix F, and pharmacies and distributors of natural HRT are listed in appendix G.

ovaries, has to be available in the body in sufficient quantity in order for conception even to occur.

Jerome Check, M.D., an infertility specialist and professor of obstetrics and gynecology at Thomas Jefferson University and Hahnemann University, says that "too often physicians will treat the infertility problem with strong medication or even surgery without checking progesterone levels first. . . . But for many women, progesterone therapy has been very effective in helping them to become pregnant and to carry the child to term. Only after this treatment is tried, should more drastic procedures be considered."[150]

An adequate amount of progesterone is crucial to a woman who is trying to become pregnant. It actually prepares the uterine wall for implantation of the fertilized egg. Without sufficient progesterone, the egg will be expelled. Progesterone treatment can also be used to induce fertility when there appears to be ovulatory dysfunction (most commonly a luteal phase defect).[151] A study was performed involving fifty women who had lived with infertility for a minimum of one and a half years. Seventy percent of the women conceived within six months while exclusively using progesterone therapy, reports Dr. Check. "The Efficacy of Progesterone in Achieving Successful Pregnancy" describes this group:

> Five patients had a history of previous spontaneous abortions; all others had primary infertility. The range of ages was 18 to 39, with an average of 31. Their average period of infertility was 2.8 years in the 35 patients who conceived, and 2.7 years for the entire group.[152]

From all the data it seems clear that natural progesterone therapy offers no risks to the patient and will be likely to benefit those wishing to conceive. Additional reports indicate that without progesterone treatment, women with luteal phase defect are at very high risk for spontaneous abortion (first trimester miscarriage). Progesterone has been found to be important in maintaining a pregnancy during the early months. Some women find it beneficial to use natural progesterone throughout the term, up until one week before their due date (see page 81).[153]

A report in the *British Medical Journal* (August 1957) described the need for progesterone supplementation for one woman, Alison, who had a tendency to miscarry, along with headaches, backaches, and exhaustion. Her progesterone treatment had to be sustained throughout pregnancy, as attempts to discontinue the progesterone brought an immediate return of her symptoms.[154]

Several studies regarding estriol's role in promoting fertility have been published. The clinical trials have shown that taking 1 to 2 mg of estriol daily on days 6 to 15 of the cycle seems to be sufficient to stimulate an increase in fertility in most cases. Doses of up to 8 mg of estriol daily were used without adversely affecting cycle length.[155] Estriol improves fertility by improving the quality and quantity of the cervical mucosa. In a study of ten infertile women, 40 percent became pregnant after using estriol.[156] As always, the addition of progesterone is recommended with any estriol treatment (see chapter 2 for details).

Jesse Hanley, M.D., encourages women with fertility problems to use a liquid extract of the herb chasteberry *(Vitex agnus-castus)*—approximately forty drops in water each morning for three months,[157] even during menstrual periods. Often a patient will then come back to her office with a positive pregnancy test. If not, Dr. Hanley observes that some herbalists recommend using *Vitex* for as long as a year and a half. Once a woman becomes pregnant, however, she advises discontinuing its use.[158]

Vitex itself does not contain hormones. Rather, it stimulates the pituitary gland's production of luteinizing hormone (LH), which in turn stimulates ovarian production of progesterone. The benefits include normalizing of a woman's cycle and reducing PMS, heavy menstrual bleeding, and even amenorrhea.[159] The authors of *The Natural Pharmacy* refer to a study that indicates this may be due to its "ability to decrease excessive prolactin levels."[160]

You can learn to chart your own most fertile time of month by your basal body temperature and changes in your saliva and cervical mucus. By keeping records in the form of a graph, you will learn your ovulation pattern. Whether you are trying to conceive or to avoid conception, this information will be of value to you.

If you take your temperature every morning before rising, you will notice that it dips and then shoots up around the time of ovulation. Likewise, your vaginal fluid will become more slippery, wet, and copious at this time, with a consistency and color similar to egg white.[161] And last, each month your saliva goes through changes because of the cyclical variation in ovarian hormones. When saliva dries, it creates a distinctive pattern that looks like frost or crystals on the windowpane, called "ferning," which is an indicator of when you will ovulate. By monitoring and recording this dried saliva pattern daily, you will begin to see a connection between the ferning patterns and your fertile days. Most women will see this pattern around mid-cycle.

One company, Body Wisdom, sells a complete kit with a small compact-shaped microscope called the TCI-31 ovulation tester. This has a round tracking disk with thirty-one slides, one for each day of the month. Also available is a video detailing all of the systems mentioned above. The video features Dr. Kathleen Fry, a gynecologist and president of the American Holistic Medical Association. For more information, see the Web site www.tci31.com or contact Body Wisdom at (800) 888-9897.

PREGNANCY AND PROGESTERONE

During pregnancy women may develop symptoms such as a rise in blood pressure, protein in the urine, excessive weight gain, headaches, or edema. Dr. Katharina Dalton explains that "these women have an underdeveloped placenta, but they can still be helped with progesterone therapy throughout pregnancy.[162] The placenta's production of progesterone is key to a healthy and full-term gestation. By the third trimester, the optimal level is 300–400 mg per day. When that occurs naturally, or when it is supported with the use of transdermal cream, many of the aforementioned conditions can be alleviated or avoided altogether.

Often the most crucial time is during the first trimester, before placental production of progesterone has been fully established. During this phase, low levels often result in miscarriage—what is referred to as a luteal-phase defect. Because it is the corpus luteum that produces our supply at a rate of 15–20 mg per day, we can see that progesterone deficiency has a profound influence during the first-trimester transition.

The purpose of supplementation during a normal cycle is to maintain optimal physiological levels; likewise during the course of pregnancy. However, if a woman is at risk for miscarriage after the first month of pregnancy, Dr. John Lee would gradually increase the dose to 60 to 80 mg per day. This amount can be continued up to the last month for maximum support and should be applied throughout the day. He goes on to suggest decreasing the dose incrementally during the last month until discontinuing use completely a week before the expected delivery date. This signals the body to raise prolactin levels, which stimulate milk production in the breasts.[163]

A study reported in the *British Journal of Psychiatry* observed that administering progesterone from the middle trimester of pregnancy for relief of the symptoms of toxemia had some unexpected benefits: "A significant improvement in educational performance was demonstrated among children [whose mothers] received progesterone before the sixteenth week" following conception; and after giving birth their mothers seemed to have greater success at breast-feeding.[164] Clinical observations involving ninety children whose mothers received progesterone were summarized thus:

More progesterone children were breast-fed at six months, more were standing and walking at one year, and at the age of 9–10 years the progesterone children received significantly better gradings than controls in academic subjects, verbal reasoning, English, arithmetic, [and] craftwork, but showed only average gradings in physical education.[165]

Dr. Katharina Dalton, who conducted these studies, first discovered the amazing benefits of progesterone through personal experience when she found that her own menstrual migraines disappeared during the last six months of pregnancy. She concluded that the high levels of progesterone during pregnancy might have made the difference. She then tested the use of progesterone on other women and found the same rapid relief of both headaches and other symptoms. She reports further that about 10 percent of women have PMS, high blood pressure, preeclampsia, and protein in the urine during their pregnancies. "These women have an underdeveloped placenta," writes Dr. Dalton, "but they can still be helped with progesterone therapy throughout pregnancy."[166]

Noting that if symptoms normally associated with PMS should return at any stage of pregnancy, a resumption of progesterone treatment would be indicated, she advises: "You could be wise to arrange prophylactic progesterone during pregnancy."[167]

Dr. Dalton is one of many scientists and doctors who have discovered that progesterone in the natural form

- protects the fetus from miscarriage;
- increases the feeling of well-being of the mother;
- increases the potential IQ of the child; and
- produces calmer, less colicky babies.[168]

To protect the fetus the body secretes ten to fifteen times more progesterone during pregnancy than at other times. Dr. Lee tells us that the placenta becomes the major source of progesterone, producing 300 to 400 mg per day during the third trimester. What a great protection we have during pregnancy with this incredible hormone! And with no known dangerous side effects.[169–171]

Dr. Dalton calls morning sickness "a sign that the ovarian progesterone is insufficient and the placenta is not yet secreting enough progesterone." She says that giving the woman extra progesterone will ease the symptoms.[172] Also, the medical archives of the year 1952 include a study of seventy pregnant women with nausea and vomiting. After receiving additional supplementation of vitamins B₆, C, and K, 91 percent of these women found complete relief of their symptoms. Says Dr. Alan Gaby, "Although this study was reported in the *American Journal of Obstetrics and Gynecology*, very few obstetricians today know about it."[173] Many herbalists have also found ginger or cloves to be quite effective and safe remedies.

Biologist Margie Profet of Seattle has proposed a theory that morning sickness evolved as a way of protecting the fetus during its first, most vulnerable stage of development. The diet of early humans often included substantial amounts of wild plants that contained strong toxins as part of their own built-in defense system. While the adult woman may have developed a tolerance for these toxins, they might have been dangerous to the fetus. Thus, it's intriguing to postulate that nausea during early pregnancy discouraged a woman from eating very much, or perhaps interfered with her keeping foods down. She thereby would avoid ingesting (or retaining) poisons and consequently passing them on to her developing child. This may have brought about "morning sickness" as a protective adaptation,[174] triggered by the hormonal changes of pregnancy.

Dr. Ray Peat adds, "Since natural progesterone has been found to reduce the incidence of birth defects, it would seem reasonable to be sure that your own progesterone has returned to normal before getting pregnant."[175]

MISCARRIAGE AND PREMATURE BIRTHS

On February 6, 2003, a groundbreaking study was publicized explaining how "progesterone prevented premature births in a surprisingly high number of high-risk pregnancies. . . ." This study was carried out in nineteen centers called the Maternal-Fetal Medicine Units Network, under the direction of the National Institutes of Health.[176] Needless to say, this news about the multiple physiological roles of natural progesterone was not surprising. But why isn't this critical information put to use, especially when we know that one in every three pregnancies in the United States ends in miscarriage?[177] Why are organizations such as the United Way willing to donate large portions of their valuable and hard-earned resources to research this common occurrence as if it's not yet understood? Why do they approach this issue without consideration for this simple, successful, and inexpensive method for assisting mothers-to-be in carrying their babies to term?

More education in this area would help to alert women to the fact that if they have had four or five miscarriages in the first six or eight weeks of a pregnancy, this is always due to luteal phase failure, says Dr. John Lee. Progesterone is needed to facilitate implantation and to prevent rejection of the developing embryo.

Dr. Lee's recommendation: "Wait till you ovulate, and then four to six days after possible conception do a blood test (for HCG) to see if you're pregnant. If you are, start the progesterone; that way you will increase your chance of having a healthy baby." Blood tests for pregnancy tend to be positive within three days of conception, whereas he says urine pregnancy tests are not usually positive until two weeks after conception.

One of Dr. Lee's notable findings is that there is an immune-suppressing effect in the uterus from higher doses of progesterone. This is important, because when conception takes place, half of the baby's chromosomes are from the male and half of them from the female. That makes the baby's tissue DNA different from the mother's because of the contribution of the father. Normally, if there's not a good tissue match, the difference will create tissue rejection. If, for instance, you try to do a skin graft or a kidney or heart transplant and the tissue isn't the same, the body will reject it. But this doesn't happen with pregnancy. Why? Because of the progesterone response in the uterus. It's a site-selective action that doesn't occur anywhere else in the body; therefore, the baby is not rejected. By giving more progesterone after conception, you thus increase the likelihood that the baby will survive.

Looking at the problem from another perspective, Dr. Lita Lee informs us that "after conception progesterone prevents miscarriages resulting from excess estrogen."[178] It is interesting to note the consistency of the research, as in Dr. Peat's study indicating that "pregnancy toxemia and tendency to miscarry or deliver prematurely are often corrected by progesterone."[179–181] Dr. Peat goes on to say, "My dissertation research, which established that an estrogen excess kills the embryo by suffocation, and that progesterone protects the embryo by promoting the delivery of both oxygen and glucose, didn't strike a responsive chord in the journals which are heavily influenced by funds from the drug industry."[182]

It is a fact that if a pregnant woman produces too much estrogen, her embryo can be suffocated (fetal hypoxia). Dr. Lita Lee cautions that during the ninth week of pregnancy, a woman can lose her baby if she is a "high estrogen producer and/or [is] consuming commercial meat, poultry and dairy products containing synthetic estrogen (DES)." However, she goes on to say that natural progesterone "has been known to protect against the toxic effects of excess estrogen, including abortion."[183] Make certain, if hormones are prescribed during pregnancy, that they are not the synthetic progestins. We now know that artificial hormones, as well as too much estrogen, can be danger-ous to the fetus during pregnancy.[184]

Dr. John Lee stresses that synthetic compounds cannot be efficiently "excreted by one's usual enzymatic mechanisms. Despite their advertisements, synthetic hormones are not equivalent to natural hormones."[185] Side effects can include fatigue, elevation of cholesterol, heart palpitations, headaches, depression, emotional disorders, weight gain, bloating, and more.[186]

MOTHERHOOD AND POSTPARTUM DEPRESSION

After the birth of a child, symptoms may develop in the mother that she can-not control—and supplementation with natural progesterone is not considered a therapeutic option by mainstream medical practice. However, if you have depression or insomnia, find that you want to sleep all the time, or have mood swings or any of the signs we've mentioned in the introductory chapter of this book, think twice and have your doctor test you for progesterone deficiency.

This deficiency may be the culprit if you are suffering from anxiety or "the blues" after the birth of your baby. Many women feel they have to resort to medication or a support group for postpartum depression. However, the pre-ventive step of taking natural progesterone immediately after childbirth might reduce their need for such measures. Dr. Dalton explains why:

> At delivery of the baby the placenta [which produces progesterone] is also delivered, and there is a sudden alteration in the levels of all hormones. The new mother must abruptly adjust to the complete absence of prog-esterone after nine months of a continuous and plentiful supply. It is sug-gested that some women find this alteration of progesterone level difficult to tolerate and react with the development of postnatal depression.[187]

It is very possible that temporary supplementation with progesterone will prevent anxiety and uncomfortable physical problems, as indicated in Dr. Dalton's *Guide to Progesterone for Postnatal Depression*. Additionally she states:

> Progesterone therapy may be combined with the patient's usual medica-tion, be it antidepressants, tranquilizers, beta blockers, anticonvulsants etc. When symptoms abate the other medication can be gradually reduced.[188]

She continues with this caution about prescribing synthetic birth control pills to such women: "Progestogens . . . are man-made oral substitutes for progesterone, and are present in all oral contraceptives. They are known to lower the blood progesterone level. Thus oral contraceptives should not be used in any women at risk of, or currently suffering from, postnatal depression."[189]

NURSING MOTHERS

Many women join LaLeche League, a support group that helps mothers who want to nurse their babies and gain information and confidence about keeping their infants healthy. Seldom are they told, however, that in excess, "estrogens may reduce the flow of breast milk," as reported in *The Pill Book*.[190] One of the reasons so many women become discouraged and switch to bottle formulas is the frustration of not being able to produce enough breast milk.

Dr. Dalton mentions extensive studies that link mammary development to the amount of progesterone prescribed to mothers during pregnancy. It was found that the women who had been given natural progesterone were able to sustain breast-feeding of their infants for at least six months after birth. Furthermore, the likelihood of success at breast-feeding was related to the dosage of progesterone previously administered.[191]

As to whether a woman needs additional progesterone while nursing, Dr. John Lee points out that it could suppress her prolactin secretion and possibly interfere with breast-feeding. Besides, Dr. Ray Peat says that human breast milk usually contains a considerable amount of progesterone.

Nutritionists tell us that productive nursing requires plenty of minerals, vitamins, proteins, chlorophyll, enzymes and beneficial fats.[192] If a woman's diet is of high quality, her breast milk will contain what the baby needs for optimal growth.[193] Fresh, whole foods, of course, are preferable to those that have been commercially processed. Udo Erasmus, a biochemist, stresses in *Fats That Heal, Fats That Kill* that the quality of the mother's milk is particularly dependent on the type of fat she is consuming.[194] Unrefined organic coconut oil will also confer benefits to both the mother and her new baby. More information on this subject can also be found on pages 181–184 as well as in appendix C. Erasmus recommends that a nursing mother include in her diet fresh seeds, extra-virgin olive oil, and fresh fish such as salmon, trout, and sardines.[195] (For more information, see chapter 6.)

HYPOTHYROIDISM

As Dr. Lee has said, low progesterone is often misdiagnosed as thyroid deficiency. Nevertheless, Dr. Peat emphasizes that thyroid hormone is basic to all biological functions and that sometimes both thyroid and progesterone supplements are needed, as "each has a promoting action on the other." To see whether thyroid supplementation might be needed in addition to the progesterone, he recommends a test called the Achilles tendon reflex, which measures muscle energy by the speed at which the calf muscle relaxes.[196]

"Without adequate thyroid," says Dr. Peat, "we become sluggish, clumsy, cold, anemic, and subject to infections, heart disease, headaches, cancer, and many other diseases and seem to be prematurely aged. . . . Foods aren't assimilated well, so even on a seemingly adequate diet there is 'internal malnutrition.'"[197] Irregular periods, often leading to needless hysterectomies, are common aspects of hypothyroidism; and breast disease, he says, is another classic manifestation. In explaining this, Mark Perloe, M.D., says, "Too little thyroid production may cause . . . increased prolactin levels and persistent estrogen stimulation."[198] In chapter 6, we discuss current food fads, such as soy products, that have a dramatic effect on lowering thyroid hormone production.

In a conversation, Dr. Peat told us that estrogen (which we can try to balance with supplemental progesterone) inhibits the release of thyroid hormone from the gland, whereas an adequate amount of thyroid hormone raises natural progesterone production and lowers estrogen. That makes it easy to see how thyroid hormone and progesterone can complement each other. He even made the interesting observation that since estrogen and cortisone weaken the blood vessels, progesterone is a good way to help prevent easy bruising.

Unfortunately, our physicians often fail to understand or explain the benefits of natural (marketed under the name "Armour") over synthetic thyroid medication. Though the formula has changed somewhat in recent years, Dr. Peat calls the natural "the most generally effective," since "many people whose thyroid gland is suppressed by stress cannot respond to synthetic thyroxine, T_4." Additionally, those whose liver function is not up to par may require the active form of the hormone, T_3, to which thyroxine is normally converted in the liver. While an excess of unconverted T_4 can be toxic, sometimes just a bit of complex carbohydrates between meals (to maintain a stable level of glucose in the liver) allows the conversion to T_3.[199] (For more information on thyroid medication and bone loss, see chapter 4 under section "Bone Loss from Common Medication.")

It's important to remember that the conventional test for thyroid activity is the blood test. Most test results return as normal, despite symptoms of an underactive thyroid. Many women often complain of feeling sluggish, exhausted, and depressed. They also have difficulty losing weight—regardless of how little they eat or how much they exercise. These individuals are suffering from clinically low thyroid activity. The following offers an inexpensive way of assessing your own thyroid function at home—a very simple test—is explained by William Campbell Douglass, M.D.: Purchase a small bottle of 2 percent tincture of iodine at your drugstore. With a cotton-tipped swab, "paint an area about the size of a silver dollar."[200] The painted spot might preferably be on the tummy or in the thigh area, so as not to alarm your friends or have to justify to your associates the reason for this strange yellow stain on your skin. This mark will disappear after 24 hours if your iodine level is normal. According to Dr. Douglass, "If it disappears in less than twenty-four hours, it means your body is deficient in iodine and has thirstily sucked it up."[201] This finding is highly indicative of underactive thyroid function.

Contrary to the advice given in most "health books," however, Dr. Peat counsels against an *excess* of dietary iodine, which might depress thyroid function. He has also done some groundbreaking research that indicates that an excess of *unsaturated* oils in our diet powerfully inhibits the thyroid. To counteract the resulting fatigue, obesity, and other effects, he advocates the regular consumption of coconut oil.[202–204] (For more information, see chapter 6.)

The thyroid secretes the hormones T_4 and T_3, 4 atoms of iodine and 3 atoms of iodine, respectively, which act on the DNA of target cells. The hypothalamus and thyroid work together. When thyroid function is low, the hypothalamus sends a message to the pituitary gland to release TSH (thyroid stimulating hormone) and raises T_3 and T_4. If you are interested in knowing whether your thyroid function may be low, take your temperature with a basal thermometer under your arm before you get out of bed in the morning. It should be 97.8 to 98.2. The key is to use nutritional support from as many sources as possible: homeopathic remedies; herbal, vitamin, and/or mineral blends; and desiccated thyroid supplements. Dietary changes are especially necessary in order to naturally restore normal thyroid function as opposed to jump-starting it with synthetic thyroid medications. Please refer to chapter 6 for more information on maintaining a healthy thyroid.

Dr. Peat has also concluded, on the basis of convincing research, that hypothyroidism (along with too much estrogen) is the main cause of multiple sclerosis (MS), and that progesterone deficiency is one of several other factors that may be involved. The mechanism appears to be that edema caused by the unbridled estrogen can result in blood clots in the brain, with associated areas of destruction of the myelin sheath of the nerve tissue.[205] Low levels of DHEA have also been linked to MS.[206]

Incidentally, dieters take note: This concerns a modern-day neurological puzzle. Lecturer Nancy Markel told the World Environmental Conference that an epidemic of MS-mimicking symptoms—and also systemic lupus—has been linked to the artificial sweetener aspartame, which has certain similarities to estrogen in that it is an excitotoxin.[207, 208]

HORMONE IMBALANCE AND THE MYELIN SHEATH

The myelin sheath, which has been described as "to nerves what plastic insulation is to electrical wires,"[209] not only serves as the protective outer layer of our nerves but rehabilitates nerves that have been injured. Myelin formation is encouraged by progesterone that is manufactured by Schwann cells in the peripheral nerves from the hormone pregnenolone.[210–212]

A decline of progesterone production in these cells will impair myelin sheath production.[213, 214] If there is interference with a woman's output of ovarian progesterone, such as by the use of any one of the variety of birth-control methods (the pill, surgery, etc.), the Schwann cells will no longer adequately promote development of the protective myelin sheath.[215–217] Nerve problems can result, such as diabetic neuropathy, multiple sclerosis, and vision disorders.[218, 219] In experimental studies, progesterone has immediately appeared at the site of nerve damage, with "a significant increase in the thickness of new myelin sheaths."[220] This is an illustration of one of the many ways supplemental progesterone can be helpful to the body.[221–223]

WHO NEEDS PREMATURE WRINKLES OR OTHER SKIN PROBLEMS?

Dr. Peat has somewhat encouraging news for those of us concerned about wrinkled skin. In spite of estrogen's promotion as a "youth drug," he says it "is known to advance the aging of collagen in all tissues that have been studied, including skin." He comments wryly that "women, like cows, will puff up with water and fat under the influence of estrogen, and wrinkles will naturally be smoothed out, but the skin itself is actually losing its elasticity faster when estrogen is used." On the other hand, he says, "Progesterone has been found to reverse the chemical changes which occur in collagen with aging"—

as well as to normalize the immune system so as to suppress reactions that may contribute to the aging process.[224]

But one should not expect miracles! This treatment seems to be more effective for some women than for others and is probably dependent on many factors, including the age at which it is begun and the degree of prior over-exposure to the sun. Dr. Peat, however, has one more bit of advice: use coconut oil in place of skin creams and lotions containing the much-touted polyunsaturated botanical oils. These latter, he says, actually promote aging of the skin by intensifying the effects of the sun's ultraviolet rays!

We know of other skin conditions as well that sometimes respond to topical progesterone therapy. Dr. Lee can document cases where his patients' acne, psoriasis (scaly reddish patches), rosacea (rose-colored, flaky areas near the nose and forehead), seborrhea (flakes and itching), and even keratoses (hardened skin cells that could be precursors of squamous-cell skin cancer) cleared up when they applied progesterone cream. This natural approach sounds wonderful compared with other options, such as surgery or antibiotics (which kill friendly bacteria, often leading to "leaky gut" syndrome and candida yeast overgrowth).[225]

MEMORY LOSS AND ALZHEIMER'S DISEASE

We often encounter articles such as one that appeared in *Newsweek* (April 1999), that would have the reader believe that there is increased brain activity and possibly better memory performance with increased estrogen. A team of Yale scientists took MRI snapshots of the brain while women were on estrogen. The researchers "interpreted" these studies (*Journal of the American Medical Association*, April 1999) to show that estrogen may lessen the risk of Alzheimer's disease because of its effect on the neurocircuitry of recall in the brain.[226]

Perhaps a more balanced view is in order. Many researchers agree that estrogen "has an excitatory effect on the brain"[227] and can enhance memory for a while. But responsible reporting should take into account the effect of possible over-excitation when estrogen is taken on a long-term basis.[228] Additionally, increasing brain cell excitability with estrogen intake doesn't necessarily mean you will have a higher IQ. Instead, this is found to cause hyperactivity, anxiety, and insomnia.[229] Furthermore, Dr. Peat explains that when estrogen dominates, it can cause an "imbalance in cellular fluid," which may eventually lead to headaches, blood clots, and even "aging and death of brain cells. . . ."[230] This occurs during both natural or surgical menopause and even when ovulation is suppressed by chemical means (birth control pills, implants, or injections of

DepoProvera). Chronically high estrogen levels can actually mar the memory. In contrast, pregnenolone, the precursor of many of our hormones (see page 186), has been found to activate memory in aging animals.[231–233]

A closer examination of the medical literature reveals evidence that among estrogen's *harmful* effects on the brain is, in fact, its action as an "excitotoxin," whereby it can stimulate the brain beyond the nervous system's ability to respond and can thus cause a debilitating energy drain and state of exhaustion. Any short-term stimulatory effect seems to be offset by accelerated long-term degeneration.[234–238] According to Dr. Peat, "the information on this is overwhelmingly clear, and the publicity to the contrary is a horrifying example of the corruption of the mass media by the drug industry."[239]

A great deal of unscientific speculation has been publicized recently to promote estrogen as a preventive for Alzheimer's disease. However, it is important to note that when women have been on estrogen replacement, a study shows that they often show a greater tendency to Alzheimer's than men.[240] Another objective study points out that "exposure to estrogen in middle-age increases the risk of Alzheimer's disease in old age. . . ."[241]

Yet the point not emphasized, but detailed in a significant Seattle HMO investigation of dementia, is that this group of women had a higher rate of *former* estrogen use (Alzheimer's has a long developmental history). They also had a much higher rate of hysterectomy (indicating an excess of estrogen), and a lower rate of use of progesterone-like compounds than the normal control group.[242–244] Nor should we fail to consider "environmental and dietary factors such as radiation, unsaturated fats, vitamin A and E deficiencies, undigested starches, excitotoxins such as aspartame, and various other food additives in the development of Alzheimer's disease as well as immunodeficiency, colitis, and fatigue syndrome."[245]

Dr. Ray Peat observes, "Ordinary estrogens are being promoted to prevent osteoporosis, heart disease, and (though they don't yet make direct product claims in this case) Alzheimer's disease and other degenerative brain diseases." If estrogen is protective against these diseases, we need to ask our doctors and pharmacists why the incidence of osteoporosis and Alzheimer's disease is so much higher in women than in men. And why is the incidence of bone fractures caused by osteoporosis increasing? This is happening even among men, who are now being exposed to more estrogenic compounds than in the past.[246] A coincidence? I think not.

Certainly, considering estrogen's top billing in the drug sales category, something is wrong or statistics such as these would not be on the increase. Are we being duped by advertising promises and distracted by prejudicial studies, only later to be faced with a host of estrogen-induced diseases? Imagine the headway we could make not only against Alzheimer's disease, but breast and prostate cancer and osteoporosis as well, if we looked beyond this over-promoted hormone (estrogen) and focused on its botanical counterpart—natural progesterone.

WHY DO I HAVE THESE MUSCLE ACHES AND PAINS?

In evaluating symptoms of illnesses common to women, I found it interesting to note how many diseases elicit complaints similar to those of PMS and menopause. For instance, a popular diagnosis given to an incredible number of female patients is *fibromyalgia*. As I was interested in the subject, I decided to attend a lecture given by a well-known rheumatologist from Emory University. In his talk he mentioned that fibromyalgia is a disease found predominantly in women. And sure enough, the huge assembly room was packed with women of all ages.

A couple of months prior to this event, I had met a woman at a senior citizens' health fair who told me she had fibromyalgia. Because I was researching a book on arthritis, I had learned that a physician from the Mayo Clinic had named this disease "fibrositis" and called it "the most common form of acute and chronic rheumatism." The report continued, "Its symptoms are similar to chemical sensitivities and chronic fatigue syndrome."[247] It turns out that other doctors and medical studies report that "a number of poorly understood conditions, such as chronic fatigue syndrome or fibromyalgia, are misdiagnosed as 'chronic Lyme disease.' Fibromyalgia occurs mostly during midlife but it may be seen at any age."[248] In reviewing an article in the *Journal of Internal Medicine*, Betty Kamen says, "There is no evidence that fibromyalgia is a disease of the muscle or a rheumatic syndrome."[249]

What caught my attention most is that the symptoms mimic all the characteristics of progesterone deficiency or estrogen dominance that we list in chapter 2: depression, fluid retention, joint and muscle pain, headaches, insomnia, poor memory, and even PMS.

So my newfound friend decided to use the progesterone cream. After approximately one month, she called me and excitedly announced that all her "fibromyalgia" symptoms were gone. She was particularly happy when her distended abdomen began slimming down and she had to buy new clothes a couple of sizes smaller. This woman was not afraid to speak up when it was necessary. So I wondered what her doctor was going to say when she told him, "Well, doctor, after using this botanical progesterone cream my symptoms just disappeared." In my mind I could just imagine what the doctor was thinking at this point. Probably that he knew of a good specialist who could help this woman with these unusual fantasies. . . .

My friend knew she was onto something. For over thirty years she had been living with these problems, and the only time she had been completely symptom-free in her married life was when she'd been pregnant (seven times). As Dr. John Lee tells us, "In pregnancy, the placenta produces 300–400 mg of progesterone a day in the third trimester." (This is when many women feel the healthiest.) This amount is approximately ten to fifteen times higher than what's normally produced in an ovulating woman.

What great protection progesterone provides us during pregnancy! It's the hormone essential for the survival of the embryo. *Could it also be essential for the survival of our good health?*

IF I'D ONLY KNOWN THEN WHAT I KNOW NOW (POSTMENOPAUSE)

Once a woman has reached the stage in her life when she no longer has natural menstrual periods, why must she be artificially thrust back into her cycle? How unrealistic that women should endure these drug-induced cycles and suffer through multiple side effects in lieu of passing through what should be a peaceful time of life. I have found that natural hormone replacement therapy will not bring on a period when taken on a regular basis, even though, in the first three months of use, a woman may notice a few days of spotting or light bleeding. If I had known back then, at the peak of menopause, what I know now, I would have put the knowledge into practice immediately.

In her book titled *The Menopause Industry: How the Medical Establishment Exploits Women*, author Sandra Coney talks about how the pharmaceutical industry has promoted the idea of menopause as an ailment because it has the drugs to medicate the symptoms. By treating menopause like a disease, we condition the body to sustain monthly periods synthetically and indefinitely—right into old age.[250]

What has been promoted by the pharmaceutical companies as a dream to preserve youth has turned out to be more of a nightmare, however. Promises of synthetically covering up natural menopause and postmenopause with estrogen have far from lived up to expectations. And the reality of this nightmare is showing up in the studies. The *American Journal of Obstetrics and Gynecology* now states that not only long-term, but short-term users of HRT carry a 40 percent risk of acquiring breast cancer.[251]

Through preventive care, it is possible that the pre-, peri-, and post-menopausal years can turn out to be very constructive ones. We can devote our energies to achieving a degree of health that allows us to reach out to others with stamina and creativity. As Margaret Mead, author and anthropologist, puts it, "The most creative force in the world is the menopausal woman with zest."[252]

SOME CLOSING THOUGHTS

The better I've begun to feel, the greater has been my desire to learn why, and to share my findings with all who would listen. The more I've read, the more excited I've become to be part of a generation that is making such progress in understanding the impact of natural botanical medicine. I realize that if we spread the word concerning the powerful and wonderful gifts of nature, perhaps others will benefit physically, mentally, and even spiritually from our newfound freedom of choice.

FOUR

Can We Circumvent Osteoporosis?

There is one thing stronger than all the armies in the world,
and that is an idea whose time has come.

Victor Hugo[1]

It was an unsettling revelation to me that osteoporosis can begin as early as fifteen years prior to the first signs of menopause—often around the middle to late thirties.[2] By the time most women reach their postmenopausal years, the majority will suffer from this disease—a fact that has made it the most common metabolic bone disease in this country.

In other words, osteoporosis starts much earlier than most people think. In fact, Dr. John Lee says a woman can "lose 20 percent or more of her bone mass *before* menopause."[3] The gradual loss of bone, perhaps 1 percent each year at first, accelerates to a rate of 3 to 5 percent per year during menopause and then reverts to about 1 to 1.5 percent a year thereafter.[4] This association of accelerated bone loss with menopause, first recognized more than fifty years ago, led medical doctors to prescribe estrogen supplements during menopause to reduce these chances. Unfortunately, however, there are some problems with this approach. Of great importance are the significant side effects that start appearing in a woman's body when supplemental estrogen, unopposed by natural progesterone, is introduced. They constitute a long list, ranging from increased blood clotting and water retention to liver dysfunction and greater risk of endometrial and breast cancer.

As if that weren't bad enough, it also turns out that this estrogen therapy doesn't really do very much good. Nevertheless, standard medical wisdom continues to support this approach and to assume that it is the most effective treatment. There is ample evidence in the medical literature that the therapy is of some limited value, at best, during the menopausal years. However, according to Sandra Cabot, M.D., "when estrogen is discontinued, calcium loss resumes."[5] So we need to look much more closely at the conventional method of treatment.

Dr. John Lee suggests that this escalating bone loss is due to decreasing levels of progesterone, caused by failure to ovulate during some menstrual cycles—for progesterone is mainly produced in the process of ovulation. In nonpregnant ovulating women, the ovaries can produce up to 40 mg of progesterone daily during the second half of the menstrual cycle.[6] During pregnancy the placenta becomes the main producer of progesterone, making ever-increasing amounts, so that by the last three months of pregnancy, it is making 300 to 400 mg a day. Failure to produce these levels of progesterone naturally can lead to trouble. Even though estrogen aids somewhat in slowing down bone loss, progesterone could be called proactive, since studies verify that its stimulatory effect on the osteoblastic cells actually encourages new bone growth.[7, 8]

The Importance of Ovulation

The onset of irregular periods is an indicator that progesterone levels are becoming depleted with respect to estrogen. When menopause is upon us (that is, when we have stopped ovulating), our progesterone level will decline to almost zero.[9] A reasonable question would be, "Why do some women experience this sooner than others?" Researchers tell us that stress, injury, poor diet, lack of exercise, and trauma all may play a role in the degree to which ovulation becomes sporadic and then tapers off at menopause.[10]

To these Dr. John Lee would add the damage done to the ovaries by any of the many human-made estrogenic chemicals in the environment (see chapter 5). Such exposure to the female fetus or very early in life may damage the ovarian follicles to the extent that in adulthood they can no longer make progesterone as they should. Follicle dysfunction induced by these so-called xenoestrogens may well be the primary cause of the progesterone deficiency that often occurs fifteen years or more before actual menopause.

In addition, as is widely reported in the press these days, the way you treat your body in general can contribute to premature bone loss. Smoking and excessive consumption of alcohol, caffeine, soft drinks, and meat protein, as well as the use of certain anti-inflammatory or antiseizure medications or thyroid hormone replacements, may all place you at higher risk. And some factors can't be avoided: thin, small-boned women and those of Caucasian descent have a higher risk of osteoporosis.[11]

In the United States, approximately 24 million people are affected by osteoporosis, at a medical cost of over $10 billion and as many as 1.5 million fractures[12] leading to disability, deterioration, and, for too many, death. Today, the annual number of fractures attributable to osteoporosis continues to escalate as our exposure to estrogen from various sources has drastically increased.[13] But, as Dr. Robert Lindsay has said, "The problem is, nobody feels the bone they're losing until it's too late. . . . Osteoporosis is without symptoms until it becomes disease."[14] According to Dr. Patricia Allen, when the "acceleration of bone loss begins, risks for coronary artery disease start to increase [and] atrophy of breast and genital tissue starts. And so most doctors now believe that a woman who is bothered by menopausal symptoms should be treated before the cessation of her periods."[15]

PROGESTERONE (NOT ESTROGEN) SUPPLEMENTS FOR HEALTHY BONES

Jerilynn C. Prior, M.D., and her associates found evidence of progesterone's possible role in countering osteoporosis in a study of sixty-six premenopausal women between twenty-one and forty-one years of age. All these women were long-distance marathon runners. It was observed after twelve months that

> the average spinal bone density decreased by about 2%. . . . However, women who developed ovulation disturbances during the study lost 4.2% of their bone mass in one year. While there was no correlation between the rate of bone losses and serum levels of estrogen, there was a close relationship between indicators of progesterone status and bone loss.[16]

Now this is news! And then *Medical Hypotheses* claims that the use of natural progesterone is not only safer but less expensive than using its synthetic formulation, Provera (medroxyprogesterone), and that *"progesterone and not estrogen is the missing factor . . . in reversing osteoporosis."*

The journal continues:

> The presence or absence of estrogen supplements had no discernible effect on osteoporosis benefits. . . . Progesterone deficiency rather than estrogen deficiency is a major factor in the pathogenesis of menopausal

osteoporosis. Other factors promoting osteoporosis are excess protein intake, lack of exercise, cigarette smoking, and inadequate vitamins A, D, and C.[17]

Dr. Majid Ali says that the use of estrogen to prevent osteoporosis is really quite "frivolous."[18] Osteoporosis is a disease we can do much to prevent. With the knowledge we presently have, it is imperative that women take active steps toward a healthier lifestyle. We must take to heart what author Gail Sheehy says in *The Silent Passage: Menopause:*

> Nearly half of all people over age seventy-five will be affected by porous bones causing the risk of fractures of many kinds. The National Osteo-porosis Foundation in the U.S. says that almost a third of women aged sixty-five and over will suffer spinal fractures. And of those who fall and fracture a hip, one in five will not survive a year (usually because of post-surgical complications).[19]

It has been estimated that twice as many serious fractures occur today than thirty years ago. How long will it take us to grasp the truth of the matter, so we can help ourselves and the aging population? "Clearly," says Dr. Alan Gaby, "there is something wrong with our bone health, something that the medical profession has not been able to do much about. There is more to preventing bone loss than calcium supplements, estrogen replacement therapy and exercise."[20]

Following the publication of the first edition of this book, a woman in her late seventies called to tell me her doctor had put her on estrogen to protect her heart and her bones. She said, "I've had three heart attacks since being on estrogen and have also been diagnosed with osteoporosis. Now, after reading your book, I understand that I can reverse and even prevent these conditions with regular use of natural progesterone."

These reminders about the decline in bone mass as we age make me think of my own family gatherings during the holidays, when we are at long last in the company of several generations of family members. Someone usually says, "Haven't you grown!" In our family we take it a step further: someone stands next to Mom, and then Mom next to Grandma—and, sure enough, there is a definite change! But it's in the opposite direction. Soon a grandchild will say, "Wait a minute, Grandma, aren't you shrinking?" It seems that these changes start earlier than we may think and are more crippling than we realize.

Is this a topic we can continue to take lightly? Not according to Robert P.

Heaney, M.D., professor of medicine at Creighton University School of Medicine in Nebraska. In commenting on the medical community's having overlooked the importance of progesterone in osteoporosis, he expressed the hope that research will "galvanize the field into taking the matter seriously."[21] Perhaps statements such as his will begin to reeducate the very doctors who think they know all there is to know about this most vital subject.

It is a mystery that so much focus has been placed on declining estrogen levels; it seems the emphasis has been on the wrong hormone. The October 14, 1993, issue of the *New England Journal of Medicine* makes it clear that taking estrogen for five or ten years after menopause will not protect a woman from having a hip fracture in her later years.[22] Why should we wait ten to twenty years for the results of the studies that are now in progress? We have already been counseled by many medical experts. Now is the time to make the change from an estrogen replacement program to one based on natural progesterone therapy.

We should ask ourselves, "Why would we use a hormone that has not worked for generations past?" The traditional and often one-sided references to estrogen decline have created a body of misinformation that has sentenced many to poor health and needless distress. Even though evidence clearly shows that progesterone stimulates active new bone formation and estrogen merely delays bone loss,[23, 24] mainstream medicine promotes an entirely different hypothesis to patients and consumers. It seems irresponsible that the medical world is not doing double-blind studies, utilizing baseline and follow-up bone mineral density tests, and natural progesterone.

However, we can be grateful to the many doctors who have searched the archives for the truth of the matter. We now have reliable evidence that despite declining estrogen levels, bone loss accelerates when progesterone levels decline, and bone minerals can be restored with natural progesterone replacement therapy.[25–28] Yet, the message women receive from their medical doctors is that "estrogen is the single most potent factor in prevention of bone loss."[29] This belief has been handed down from one generation to the next. But now, when it's been found that estrogen (ERT) is not as effective as originally alleged and bone fractures occurred in spite of such therapy, other drugs were prescribed in combination with estrogen or alone, such as Evista (Raloxifene), Bisphosphonates (Alendronate), Calcitonin, Fluoride, etc.[30] For contraindications regarding Fosamax see pages 114 and 115. Fortunately, recently published studies and books are now challenging these medical theories and bringing more light to the subject of preventing osteoporosis (see appendices D, E, F, and G).

A case in point is the book *Preventing and Reversing Osteoporosis*, written by medical doctor Alan Gaby. I became so absorbed in it that I could not put it down—nor will you, when you find that, yes, osteoporosis *can be reversed*. Much of what Dr. Gaby says would be beneficial to many and should be shared. He cautions that despite the preventive measures of calcium supplementation and exercise, and despite medical intervention with estrogen therapy, osteoporosis is getting worse: "At least 1.2 million women suffer fractures each year as a direct result of osteoporosis. . . . Fractures seem to be increasing, . . . and this difference cannot be explained by the aging of the population."[31]

Let us hope that more medical doctors are getting away from the mainstream of drug therapy and are discovering natural remedies that seem to work more efficiently for such problems in the long run. Dr. Gaby, for instance, with over two decades of medical research and clinical practice, writes that many of the most significant advances and effective treatments have been those discovered or administered outside the auspices of the traditional medical community.

Dr. John Lee comments that modern medicine "strangely persists in the single-minded belief that estrogen is the mainstay of osteoporosis treatment for women." Strange, indeed, that doctors should think like this, when even medical textbooks such as *Harrison's Principles of Internal Medicine* (12th edition, 1991) and *Cecil's Textbook of Medicine* (18th edition, 1988) don't back up this theory.[32] Along the same lines, Dr. Lee also quotes the 1991 *Scientific American Medicine:*

> "Estrogens decrease bone resorption" but "associated with the decrease in bone resorption is a decrease in bone formation. Therefore, estrogens should not be expected to increase bone mass." The authors also discuss estrogen side effects including the risk of endometrial cancer which "is increased six-fold in women who receive estrogen therapy for up to five years; the risk is increased 15-fold in long-term users."[33]

PROGESTERONE CREAM FOR OSTEOPOROTIC PATIENTS

Although there are many forms and ways to take natural progesterone, Dr. Lee acquaints us with the transdermal method. By carefully observing his patients over the course of fifteen years, he proved the effectiveness of transdermal progesterone cream. His work confirmed its safety and its remarkable benefits to his osteoporotic patients who had a history of cancer of the uterus or breast and to those who had diabetes, vascular disorders, and other conditions.

Dr. Lee had hoped that the progesterone would strengthen his patients' bones. To his surprise, it did; their bone mineral density tests showed progressive improvement and the number of his patients suffering osteoporotic fracture dropped nearly to zero.[34]

Dr. Lee is perplexed at "the reluctance of contemporary medicine to adopt the use of natural progesterone." It's his impression, however, that "the news is spreading and change is on the way." In the publication *Natural Solutions*, Dr. Lee voices true dismay with his orthopedic colleagues who chose not to use the progesterone cream in their patients' care "but did put their own wives on the cream."[35]

Dr. Lee points out that the "conventional treatment of osteoporosis with estrogen, with or without supplemental calcium and vitamin D, tends to delay bone mass loss, but not reverse it."[36] His investigation into using transdermal progesterone cream instead of a synthetic estrogen replacement treatment demonstrates that "osteoporosis subsided, musculoskeletal strength and mobility increased, and monthly vaginal bleeding did not occur."[37] Most striking were the results of the dual-photon densitometry test (DEXA), which measured a 10 to 15 percent increase in bone mineral density, most notably in women who had experienced menopause twenty-five years earlier.[38]

After years of researching transdermal progesterone supplementation, Dr. Lee observed in his patients "a progressive increase in bone mineral density and definite clinical improvement including fracture prevention. . . ." He concluded that "osteoporosis reversal is a clinical reality using a natural form of progesterone derived from yams that is safe, uncomplicated and inexpensive."[39] Unfortunately, by the time many of us are ready to deal with the impact of osteoporosis it has already done considerable damage, as it is symptomless until the fractures begin. If you think that you can afford to wait to deal with brittle bones until after you get through the inconvenience of hot flashes and night sweats, you need to think again.

It is an enigma to me that our nation's supposedly up-to-date medical researchers continue to be oblivious to the evidence that progesterone stimulates new bone formation by the osteoblasts, the bone-building cells.[40] Think of the many aging women who could benefit from this information and be freed from unnecessary pain and spared their disability. As Gail Sheehy observes, osteoporosis "often leaves older women frail, susceptible to falls and broken bones. . . . [It] makes it painful merely to sit." Many elderly osteoporotic women die of secondary infections following hip surgery.[41] These infections are what makes osteoporosis victims subject to death, not the osteoporosis itself.

Reading about this reminded me again of my mother's fragile condition as her hip bones grew so weak she could hardly get out of a chair. The longer she sat in one place, the more pain she felt. Before long she had to depend on a wheelchair to get around, and in an even shorter time she yielded to a hospital bed in our home. We felt blessed that she at least did not have to enter a nursing home, as so many do.

BONE MINERAL DENSITY TESTS

Establishing a baseline bone mineral density (BMD) is of vital importance for all women as they make the transition from monthly ovulatory cycles to the early menopausal stage that heralds the onset of accelerated bone loss. Currently, the most precise test with the least radiation dose is dual X-ray absorptiometry (DEXA or DXA), which yields an accuracy of 98 to 99 percent on a study of the lumbar spine and hips.[42] Another highly reliable scan is the dual photon absorptiometry (DPA) test, which is 95 to 98 percent accurate and uses photons (high-intensity light beams) to determine the density of your bone. The importance of such testing cannot be overemphasized, as osteoporosis is asymptomatic in its earlier stages. Multiple scans, several years apart, from the mid-forties (baseline evaluation) to the mid-sixties will give women an accurate picture of their BMD status as well as feedback regarding the efficacy of the HRT program they are using. (Please see chapter 7 for additional diagnostic resources.)

Dr. Lee has found these tests extremely useful. One woman in her seventies consulted him for her advanced osteoporosis and spinal compression fractures:

> She had previously avoided hormone therapy because of a long history of fibrocystic breasts prior to menopause. With natural progesterone applications, her BMD (bone mineral density test) rose gratifyingly, her back pains disappeared, and she resumed normal activities such as hiking, boating, gardening, etc.[43]

The women who received the best results from the progesterone studies were those who seemed to need it the most. In other words, as progesterone was administered to women with all levels of bone loss, regardless of age (whether seventy or thirty-five), those with the lowest initial bone densities had the greatest increases in bone mass.[44]

I'm pleased to say that I myself can be counted among the success stories. I happened to attend a health fair and had the chance for on-the-spot bone mineral density testing. The mini DEXA screening test assesses the BMD of the middle finger or the heel of the foot.

Apprehensively I took advantage of this opportunity, fearing the worst because of my age (64) and my family history. But after years of adhering faithfully to the many nutritional guidelines I'd learned about while researching this book (including the use of progesterone, of course), I had to know what effect my own lifestyle choices were having on my bone mass.

To my great surprise and relief, tests on both my finger and my foot confirmed that my bone density was better not only than that of most women my age, but of normal, healthy women who are much younger! Here is my scoring:

Bone Mineral Density (BMD)

Age-Matched BMD: 117%
(17% higher than others of similar age)

Young Healthy Normals (YHN): 109%
(9% higher than others who are considered to be young healthy normals)

Dr. Lee cautions against relying on the hair analysis testing some laboratories do supposedly to diagnose osteoporosis. The reason is that at this point in the resorption process, calcium will naturally register high—because all the calcium that has been released from the bone is now circulating in the bloodstream and is being picked up by the hair. When the lab reports you have a good level of calcium and there is no need to worry about osteoporosis, be wary; he says it is wrong to use this test to measure whether or not osteoporosis is present and extra magnesium and calcium are needed.

HOW OLD IS TOO OLD FOR PROGESTERONE?

A study was conducted with a hundred patients who ranged in age from thirty-eight to eighty-three years. They were all menopausal or postmenopausal. The majority of these women had already noticed a loss of height due to compression fracture of the spinal vertebrae from age-related bone thinning. Dr. Lee calls this "a cardinal sign of osteoporosis." A number had also experienced fractures of other skeletal bones, such as hips or ribs. We read in *Medical Hypotheses:*

> Since the U.S. medical insurance does not include payment for dual photon bone density tests . . . ,* only 63 of the patients were [covered for]

* Some insurance plans now offer coverage for osteoporosis testing. Unfortunately, they may require your doctor to certify that you are estrogen-deficient, with no consideration of progesterone levels.

serial testing. Thus, 37 patients could be followed only by clinical signs, i.e., relief of osteoporotic symptoms and reduction in expected fracture incidence. Even so, the benefits from the treatment program [see below] were so obvious to these patients that no problems with patient compliance arose. No side-effects or adverse alterations in blood lipids were observed. Each patient was followed a minimum of 3 years.[45]

Of the hundred patients in this group, the report states that "height loss was stabilized" and there was an associated relief from osteoporotic pains. The amazing findings of the test given to determine bone density measurements of the lumbar vertebrae (serial DPA) included (1) reduction in fracture incidence and (2) increase in bone density. Most of these women were responding to a transdermal progesterone dose of only 240 mg per month or 10 mg per day. In the sixty-three women given natural progesterone, the benefit proved to be extraordinary—showing that in three years, instead of losing 4.5 percent of bone as expected, some subjects actually increased their bone density by 15.4 percent, regardless of their age. This report confirms that the greatest relative improvement was made by those with the lowest bone density to begin with.[46]

Further, the study refuted the myth that osteoporosis is irreversible for older women, or even that it is more difficult to correct. Indeed, test subjects over the age of seventy (the oldest was eighty-three) showed somewhat better results than those under the age of seventy. The former responded to the progesterone therapy regimen with an average increase in bone density over the three-year period of 14.4 percent, while the younger women showed an increase of just 14.0 percent.[47]

Many similar studies can be found in the *International Clinical Nutrition Review*. In them, not only were the benefits to skeletal strength observed, but patient complaints such as gastric irritation, joint stiffness, moodiness, and headaches were also relieved. Aside from the safety and effectiveness of using a natural progesterone, it has proven to be extremely cost-efficient—about one-tenth the cost of the same dosage of medroxyprogesterone (Provera), and it comes with no side effects.[48]

We need to reiterate, then, the important point that Dr. Lee makes in the *International Clinical Nutrition Review*. Natural transdermal progesterone cream, he says, "is the missing link in healthy bone building in postmenopausal women." Concerning osteoporosis he says, "Reversal has been demonstrated by the bone density tests and by the clinical results. This cannot be said of any other conventional therapy for osteoporosis."[49]

The conclusion of twelve different reports is that progesterone deficiency rather than estrogen deficiency is one of the main factors in the development of menopausal osteoporosis. Dr. Lee found the best overall results when his patients combined use of the natural progesterone with optimal nutrition. Women were given a "low protein, high vegetable diet, modest exercise and vitamin supplementation." Dr. Lee recommended supplemental estrogen in the form of estriol only when his patients experienced hot flashes, cystitis, or vaginal dryness that did not subside after three to six months of natural progesterone treatment.[50] (Also see chapter 3 and appendix A.)

Dr. Lee informs us that "age is not the cause of osteoporosis; poor nutrition, lack of exercise, and progesterone deficiency are the major factors."[51] He says osteoporosis seems to be more common in "white women of northern European extraction who are relatively thin" or who smoke cigarettes, are under-exercised, are deficient in vitamins A, D, or C, calcium, or magnesium, or whose diet is meat-based rather than vegetable- (especially alkalinizing greens) and whole grain-based.[52] Dr. Gaby confirms some of these observations on the basis of numerous studies. It was found that the most comprehensive program (one that included proper diet, botanical progesterone, and a broad spectrum of vitamins and minerals) produced an astounding 11 percent increase in bone mineral content in postmenopausal women in less than one year. Any one aspect of treatment used alone could never have come close to bringing such improvement in such a short period of time.[53]

Jonathan V. Wright, M.D., an expert in nutritional biochemistry, applauds Dr. Gaby for going "beyond the calcium craze to a holistic approach to healthy bones." He says, "What's good for the bones is good for the heart, the skin, the breasts, the stomach, and even crucial for future generations."[54]

We need to take these experts' advice and question the end result of the extra protein we eat. "A nutritional program that is more than 30 percent protein increases calcium excretion," says Serafina Corsello, M.D., "because metabolism of the protein acidifies the body, which then tries to achieve normal alkaline balance by excreting calcium."[55]

MEAT PROTEIN, PHOSPHATES, AND BONE LOSS

Both kidney stones and kidney failure are an indication that acidosis may be silently weakening our bones as well as impacting the kidneys. In the periodical *Health Science*, we learn that meat eaters have a much higher rate of osteoporosis than vegetarians, even though vegetarians have a lower calcium intake. The conclusion from this research is that the best prevention for osteoporosis is a relatively low-protein diet and plenty of fresh fruits and vegetables. This may provide enough calcium without the need for dairy products. In fact, who would believe that a half cup of sesame seeds contains 870 mg of calcium?[56]

According to Joel Fuhrman, M.D., protein from meat also contains a large quantity of disulfide bonds, which, "while undergoing oxidation when broken down, create sulfate and hydrogen ions that further increase the acid load in the blood. To neutralize this acid load, the body calls on its bony stores of calcium to provide basic [alkaline] calcium salts. . . . In addition, urea and other waste products from excess protein digestion cause the kidney to work harder and excrete more fluid and with this increased function more calcium is lost in the process."[57] Under these conditions the kidney is not able to reabsorb calcium before it is evacuated, and the consequence is more calcium lost via the urine.

Dr. Fuhrman cautions that calcium loss is stimulated in a variety of ways. For instance, with cigarette smoking, the nicotine disrupts hormone communication to the kidneys, curtailing calcium reabsorption. Antacids (with aluminum added), diuretics, and antibiotics also contribute to the loss.[58] And most significant, affecting young and old alike, are soft drinks. Read the labels before you quench your thirst. Many sodas contain not only caffeine but sodium and phosphoric acid—all of which contribute to bone loss in different ways.[59] As Dr. Fuhrman tells us in *Health Science:*

> Phosphates have been shown to increase the release of parathyroid hormones, which mobilizes skeletal calcium reserves. The phosphoric acid found in carbonated drinks is particularly damaging, and is more powerful in inducing calcium excretion than is the phosphorus contained in natural foods.[60]

People who habitually drink soda are oblivious to the fact that many brands contain this dangerous ingredient. Unknown to most consumers, the phosphoric acid is insidiously robbing calcium from our teeth and bones. Phosphates are even added to processed foods such as cheeses and meats. If soda drinkers also eat too much meat (high in phosphorus), they are adding to an already serious problem.[61] This aspect of malnutrition may be causing unsuspected bone loss as well as other degenerative disorders in many thousands of Americans. To moniter how much calcium is being lost in the urine, please see chapter 7, pages 191–192, where we talk about a home urine test kit.

The widespread use of phosphate additives in processed foods can create a phosphorus overload that disrupts the body chemistry, especially when the typical American diet also includes plenty of other sources of this mineral.[62]

A sampling of foods relatively high in phosphorus includes processed meats, turkey, ham, pork, fried potatoes, crackers, legumes, nuts, salmon, eggs, brewer's yeast, asparagus, and whole grains.[63, 64] *The Herb Quarterly* suggests avoiding the following to prevent osteoporosis: dairy products, coffee, alcohol, salt, and sugar; and that eating "a diet rich in dark-green leafy vegetables, nuts, seeds, tofu, [and] molasses"[65] will assist in reversing osteoporosis.

THE IMPORTANCE OF pH BALANCE

A key benefit to eating plenty of raw vegetables is their effect on the body's acid-alkaline (pH) balance. When certain foods (such as dairy products, meat, cooked foods, coffee and tea, and refined flour, sugar, and table salt) are metabolized, they create an acidic effect in the body.[66] Others, such as many fruits and vegetables, as well as some whole grains, have an alkaline effect when metabolized.

Joel Robbins, M.D., N.D., D.C., lectures his patients that the secret to health is to try to consume approximately 80 percent of our diet in "alkaline" foods and 20 percent in acid-producing foods. When the alkaline percentage drops below 80, we lack sufficient catalyst minerals to keep the cells healthy. The body, in its innate wisdom, thus compensates by robbing from other areas, such as the bones, to neutralize the excess acidity. That's why an acid-alkaline imbalance plays such a large role in the onset of the osteoporotic process.[67]

Dr. Robbins says it's unfortunate that of the foods we commonly eat, far more than 20 percent cause an acidic response when metabolized. But if we concentrate on keeping the alkaline percentage in the 80s, we will ensure that there will be enough nutrients to balance the 20 percent of acid-producing food we may wish to consume, including meats and other foods.[68] Dietary supplements such as wheatgrass, green barley, and kelp are high in minerals and chlorophyll[69, 70] and go a long way to help restore the body's pH balance.

According to the *American Journal of Clinical Nutrition*, studies involving sixteen hundred women disclosed that those who eat "a vegetarian diet for at least 20 years have 18 percent less bone mineral by age 80, whereas meat eaters have 35 percent less bone mineral."[71] Other interesting statistics have appeared in many nutritional reviews, such as this one from the Center for Women's Health at Columbia-Presbyterian Medical Center in New York: A diet containing more vegetables and fewer of the harmful kinds of fats[72] (such as hydrogenated and polyunsaturated oils) has been associated with fewer female disorders identified with PMS or menopause.[73–75] However, if you do include meat in your diet, take a little time to ask your grocer to purchase your meat from one of the free-range and organic meat producers listed in appendix E. Most of these brands of meat are free of antibiotics, growth hormone stimulants, herbicides, and pesticides.

THE CALCIUM MYTH

Many American women are being told by their physicians that one of the most efficient and inexpensive ways to supplement their calcium intake to prevent osteoporosis is with ordinary antacid medications (such as Tums). These mainly contain calcium carbonate, which may be inexpensive but is also one of the forms most poorly absorbed by the body.[76] According to John Mills, Total Quality Manager at the Highland Laboratory (Mt. Angel, Oregon), if your stomach is not functioning normally the calcium carbonate in the antacid will not remain dissolved long enough to be absorbed in the intestine and then be conveyed to where it is needed in the body (bones, teeth, and muscles). It will pass through the intestines without being assimilated, contributing to constipation.[77] (A more usable form of calcium is discussed below.)

Antacids in general may temporarily relieve symptoms of indigestion, but they do more harm than good in the long run as they may "contain aluminum, silicone, sugar, and a long list of dyes and preservatives, none of which will help you and may even harm you," reports Dr. John Lee.[78] He warns us, regardless of what your pharmacist or doctor says, not to try to obtain extra calcium by taking antacid tablets, as their side effects may far outweigh any benefits you would gain from their use.[79]

Other well-intentioned measures in common practice are also suspect. John McDougall, M.D., notes cases in which people took calcium without understanding what else contributes to its absorption or loss. Consumption of too much protein can result in excessive calcium excretion and cause the body's calcium reserve in the bones to be at risk. "Experiments have shown that when subjects consumed 75 grams of protein daily, even with an intake as high as 1400 milligrams of calcium, more calcium was lost in the urine than was actually absorbed."[80]

THE CALCIUM BOOSTERS

Bones are dependent upon much more than just calcium. In his book on preventing osteoporosis, Dr. Gaby explains in detail:

> Magnesium is necessary to promote normal bone mineralization; silicon, manganese, and vitamin C are also essential for proper formation of cartilage and other organic components of bone; vitamin K is needed to attract calcium to the bones. It plays a role in remodeling and repair; vitamin D is necessary for absorption of calcium from the diet; zinc and copper are involved in repair mechanisms, presumably including those that occur in bone.[81]

Today we are finding that due to low levels of vitamin D, calcium is not being utilized properly. A vitamin D deficiency can decrease insulin levels as well as increase its resistance—both of these factors are linked with diabetes and cardiovascular problems. Dr. David Williams states that "any amount of vitamin D intake under 800 I.U. [isn't] enough to prevent a vitamin deficiency." This is another important consideration in preventing osteoporosis and other related diseases. It is interesting to note that this amount is almost twice as much as the daily amount recommended by the U.S. Food and Nutrition board.[82]

THE IMPORTANCE OF MAGNESIUM

The importance of magnesium is easy to underestimate. As Dr. Lee says, "If magnesium is deficient, calcium is less likely to become bone and more likely to appear as calcification of tendon insertion points . . . leading to tendinitis, bursitis, arthritis, and bone spurs."[83]

Magnesium plays a fundamental role throughout the body as an enzyme catalyst for the skeletal uptake of calcium and potassium.[84, 85] It's an essential partner of calcium and can be taken as a supplement in at least equal amounts.[86] And since stress, such as that brought on by drugs or by physical or emotional strain, is known to deplete magnesium, many practitioners recommend an even higher magnesium-to-calcium ratio.[87] Dr. Gaby's findings suggest that "boron has a powerful influence on the metabolism of calcium, magnesium and some hormones."[88]

Sucrose and refined carbohydrates will also deplete us of the minerals we may think we are getting from our diet,[89] as well as alter the mineral ration in the blood.[90] High glucose ingestion (from refined carbohydrates) interferes with mineral metabolism by reducing calcium resorption in the kidneys and increasing its urinary excretion. This in turn leads to a magnesium deficiency and eventually affects the health of the bones.[91–93]

It is advised by some that if we choose to take calcium supplements, we should take twice as much magnesium as calcium on a daily basis (approximately 800 mg of calcium and 1,500 mg of magnesium).[94] Dr. Gaby says that magnesium has been a forgotten mineral and that at least a one-to-one ratio of magnesium to calcium (if not two-to-one) would lead to stronger bones and less inappropriate calcium deposition in places where calcium does not belong.[95] When he put his patients with premenstrual syndrome on only 400 mg of calcium plus 800 mg of magnesium, he saw improvement as well.[96]

Dr. Guy Abraham, a gynecologist in Torrance, California, also reversed the calcium-to-magnesium formula in a trial of twenty-six postmenopausal women. They were given daily supplements of 600 mg of magnesium (oxide) and 500 mg of calcium (citrate). The women were also on a high-vegetable, low-protein diet and their supplements included C, B complex, D, zinc, copper, manganese, and boron. After eight to nine months the women's bone mineral density increased 11 percent with these higher amounts of magnesium.[97]

David Smallbone, M.D., of Buxton, England, further increases the amount of magnesium for women who are under a lot of stress (1,800 mg magnesium with 1,600 mg calcium).[98] He also suggests taking calcium before bedtime.

Sodium, too, should not be overlooked. Dr. Bernard Jensen says that it's the elemental sodium from vegetables that we need, and that another excellent source is whey,[99] not the overused table salt that only causes further metabolic imbalances. While an excess of sodium in the body may lead to calcium depletion, however, it is also not unusual to be lacking in this vital mineral, one of whose functions is to neutralize body acids. When we are deficient in sodium, calcium is pulled out of solution for this purpose and often ends up in the joints and tissues instead of supporting our osseous framework.

In all, there are seventeen minerals that Nancy Appleton, Ph.D., a well-known author and nutritional consultant calls "essential in human nutrition. If there is a shortage of just one of these," she writes, "the balance of activity in the entire system can be thrown off."[100] James Balch, M.D., and Phyllis Balch, C.N.C., state in *Prescription for Nutritional Healing* that "a proper balance of magnesium, calcium, and phosphorus should be maintained at all times,"[101] along with the various other minerals and vitamins that work synergistically with one another as catalysts and promote the assimilation of nutrients. This, according to the Balchs, "is why taking a single vitamin or mineral may be ineffective, or even dangerous."[102]

It's becoming abundantly clear, then, that concentrating on calcium alone can cause serious problems. Dr. Morton Walker, too, knows that for calcium to be properly metabolized, the right amounts of magnesium, phosphorus, and vitamins D (the "sunshine vitamin"), C, and A must also be present.

When properly absorbed, he says, calcium is the nutrient that "helps to overcome cramping in the legs and feet."[103]

To prevent brittle bones, Dr. Carlton Fredricks recommends cod liver oil as an excellent food source for high quality vitamin D. It is suggested by Dr. Raymond Peat that vitamin E should always be taken with D as the vitamin D in cod liver oil somewhat increases one's need for vitamin E.[104, 105] Researcher and author Elaine Hollingsworth says that "vitamin D in the form of cod liver oil . . . contains all of the Omega-3 and vitamin A that is needed each day."[106] It's important to learn that the best brands are those that obtain their cod liver oil from codfish in the deep, unpolluted waters near Norway.* Krispin Sullivan, a clinical nutritionist, says that Norwegian cod liver oil is naturally rich in vitamin A, vitamin D3, EPA, and DHA. Only codfish caught during the winter and early spring are used, as the liver oil content is highest at this time of year.

Sullivan says that "in Northern California 80% of clients tested in winter months have serious D deficiency . . . This problem increases dramatically in more northern latitudes." Even in Southern California a lack of vitamind D is possible due to so many people avoiding the midday sunlight and slathering themselves with sunscreens. For more information on the dos and don'ts of vitamin D, how much to take and what to take it with, take a look at the Web site www.carlsonlabs.com or call (800) 323-4141.

Referring to a study in *Acta Endocrinologica*, Dr. Gaby comments that the mineral zinc "enhances the biochemical actions of vitamin D, which is itself involved in calcium absorption and osteoporosis prevention. Because of its essential role in DNA and protein synthesis, zinc is required for the formation of osteoblasts and osteoclasts, as well as for the synthesis of various proteins found in bone tissue." In another investigation drawn from *Acta Medica Scandinavica*, Dr. Gaby tells us that "zinc levels were found to be low in the serum and bone of elderly individuals with osteoporosis. . . . The most efficiently absorbed types of zinc," he advises, "are zinc picolinate, citrate and chelated."[107]

Dr. Lee adds that "zinc is essential as a co-catalyst for enzymes which convert betacarotene to vitamin A within cells. This is especially important in building the collagen matrix of cartilage and bone. As with magnesium, zinc is one of the minerals lost in the 'refining' of grain. As a result, the typical American diet is deficient in zinc and modest supplementation (15–30 mg/day) is recommended."[108]

---

* Check the ingredients lebels on the cod liver oil and vitamin E capsule bottles to make sure that they do not also contain soy. (See chapter 6 for more information on soy.)

Other nutrients with an important role in calcium absorption include silica and pectin.[109] Found in unpeeled apples, citrus fruits, the cabbage and broccoli family, and many other fruits and vegetables, pectin transports calcium molecules to the large intestine for slow absorption into the body (as well as neutralization of potentially cancerous toxins). The authors of *The Calcium Connection*, Drs. Cedric and Frank Garland, also stress the importance of drinking plenty of water to help dissolve and absorb dietary or supplemental calcium.[110]

Concerning calcium and hormones, Gail Sheehy advises that just taking calcium is not enough and that exercise *by itself* is also ineffective in preventing bone loss.[111] The combination of weight-bearing exercise, proper diet, and the appropriate kind of calcium (see "Misconceptions about Calcium and Diet," this chapter), along with natural hormone replacement therapy, has been shown to increase bone mass and decrease symptoms of insomnia and hot flashes. Citing a study from the Netherlands, Gail Sheehy also notes that "vitamin K has been found to inhibit the precipitous loss of calcium in postmenopausal women by up to 50 percent. . . . Dark green leafy vegetables like broccoli and Brussels sprouts are sources of vitamin K."[112]

We might want to think twice before a "professional" directs us to calcium supplements alone and consider Nancy Appleton's warning about the possible harmful aspects of calcium supplementation. "Excess calcium," she says, "can be redistributed in the body and is often deposited in soft tissues, possibly causing arthritis, arteriosclerosis, glaucoma, kidney stones and other problems."[113]

Furthermore, says Ruth Sackman in *Cancer Forum*, "Fragmented supplements [e.g., calcium that has been separated from other natural components of food] can actually cause a deficiency of the very supplement that is being used because it robs the body's storage areas (bones, nails, muscles, hair, etc.) in order to reconstruct the natural complex found in nature. To avoid the risk of bone loss from calcium deprivation, why not use foods rich in calcium?" From raw almonds to dried beans to parsley, many valuable foods are identified by books on nutrition.[114] Dr. Lee, pointing out that "cows get the calcium for their bones and their milk from plants they eat," says that among the best sources of dietary calcium are fruits and, especially, broadleaf vegetables.[115] For example, one cup of collard greens contains 289 mg of functional calcium, one cup of kale 210 mg, and one cup of spinach 200 mg. From a four-ounce serving of scallops we can get 110 mg, and as much as 500 mg from sardines.[116]

THE IMPORTANCE OF MINERAL BALANCE

When women are told to take high doses of only calcium, it's a real cause for concern. Calcium supplements taken without the necessary co-minerals have the potential to cause harm and even contribute to osteoporosis,[117, 118] the very disease one is trying to prevent. Minerals, vitamins, and enzymes perform synergistically with each other,[119, 120] and "work as catalysts, promoting the absorption and assimilation of other vitamins and minerals."[121] Indeed, Nancy Appleton says that such imbalances can cause arthritis, kidney stones, or gallstones.[122]

In the past, however, when I did use a calcium supplement I deliberately chose one without phosphorus as an ingredient, and I noticed that this mineral is generally not included in commercial daily multivitamin/mineral products or most calcium/magnesium supplements. I assumed I was getting enough from my diet, which included foods rich in this mineral. By the same token I had tried to avoid those that are high in phosphoric acid, knowing that its metabolites may upset the mineral balance.[123] One authority even states that we need at least 2 to $2^1/_2$ times as much dietary calcium as phosphorus,[124] yet the Recommended Dietary Allowances (RDAs) for adults have for years called for approximately a one-to-one ratio of calcium to phosphorus.[125]

We learn that an excess of phosphorus can create a calcium deficiency by binding calcium in the gut and rendering it useless, just as it can also bind up other important minerals.[126] Studies reported in the *Journal of Nutrition* confirm that high intakes of phosphorus (or its metabolites) may lead to overstimulation of the parathyroid gland, impaired synthesis of the active form of vitamin D, and (especially in older women) a disruption of calcium homeostasis, all of which eventually lead to bone loss.[127] However, if one's dietary phosphorus intakes were lower than the normal, and then if one's calcium intake were increased without a change in the phosphorus level, the surplus calcium could become toxic,[128] says Dr. Appleton.

Even though the typical American diet contains an excess of phosphorus (perhaps the reason the majority of supplement products do not include this mineral), it seems that certain types of diets may actually be deficient in phosphorus. As a guideline for modifying or supplementing your diet, Dr. Appleton provides a home test kit (P.O. Box 3083, Santa Monica, CA 90403) for determining your own calcium/phosphorus status, which can be used as an indicator of your mineral ratio.

Although many more objective studies are needed, especially concerning the calcium/phosphorus ratio, I believe that if one is to take mineral supplements, the research supports including all the minerals as needed and in their correct ratio for proper calcium absorption. Incidentally, it's worth noting that since many "trace" minerals can be toxic in nonphysiological doses, a natural source such as sea vegetable capsules or green food extracts, like spirulina, barley green, chlorella, or sea vegetation, taken as directed, may be one way of obtaining a safer balance.

All this investigation has made me focus on the likelihood that, in addition to osteoporosis, joint disorders such as temporomandibular joint syndrome (TMJ) and bone spurs might also be exacerbated by an imbalance in the mineral ratio. My research into this subject has uncovered a wealth of important information on joint health, which motivated me to write *Preventing and Reversing Arthritis Naturally* in order to explain how, once again, the quality of our lives depends upon the nutritional choices we make.

HIGH RISK OF BONE AND SPINAL FRACTURES

It's important to understand what our bodies need, since it is currently predicted that one out of every three women will eventually suffer from low bone mass and structural weakness leading to fractures and possible skeletal deformity.[129] Women face at least a 15 percent risk of hip fracture. The annual cost of this trauma, which could be reduced by preventive efforts, is estimated at $7.3 billion in the United States—an amount that is rising each year. We need to focus on what we can do to circumvent such statistics in our lives—to achieve a healthy state of mind and body so as to have the energy to pursue our creative passions and goals to their fullest.

These figures constitute a national tragedy, considering that many of these women were faithfully subjecting themselves to synthetic HRT (with all its side effects)—and to what end? Their hips fractured just like those of the women who chose not to use any estrogen at all. This will seem even more of a crime when you read the following discussion of the role progesterone plays in bone formation.

This report, dealing with the prevention of osteoporosis, comes from the *Canadian Journal of OB/Gyn & Women's Health Care*. The authors, of the Division of Endocrinology and Metabolism at the University of British Columbia in Vancouver, state:

> Progesterone acts on bone, even though estrogen activity is low or absent. Because progesterone appears to work on the osteoblast to increase bone formation, it would complement the actions of estrogen to decrease bone resorption.[130]

The authors go on to explain that progesterone fastens to receptors on the osteoblasts (the bone-building cells) and "increases the rate of bone remodeling."[131] It is interesting to note once again that the role of estrogen is to slow down bone loss, while natural progesterone actually promotes bone production. Dr. Lee concludes from several studies that (1) estrogen slows down the dissolving of bone by the "osteoclast" (bone-resorbing) cells, (2) natural progesterone stimulates the formation of new bone, and (3) certain progestins may also cause the osteoblasts to create a limited amount of new bone.[132]

However, some studies have shown that the synthetic progestins normally prescribed by our doctors may actually diminish our supply of natural progesterone.[133] Many of our gynecologists do realize the destructive effect these synthetic progestins have on the body. This may be a major factor in why they prescribe estrogen alone.

BONE LOSS FROM COMMON MEDICATIONS

I believe we must always be on guard against any over-the-counter or prescription drugs that speed the dissolving of bone—a process called resorption. Trien Susan Falmholtz, in her book *Change of Life*, speaks about various commonly prescribed drugs that are known to lead to the dreaded condition of osteoporosis. These include thyroid replacement drugs such as synthroid; "heparin (an anticoagulant); cortisone preparations (such as prednisone); aluminum-containing antacids; anti-convulsants; and the antibiotic drug tetracycline."[134]

At the University of Massachusetts, a research project centered on the use of levothyroxine for treating thyroid problems. In certain circumstances this commonly prescribed hormone was found to cause as much as 13 percent bone loss.[135] A thyroid specialist I spoke with, however, says that this report has been quoted out of context and blown out of proportion. The main point to keep in mind is that dosages should never be prescribed in excess of demonstrated need, or for the wrong reason (such as for weight loss, when the gain was not caused by a thyroid deficiency).

Another example is giving thyroid medication simply for a low basal body temperature (a test often used by adherents of Dr. Broda Barnes), without other clear evidence of thyroid insufficiency. This type of test is also used for fertility problems to determine the time of ovulation and thus reflects a woman's progesterone level. Progesterone and thyroid are very much interrelated, but in some cases all that is needed is natural progesterone to correct an abnormally low body temperature. Dr. Peat believes that the mechanism by which progesterone raises the temperature prevents estrogen from blocking the action of thyroid hormone, because only in women is progesterone thermogenic.[136]

Dr. John Lee makes the point that a doctor who does not understand progesterone deficiency may give thyroid medication to someone who doesn't need it. This excess thyroid will increase the rate of bone resorption. However, when thyroid hormone is replaced for the purpose of restoring it to normal, it doesn't cause bone loss. In fact, the right dosage will improve bone density. As Dr. Lee explained to me, "It's not the thyroid that should be feared; it's the doctor who gives thyroid when you don't need it."

Noting another medicinal hazard, Dr. Alan Gaby describes a study of twenty patients who were scheduled for brain surgery. Some of them were given Maalox 70 to prevent stress and ulcers. This antacid is rich in aluminum, and the research team found, after analyzing brain and bone tissue, that this toxic substance had been absorbed into the body and deposited in the osseous tissues resulting in increased bone resorption. Dr. Gaby recapitulates information from the studies, saying that "the accumulation of aluminum in bone appears to reduce the formation of osteoid [areas of new bone], while at the same time increasing the amount of bone resorption. The result of this dual action of aluminum would be to accelerate bone loss."[137]

BE WARY OF WONDER DRUGS

This is a good place to say just a word about the dangers of taking the latest "miracle" drug to prevent bone loss. We are always reading or hearing in the media about experimental drugs, new hormones, or even new compounds that activate bone growth. Highly advertised drugs come onto the market quickly and sometimes, fortunately, leave with just as much speed.

In case you have been considering the drug of the day, Fosamax, for osteoporosis, please reconsider. First of all, Dr. John Lee reports that when women take Fosamax, "The old bone remains in place and over time begins to crumble, and eventually this is likely to cause the fracture rate to sharply increase."[138] Like estrogen replacement therapy, Fosamax only helps to slow bone breakdown and does not stimulate the buildup of new bone. This temporary saving of the bone (even registering as an increase on BMD tests) only appears to be preventing osteoporosis; in reality it's a temporary crutch and an advertising gimmick that took years to promote. Over time, the preservation of our older, more brittle bone will take its toll.

Clinical trials show that after approximately five years the "apparent" bone density retention reverses itself and the fracture rate increases, even over that of women taking a placebo.[139] In the case of Fosamax, in spite of misleading statistics in the product advertisements, not only does this drug not lessen the chances of hip fracture, but it actually increases the risk of wrist fractures.[140–142]

We need to consider the potential side effects from the use of Fosamax as well. These include musculoskeletal pain, headache, and gastrointestinal problems, especially ulceration of the esophagus and stomach that may result in permanent damage. This drug comes with explicit instructions that you must not lie down for thirty minutes after its ingestion. As consumers of such products, we women are beginning to question why we are encouraged to take a drug that invites such risks and whose supposed benefits are not even guaranteed!

Dr. Lee goes on to tell us that "Fosamax also causes deficiencies of calcium, magnesium, and vitamin D, all essential to the bone-building process,"[143] and that "rats given high doses [of Fosamax] develop thyroid and adrenal tumors."[144] According to Amy McWilliams, Pharm.D. and Jason Sauberan, Pharm.D., we have insufficient data about its long-term adverse effects or its use in osteoporosis prevention, and Fosamax should not be used if you are deficient in calcium or vitamin D. Note that it unnaturally inhibits the osteoclasts and has not been shown to reduce the risk of cardiovascular disease.[145]

Our doctors and the advertising media are also now heavily promoting another drug to postmenopausal women supposedly to combat osteoporosis. Evista (raloxifene hydrochloride) is known as a "selective estrogen receptor modulator (SERM)" and comes with a multitude of what Samuel S. Epstein, M.D. refers to as "reckless claims."[146] SERMs have gained acceptance on the sole basis of their impact on the estrogen receptors, without regard to their unknown long-term effects. Another concern is the fact that the estrogens they are attempting to control are known to operate via various metabolic and neurological pathways and not just through the estrogen receptors.[147, 148]

In the "Information for the Patient" leaflet that comes with Evista are noted the adverse events that occurred during clinical trials: breast pain, vaginal bleeding, flatulence, hot flashes, infection, abdominal pain, and chest pain.[149] Other pharmaceutical literature cautions about liver problems, blood clotting in the veins, leg cramps, chest pain, coughing up blood from the lungs, and eye disturbances from Evista (due to possible formation of blood clots).[150] Breast and uterine cancer studies were conducted over a period of only three years or less, and the manufacturer even states that the drug "has not been adequately studied in women with a prior history of breast cancer."[151] Additionally, like many synthetic drugs, Evista is formulated in a base containing substances such as aluminum, carnauba wax, preservatives, and artificial coloring. Many of these compounds not only cause allergic reactions but may also be carcinogenic.

Nor does the company warn of the "serious risks of ovarian cancer," says Dr. Epstein, who notes that its premarket clearance study "clearly shows that Evista induces ovarian cancer in both mice and rats. Furthermore, carcinogenic effects were noted at dosages extending well below the recommended therapeutic level."[152] This critical information, along with an admission that Evista's effect on fractures is not yet known, is absent from both the full-page colored ads and the "Warnings" to patients and doctors. Dr. Epstein believes the manufacturer owes free, lifelong ovarian cancer screening to the over 12,000 women who participated in the clinical trials with uninformed consent. He concludes, "This drug should be withdrawn from the world market immediately."[153]

The ongoing parade of fashionable new drugs orchestrated by the drug companies will no doubt continue in the coming years, with the ones we are now talking about being replaced by others because these will have been found to be harmful, and, in the long run, futile attempts at treating or preventing osteoporosis. History reveals over and over that the whole business of developing new drugs is about profit, not about health.

We can always take our cue from the manufacturer's recital of potential effects. Unless facing an emergency situation, we'd do well to consider the risks and look long and hard at all available alternatives. As Dr. Udo Erasmus reminds us, "Drugs are foreign to the body and therefore all drugs are toxic."[154] Perhaps we also need to remember Hippocrates' wise advice advocating letting food be our medicine and medicine be our food.

In exploring the importance of enzymes and vitamins to aid in the digestion of meat protein so that calcium will not be lost in the blood, I came across some information regarding salmon calcitonin that at first reading seemed to make it another good choice for those who are suffering from severe bone loss. Few physicians seem to be aware of salmon calcitonin, which slows calcium resorption. Calcitonin is "found in humans (as well as in salmon, pigs, eels and sheep),"[155] according to an article in *Prevention* magazine. The author, Sydney Bonnick, says that calcitonin is a hormone that is manufactured by the thyroid gland. Its function is to deter the movement of calcium from the bone to the blood. Calcitonin has even been found to "relieve pain from fractured bones, and [it] may actually stimulate the formation of new bone."[156]

The reason it is not used more readily for those suffering from osteoporosis is that it is extremely expensive, costing approximately $2,700 per year; and it is quite inconvenient to administer via intramuscular or subcutaneous injections.[157] In the United States it is currently delivered by means of a daily injection of 100 I.U.[158] Although the synthetic versions of calcitonin, such as Calcimar, have been approved by the FDA for the treatment of osteoporosis, the literature on these products discusses possible severe allergic reactions, including anaphylactic shock, as well as nausea, vomiting,[159] and other possible side effects.

Volunteer Study Groups

The above studies should make us more cautious when we hear about osteoporosis study groups that provide free medication. The other day such an experiment was announced on the radio, touting a miraculous "breakthrough in medicine" that sounded like the wonder drug of the century for the prevention of osteoporosis.

Curiosity had gotten the better of me. Being most interested in the subject, I had to call the toll-free number and ask the name of the drug. The person who answered said, "You are probably well aware that estrogen is needed for all women suffering from osteoporosis." She went on to say that estrogen is essential for the building of bones, and without its use we will increase our chances of osteoporosis. She then invited me to become part of this study group that, as it turns out, was for raloxifene. Learning that it was a synthetic drug quickly ended my curiosity—but not my desire to want to reach those who would say "yes" to this proposal.

All of this highlights the potentially catastrophic consequences of not being informed about natural health care. Not long ago I met a woman in my workplace who must have been in her sixties. She was walking with a lot of difficulty. I was telling her what I'd learned about hormones and osteoporosis. She said to me that she had always refused to take pills of any kind; in fact, she was quite vehement about this. She told me that ten years earlier she'd had a hip replacement, and because her other hip was now showing the same signs and giving her trouble, she had been asked to be a candidate for a national double-blind osteoporosis study group.

I felt so sad for her, because she'd been so determined to stay healthy by not taking any medicine—and now here she was, desperately taking pills every morning and evening. She was not even allowed to know whether she was taking a placebo or an active substance. She was living day to day with little hope—only the fear that her other hip would also need to be replaced. She looked at me and said, "What you're saying about hormone deficiency is interesting, because all my problems started when I was in my forties, right after my hysterectomy."

I thought to myself, "For twenty years she has had no hormone replacement therapy." This woman, prior to her hysterectomy, had been very active and pain-free, and I could tell she had so much inner drive and energy that she was no longer able to express. I tried to picture in my mind what she would have been like now had she received natural hormone therapy before all these permanent changes occurred. Her devastating situation deeply influenced my determination to write this book.

Another account that fueled my interest in sharing this needed information came from a dear friend in her seventies. She was a former surgical nurse and, needless to say, had always been health conscious, trying to follow her doctors' orders to the letter. Well, my friend had just heard from her orthopedic surgeon the shocking news that she had quite a lot of bone loss. He proposed that she be thinking about a hip replacement. She recalls driving home with tears of disbelief at this news thinking: "How could this be, when I've always taken preventive cautions so as to avoid this dreaded diagnosis of osteoporosis?"

She finally telephoned me and said, "I don't understand why I'm having bone loss. I've been taking my estrogen for over twenty-five years, thinking that this was good for my bones." How do you tell a nurse that she has been on the wrong hormone all these years? And that estrogen's role is only to slow down the bone breakdown, while progesterone is the hormone that plays the major role in building bone mineral density? As she read a draft of this chapter and learned of the importance of progesterone as it works on osteoblast cells to increase bone mass, she related her ambivalent feelings. On the one hand, she felt robbed of her health because she had used the wrong hormone for so long; but on the other, she was relieved to realize her problems could be reversed.

If we recognize the signs of hormone imbalance and understand how and why hormone replacement therapy can correct such an imbalance, we'll be spared a lot of grief in years to come. Who wouldn't get tired of going from one doctor to another for headaches, fatigue, heart palpitations, hot flashes, heavy bleeding, irregular periods, spotting, anxiety, moodiness, night sweats, depression, or just feeling rotten? Many doctors still don't recognize that many of these problems are related to menopause or other stressful times—such as after childbirth or hysterectomy.

Just like the woman in the story above, many of us simply endure these symptoms and learn to live with them by keeping busy, trying to eat right, and so on—completely unaware of the harmful effects of progressive progesterone deficiency. Medicine is triumphant in emergencies and trauma, but it often falters in the management of degenerative diseases and preventive health care. The very drugs your doctor prescribes may mask an underlying hormone deficiency. Sooner or later, when the symptoms get bad enough, you may have to supplement Mother Nature's gifts with what she is no longer adequately providing. Why not use a natural progesterone product instead of taking such risks?

How Many Tragedies Will Strike Before We Take a Stand?

No wonder osteoporosis is so prevalent. Have we indeed been given the wrong hormone—a hormone that medical doctors have been prescribing for over five decades? Since 1942, when estrogen was approved by the FDA for production by Wyeth-Ayerst Laboratory and introduced to the market, it has been demonstrated to be of little worth in the prevention of osteoporosis. It seems that women have been under a theoretical HRT system that has been extensively prescribed without necessary checks and balances. No wonder osteoporosis is called "the silent killer." There comes a time when we may become too old to feel comfortable voicing complaints, and our bone loss, fractures, and joint problems continue as a generational plague.

Fluoride: Hard to Avoid

Try as we may to create all the right conditions to avoid osteoporosis—the right kind of hormones, the right kind of calcium, and the nutrients needed for its assimilation—we might also want to be more aware of a chemical that is added to our water and of its effect on bone mass. The threat posed by fluoride may very well obliterate all our good intentions.

The *Holistic Dental Digest* tells us that in addition to devitalizing the tooth enamel and possibly leading to periodontal disease, fluoride actually causes the bones to become more brittle and weak—even though they *appear* denser on X-ray films similar to the illusion created by estrogen and Fosamax. One study reports that "the risk of fractures for women in high-fluoride communities [is] more than double."[160]

Another study reviewed in the *Journal of the American Medical Association* found that fluoridation increases the rate of hip fracture by about 30 percent in women and 40 percent in men.[161] Despite false claims by some public health officials to the contrary, there are no legitimate studies to indicate any hip fracture protection from fluoride. Fluoride is toxic to bones in any amount, including the level found in fluoridated water.[162]

It is also harmful to the thyroid and is a known cause of cancer and other diseases. Japanese researchers reported in 1982 that "sodium fluoride, which is being used to prevent dental caries [cavities], produces chromosomal aberrations and irregular synthesis of DNA." The latest studies in the United States confirm the frightening truth that "malignant transformation of cells is induced by sodium fluoride."[163]

Over three decades ago we were warned of these dangers in *The American Fluoridation Experiment* by Frederick B. Exner, M.D., an X-ray diagnostician, biologist, chemist, physicist, and pathologist.[164] And the American Medical Association published data in the *Archives of Environmental Health* in February 1961, showing that fluorides have been found in diseased tissue from tumors, the aorta, and cataracts.[165]

Yet, from that day to this, says *Cancer Forum*, the U.S. Public Health Service has encouraged the Environmental Protection Agency to keep assuring American citizens that fluoridation is effective and safe, in spite of the fact that there is "not a shred of scientific evidence to support that claim."[166] It would be in our best interest to mount a national letter-writing campaign to convince Congress and the EPA to remove this hazard from our public water supply.

MISCONCEPTIONS ABOUT CALCIUM AND DIET

When we are trying to sort out the facts on how to maintain an adequate calcium level, let's acquire our information from unbiased sources rather than from those associated with the dairy, cattle, and poultry industries. A dramatic example appears in *Health Science*, where Dr. Joel Fuhrman states: "If your calcium intake is very high but you constantly excrete more calcium than you absorb, you are in a negative balance and osteoporosis will result in time. On the other hand, if your calcium intake is relatively low but your body is efficient at absorbing it, you are in a positive balance and your skeleton will not be stripped of its calcium stores."[167] Drs. Cedric and Frank Garland *(The Calcium Connection)* and Nancy Appleton, Ph.D. *(Lick the Sugar Habit)* agree that excessive dietary sugar intake increases calcium excretion in the urine, upsetting the body's mineral balance.[168]

From an academic viewpoint, when we refer to calcium and other minerals in our chemistry classes, the words "organic" and "inorganic" have a strictly applied definition. However, writers on nutrition use the term *organic* more loosely to mean *alive* or *bioavailable*. It is in this sense that numerous studies have been made regarding organic and inorganic minerals and their use to, or abuse of, the body.

Dr. M. T. Morter Jr., cautions against depending on unreliable types of calcium. He is convinced that the body cannot dissolve the strong "ionic" bonds of "inorganic" calcium, such as dolomite or oyster shell. Nor, in spite of dairy industry advertising, can it utilize the calcium found in cow's milk; because unless the milk is consumed raw, its calcium has been altered by the pasteurization process into a hard, unusable form, which will be deposited in the wrong areas of the body. Dr. Morter points out that women who consume large amounts of dairy products are actually among the high-risk groups for osteoporosis.[169]

Along this same vein, Norman W. Walker, D.Sc., in his book *Fresh Vegetable and Fruit Juices*, gives us some excellent thoughts to live by concerning oxalic acid and its relation to calcium assimilation:

> When food is raw, whether whole or in the form of juice, every atom in such food is vital [i.e.,] ORGANIC and is replete with enzymes. Therefore, the oxalic acid in our raw vegetables and their juices is organic, and as such is . . . essential for the physiological functions of the body. . . . The oxalic acid in cooked and processed foods, however, is definitely dead, or INORGANIC, and as such is both pernicious and destructive. Oxalic acid readily combines with calcium. If these are both organic, the result is a beneficial constructive combination, as the former helps the digestive assimilation of the latter, at the same time stimulating the peristaltic functions in the body.[170]

Please note that this advice may be contrary to what you have read elsewhere, but it really makes sense—and its author has much experience as well as credibility. Dr. Walker, after all, lived to be one hundred and nine years of age by practicing what he preached; his wife died in her nineties. He is the only person I've known to explain the distinction between *raw* and *cooked* foods containing oxalic acid:

> When the oxalic acid has become INORGANIC by cooking or processing the foods that contain it, then this acid forms an interlocking compound with the calcium even combining with the calcium in other foods eaten during the same meal, destroying the nourishing value of both. This results in such a serious deficiency of calcium that it has been known to cause decomposition of the bones. This is the reason I never eat cooked or canned spinach.[171]

Dr. Walker tells us that the most plentiful quantities of organic oxalic acid are found in fresh raw spinach, kale, collards, mustard greens, turnips, Swiss chard, and beet greens.[172] Other sources include almonds, asparagus, and parsley.

Many of these same foods are high in calcium as well, and indeed, the first source we should look to for our calcium requirements should be our daily diet. But as we've seen from Dr. Morter's views earlier, the customary idea of milk as one of the most important sources of calcium is coming into much debate these days. In fact, you will assimilate more calcium from ingesting kale than from drinking milk, according to Frederik Khachik, a researcher at the U.S. Department of Agriculture.[173]

It would seem that the very foods we are told to consume for calcium are those that often cause allergies and other serious problems. By way of illustration, cardiologist Kurt Oster conducted extensive research into the xanthine oxidase in homogenized cow's milk. This substance was shown to damage arteries and promote atherosclerosis. He found no such correlation associated with the intake of butter or cheese, presumably because they contain little or no biologically active xanthine oxidase. Oster makes a reasonable case that one of the causes of atherosclerosis is the consumption of homogenized milk.[174]

There are valid concerns, too, about skim milk. Butterfat actually provides an excellent source of vitamins A and D, is anticarcinogenic, and allows the minerals and other nutrients in milk to be absorbed and utilized. One researcher observes, "The plague of osteoporosis in milk-drinking western nations may be due to the fact that most people choose skim milk over whole, thinking it is good for them."[175]

Synthetic vitamin D, added to replace the natural, is toxic to the liver. Nonfat dried milk, which is added to 1 percent and 2 percent milk and to nonfat commercial yogurt, contains heart-damaging rancid cholesterol and high levels of nitrites and galactose (milk sugar linked with development of cataracts, glaucoma, and ovarian cancer). Thus, for several reasons, whole milk products may be preferable.[176]

A further commentary on milk comes from *How to Get Well,* a useful health book that provides practical information on nutrition and drugless treatment. Dr. Paavo Airola writes:

> Today's pasteurized supermarket-sold milk is loaded with toxic and dangerous drugs, chemicals and residues of pesticides, herbicides and detergents—such milk is not suitable for human consumption. If you are

fortunate enough to get *real* milk, fresh, raw, "farmer" milk from healthy cows fed organic food, then you can add milk to your diet.[177]

To his list we might add the synthetic hormones that are often present in commercial milk products. Dr. Airola says that the preferred way of consuming milk is as acidophilus milk, yogurt, or other soured (predigested) forms, because they "help to maintain a healthy intestinal flora and prevent intestinal putrefaction and constipation."[178] Look for plain, unsweetened yogurt (preferably organically produced) with active lactobacillus cultures or for cultured buttermilk. In some places unhomogenized commercial yogurt is available; homemade whole milk yogurt would be even better.[179]

However, if you do decide to use a calcium supplement (particularly after menopause), many authorities recommend one such as calcium citrate[180] over the more common calcium carbonate. The latter can be hard to assimilate, especially in older persons and those deficient in hydrochloric acid. But remember also the importance of magnesium and the trace nutrients mentioned earlier in the chapter, which facilitate calcium uptake by the bone.

And as another option, microcrystalline hydroxyapatite (MCHC), which the *Textbook of Medical Physiology* refers to as the "primary form of calcium in our bones,"[181] is a highly-absorbable compound that has been found effective in improving bone density. Because it contains a variety of minerals, vitamins, and proteins, it is becoming valuable therapy in the use of preventing osteoporosis.[182–184]

BUILDING BONE WITH B VITAMINS

And what else do we need to know about the health of our bones? Dr. Alan Gaby discusses the influence of vitamin B_6, pointing out that "this vitamin is a cofactor for the enzyme lysyl oxidase, which crosslinks proteins and connective tissue. Adequate vitamin B_6 is therefore required to provide tensile strength and structure to collagen . . . in bone tissue." He also mentions a study by Nelson, Lyons, and Evans, which "suggests that vitamin B_6 enhances the production or the effectiveness of progesterone. To the extent that progesterone is important for bone health, adequate intake of vitamin B_6 is also essential."[185] Studies confirm that low levels of this vitamin can create abnormal bone growth as well as create the risk of developing osteoporotic bone disease.[186, 187] Today the effects of much of modern technology are creating environmental chemicals that are causing a deficiency of B_6 and thus disrupting the necessary biochemical interactions that this nutrient provides for our body.[188]

THE IMPORTANCE OF WEIGHT-BEARING EXERCISE

The Center for Women's Health at Columbia-Presbyterian Medical Center surveyed women who exercised three or more times a week and found that they reported fewer osteoporotic symptoms than those who exercise twice a week or less.[189] But what kind of exercise would help us prevent osteoporosis? The importance of an exercise program is discussed in Dr. Gaby's book *Preventing and Reversing Osteoporosis*. He states that weight-bearing exercise, which forces the body to work against gravity, helps in building bone density. For older women, swimming may be most appropriate, as there is less risk of injury.[190]

Dr. Gaby observes that urinary calcium excretion was found to be quite extensive in astronauts following their time in space. Furthermore, patients restricted to bed for back pain demonstrated rapid bone loss: "bone mineral content of the lumbar spine decreased at an astounding 0.9% per week." Dr. Gaby emphasizes, therefore, that "physical activity plays a crucial role in maintaining bone mass."[191]

The role of exercise in preventing and reversing bone depletion cannot be overstated, nor can exercise alone make all the difference. As we have mentioned again and again, it is the combination of factors that has the greatest impact on our total health and specifically on our bone mineral density. In planning your exercise program, remember that it, like dietary changes, needs to be incorporated into your daily routine—for the rest of your life. Just as crash diets yield only temporary weight loss, sporadic exercise is not going to have any significant impact on your bone density.

Your body will give you clues as to the right kind and amount of exercise for you. Dr. Ray Peat points out in *Nutrition for Women* that women athletes are sometimes chronically deficient in progesterone (and may miss periods), probably because the stress of hard exercise causes the conversion of progesterone to cortisone.[192] He also observes that excessive stress and so-called aerobic exercise that leaves one breathless are common causes of hypothyroidism[193] and may contribute to premature aging. Thus, we must find that happy medium.

Here are a few guidelines to keep in mind when planning an exercise program:

- Start slowly and steadily; the no-pain/no-gain motto does not apply. If a twenty-minute walk causes back pain, for example, don't stop altogether; just cut the total time in half for the next week or two. Find your comfort level and build gradually from there.

- Aim for a thirty- to forty-five-minute work-out period at least three times per week.
- Include a combination of aerobic exercise (walking or jogging), strength training with light to moderate weights, and a stretching or yoga routine for flexibility. This provides variety and helps you avoid boredom.
- Check out books, tapes, and videos at your local library, bookstore, or video store; this way you can expose yourself to a wide variety of trainers and instructors.
- And for chronic exercise avoiders, here's a no-excuse, no-reason-not-to, simple-as-can-be weight-bearing exercise—the bone bounce: simply rise up on your toes and let yourself drop down on your heels, making sure you feel a vibration in your hips. You can vary the intensity as needed by varying how high you rise up off the floor. Start small and work up to two hundred to three hundred times or for two to three minutes per day.
- Finally, you're never too old or too young to start an exercise program; just remember to begin slowly, build gradually, and check with your health care providers if you have any medical, neurological, or musculoskeletal complications. Even seventy-year-olds in wheelchairs have improved their flexibility and overall fitness with light weightlifting.
- Most of all, be creative, make it fun, and stay with it.

WHERE DO WE GO FROM HERE?

It is not difficult to be overwhelmed by the health decisions that confront us. Modern-day medicines include never-ending lists of names for "new and improved" synthetic drugs and hormones. (See appendix B for a sampling of the many synthetic hormones commonly prescribed today.) Because the terms for the complex chemicals we are consuming are often incomprehensible, we too often rely completely on our medical doctors for treatment decisions.

What a contrast, and what an awakening, to discover information that is understandable! It seems almost too simple to be true—but then, isn't truth often found in the simpler forms of nature?

What we have learned so far may require some assertive action. With these alternatives to artificial hormones we now have an opportunity to become less dependent on drugs that lead us away from a sound body, mind, and soul. Prepared, we can responsibly choose a path less traveled—one that may lead to a better quality of life.

In appendix E, you will find a form letter you can give to a prospective doctor explaining your concerns about synthetic hormones. He or she should know how you feel about toxic drugs and the unwanted side effects of the synthetic hormones that cause so much distress. It is imperative that your health provider understand that your body *does require*, and *can assimilate*, natural progesterone.

It is important to note that the cream used in Dr. Lee's studies specifically contained USP progesterone, which is referred to as "natural" progesterone in most of the current literature. We are often asked if there is any difference between this and the many wild yam creams available today. The answer is that, to date, no large-scale clinical studies have been done to validate the use of wild yam extract without USP modification.

With respect to the treatment and prevention of osteoporosis, so far only USP progesterone has been clinically tested and evaluated. However, for the treatment of many of the other debilitating and draining symptoms of PMS and menopause (cramping, irritability, hot flashes, fibroids, etc.) patient after patient reports relief using a product containing the sterol from either the wild yam (diosgenin) or soybean (stigmasterol) without conversion to the USP progesterone. (See appendix A for more information). Some women have found that alternating the two types (or using a cream that combines both) gives the best results. (See appendix G.) Others alternate the cream with sublingual drops or tablets.

༄

Dr. Judi Gerstung is interested in assessing long-term response to various treatments for increasing bone mineral density. If you would like to assist her with this project, please send a brief description of your health care program, a copy of your initial bone mineral density test, and results of any follow-up studies to: Dr. Judi Gerstung, c/o Inner Traditions International, One Park Street, P.O. Box 388, Rochester, VT 05767.

The Risk of Cancer

The only known cause of uterine cancer is excess estrogen due to inadequate progesterone or to estrogen replacement without the concomitant use of natural progesterone.[1]
C. Norman Shealy, M.D., Ph.D.

We've been waging the war on cancer for many decades, and what do we have to show for it? Despite the vast sums of money that are spent on developing new drugs and new technologies, casualties continue to mount. Dr. Allen Astrow, a cancer specialist at St. Vincent's Hospital and Medical Center in New York, tells us that even with all the advances in our knowledge of the molecular mechanics of tumor formation and development, "mortality rates from cancer in the U.S. are rising."[2, 3]

Once we begin to understand the reason cancer exists, we will see why the war against cancer was lost years ago and why we need to get off this battlefield. Dr. John Lee alerts us to the research of Schippers et al., which shows that "cancer cells, far from being foreign invaders, are an intimate part of ourselves, essentially normal cells in which proportionately small changes in genes have led to changes in their behavior. The treatment strategy should be to reestablish intercellular communications." It's called *rebalancing*.

I was able to understand the process of rebalancing the body a lot better after reading Dr. Richard Passwater's research on human cancers and our environmental carcinogens. Thousands of new chemicals are added to the environment every year.[4] A study by the Department of Biological Sciences at the University of Idaho showed that many environmental pollutants contain estrogenic compounds that are suspected of increasing the occurrence of endocrine interference and reproductive failure in humans and other species.

According to Dr. Raymond Peat, in a personal communication, "environmental carcinogens—phenolics, aromatic-hydrocarbons, chlorinated-hydrocarbons, PCBs, dioxins, soot, even X-rays—are in general estrogenic." Although the public is only beginning to be aware of this deadly connection, especially to breast cancer, it has been published widely in scientific journals and articles on health research.

HORMONES, GENETIC MUTATIONS, AND CANCER

The topic is controversial and in many respects frightening. Yes, it seems that a large number of the chemicals we encounter in our daily lives, such as pesticides, solvents, industrial contaminants, and components of detergents and plastics, actually mimic the estrogen molecules found in living organisms. Because these harmful estrogenic substances latch onto or sometimes enter our living cells, which contain receptors, they can either give the cells a greater than normal hormonal "charge" or block activity of the body's own estrogen by jamming the receptors.

Why is this so serious? Recent studies cite the effects of such environmental contamination: a dramatically rising breast cancer rate in the United States, a possible decline in sperm quality plus low testosterone levels in men, abnormal penises and reduced motor and language skills among boys whose mothers were exposed to estrogen-like toxins, and other ills. Not only are humans threatened, but some animal populations (marine birds, panthers) are perhaps very close to extinction. Because of the estrogenic pollutants, sea gulls and alligators have been found with abnormal reproductive organs and a low reproduction rate, with nesting impulses observed among males and aggressive behavior in females.[5,*]

Instead of degrading like other poisons, substances such as DDT, PCBs, and dioxin accumulate over the years. Since some of these fat-soluble chemicals are sprayed on plants and eaten by animals, they especially affect those at the top of the food chain: humans. What does that bode for the next generation?

According to the journal *Pediatrics* published by the American Academy of Pediatrics (April 1997), "Environmental estrogens occur from the breakdown of chemicals in products ranging from pesticides to plastic wrap."[6] These in turn imitate the hormone, estrogen. We are now finding that young

---

* To read more about this, see Thoe Colborn's "Developmental Effects of Endocrine Disrupting Chemicals in Wildlife and Humans" in *The Journal of the National Institute of Environmental Health Sciences*, Vol. 101, No. 5, October 1993.

girls are reaching puberty earlier than ever, some even developing sexually by the time they are eight years old.[7] Ovarian, breast, prostate, and testicular cancer—all hormone-driven—have increased sharply in recent years.

Now the Environmental Protection Agency and several other organizations are looking into the impact of estrogen-mimicking chemicals on both reproduction and cancer, in an attempt to either confirm or deny this compelling theory. Every day studies are brought forth that make this simpler to confirm.

For instance, from a March 21, 1998, article in *Science News* ("Drugged Waters: Does It Matter That Pharmaceuticals Are Turning Up in Water Supplies?"), we discover that estrogens passed on in human waste are not being removed by sewage treatment plants. As a result, they are accumulating in our water supply and are having a serious impact on the reproductive patterns of exposed wildlife (and quite possibly human life as well).[8] These rather shocking results of tests on water taken from Lake Mead in Nevada showed estradiol levels to be quite high.[9] Given that synthetic estrogen is one of the top-selling drugs in this country, the fact that it is a major source of environmental contamination of many of our lakes, rivers, and streams should come as no surprise.

The insidious nature of the xenoestrogens (environmental estrogen mimickers) becomes clear when they strike close to home. I myself know of a bright young college student, ironically an environmental health science major, who by the age of twenty-three had endured multiple surgical procedures and faced uncertainty about whether she would ever be able to bear children—all as a result of exposure to the pesticide Safrotin, which had been sprayed, improperly, inside her dormitory room.

Five months after an unpleasant and violent initial reaction, the hormonal effects of this neurotoxic chemical had begun their toll: midmonth bleeding, excruciating cramps, diarrhea, and urinary pain. Before finally arriving at the diagnosis of severe endometriosis, a series of doctors put this young woman through a terrible ordeal of testing, exploratory surgery, and ineffective treatment. Then they gave her undesirable options such as synthetic birth control pills to try to normalize her cycles, more surgery to determine the extent of damage to her ova, and treatment with a drug that would induce menopause.

This was an extreme example of what we are all faced with today. In 1998, for example, *Science News* published an alarming report about some of the estrogen-mimicking products in our environment.[10] BHA (a preservative that's added to food), BBP (which makes plastics flexible and preserves paper food-packaging materials), and DBP (found in food wraps, certain insect

repellents, etc.) are just a few of the powerful pseudoestrogens that are causing endocrine disorders in both men and women. BPAs are yet another component of some plastic wraps and plastic-lined cans.

Dioxins turn up in tampons, shampoos, skin creams, and drinks from
those plastic-lined cans.[11] And more and more we are finding that dioxins
have directly contaminated our food supply. In June 1999 the Associated
Press released an announcement by the Belgian Minister of Health regarding exceedingly high levels of dioxin in chicken that had been measured at
1,000 times the "accepted" limit. This followed earlier distribution of 175,000
pounds of dioxin-contaminated animal feed to poultry, beef, and pig farms in
that country.[12]

The Tampon Safety and Research Act provides an investigation into the
dioxin in tampons. *Women's Health Advocate* sums up the concerns about
bleached tampons:

> Chlorine is used to bleach paper pulp, which provides the rayon used in
> most tampons. This process produces dioxin, a probable carcinogen
> that's suspected of acting like estrogen in the body.[13]

Author McQuade Crawford is a member of the American Herbalists
Guild and Britain's National Institute of Medical Herbalists, president of the
American College of Integrative Medicine in Albuquerque, and a practicing
herbalist in California. Her studies show that chlorinated compounds such as
dioxin are creating a variety of endocrine and reproductive problems, causing
infertility and even cancer.[14] She encourages women to avoid the use of
bleached feminine hygiene products, as well as reducing consumption of animal products exposed to pesticides and synthetic hormones.*

Meanwhile, many consumers are looking for unbleached, all-cotton tampons and pads (which more and more health food stores carry) or those that
are bleached with hydrogen peroxide. Insist on organically produced cotton
as, ironically, cotton is one of the most heavily sprayed agricultural crops.

In view of the potentially tragic health consequences, Dr. John Lee feels
we should be alarmed about our exposure to these foreign estrogens (or
"xenobiotics") derived from petrochemicals. Indeed, he says there is a corre-
sponding epidemic of progesterone deficiency among women in the indus-
trialized nations (North America and Western Europe), influenced in part by

---

* For information on meats that are free of antibiotics, hormones, growth stimulants, herbicides,
and pesticides, see appendix E.

environmental contamination and our processed food supply, whereby we do not get the progesterone in our diets that people in the less developed countries obtain from raw, natural foods.[15]

Referring to the fascinating work of Dr. Peter Ellison for the World Health Organization, Dr. Lee says:

> The estrogen levels in America today tend to be quite a bit higher than in other countries. With menopause the fall of estrogen is greater in the U.S. and other industrialized countries than in the more agrarian "Third World" countries. Progesterone levels are remarkably stable in agrarian countries whereas, here in the U.S., women's progesterone falls to levels quite close to zero, even lower than that found in men.[16]

ESTROGEN OVERKILL

At the March 1998 National Cancer Institute Symposium, twenty-six renowned cancer researchers explained the role of estrogen metabolites in the prelude to breast and prostate cancer.[17, 18] This event, the topic of which was "Estrogens as Endogenous Carcinogens in the Breast and Prostate," shed new light on estrogen's effect on our health.[19]

In short, all of us are in danger of estrogen excess. Consider the sources: (1) Estrogen is secreted in substantial amounts by the ovaries and adrenal glands in the form of androstenedione (an estrogen precursor).[20] (2) Medical doctors prescribe estrogens for numerous clinical conditions at many different stages and ages in a woman's life cycle—for menstrual problems, infertility, PMS, birth control, and postmenopausal symptoms. A big concern is that we are thereby adding more estrogen to an already estrogenic environment, setting our bodies up for a multitude of disorders and diseases. (3) Not only are natural estrogens present in many plant foods (phytoestrogens), but if we eat meat and dairy products that are not organically produced, we may also be ingesting foods daily that contain synthetic estrogen (DES)[21] or the estrogenic growth hormones that are injected into cattle and poultry. Along with feed additives, antibiotics, pesticides, and drugs, these hormones are given to animals with little or no federal regulation.[22] (4) And finally, we live in a chemically saturated environment, which is a source of additional undesirable estrogen.

With the cards stacked against us like this, most of us will undoubtedly experience what Dr. Lita Lee has referred to as "estrogen overload."[23] The host of contributing factors makes it fairly easy to understand how estrogen can permeate and eventually gain the upper hand in the body, doing significant damage without its essential partner, progesterone, to balance and oppose it. Even herbal estrogens, especially when taken alone, can contribute to this type of hormonal imbalance.

Our human cells take an amazing amount of abuse (not without consequences) from artificial preservatives, colorings, and flavorings and the other chemical additives in our foods. Many of these additives, along with the preservatives and chemical wastes that end up in our food, air, and water, are now classed as xenoestrogens and are wreaking havoc in animals and humans alike.[24]

The link between even our body's endogenous estrogen and cancer cannot be overlooked much longer. Studies are increasingly implicating estrogen in the development of cancer of the breast, uterus, ovaries,[25] and also the prostate.[26–28] Furthermore, researchers working with cell cultures are now studying the mechanisms by which estrogen metabolites can initiate cell damage by binding to DNA. Epidemiologists report that "women who have reduced amounts of the enzymes that help sop up those reactive estrogen byproducts are at higher risk for developing breast cancer."[29]

All of this information should be front-page news. David Longfellow, a chemist with the National Cancer Institute and organizer of the 1998 National Cancer Institute Symposium insists that the "carcinogenic" nature of estrogen in both men and women should be a focus of our research efforts. The urgency is mounting, as each year—in the United States alone—we see approximately 240,000 new cases of breast, uterine, and ovarian cancers.[30] How much longer are we going to acquiesce to the worn and dispassionate cliché about "weighing the benefits against the risks" of a hormone that is clearly creating such havoc?

SPECIFIC ESTROGENS AND CANCER

Many experts have observed a direct link between ovarian,[31] breast, and uterine cancer and high levels of particular estrogens in the body—specifically the estrogens known as *estradiol* and *estrone*.[32] The other common estrogen, *estriol*, is thought by some (although the matter is controversial) to have a positive effect on postmenopausal[33] or younger women. This was brought home to me by an eye-opening piece of information I came across during my search for natural hormones. The statement in Dr. Julian Whitaker's newsletter *Health & Healing* still sticks in my mind:

> There are three forms of estrogen: estrone, estradiol, and estriol. It was shown almost 10 years ago that estrone and estradiol were the primary

cancer culprits, while estriol was actually associated with a reduced cancer incidence. Premarin is composed primarily of estrone and estradiol.[34]

Let's review that comment again: Dr. Whitaker states that estriol was actually associated with a reduced cancer incidence. It now appears that this relative "reduction" in cancer makes it the "safer" estrogen. In other words, women are now supposed to believe that using a hormone that is "less risky" makes it safe.

Almost everyone, including the media, continues to focus on some type of estrogen as the cure. This is occurring due to the unfortunate fact that estrogen products still sell. Just consider the emphasis on soy that we have witnessed for over a decade now. Soy has been promoted as the safe phytoestrogen. And now the "danger of soy" is finally gaining the consumer's awareness.[35] Why the danger you may ask? Because it acts as an estrogen! It stimulates cellular overgrowth and it suppresses normal thyroid functioning just to name a few similarities. If soy can do that, why won't estriol? Why won't bioidentical estriol continue to add more estrogenic exposure to our already over-exposed tissues?

A very profound and relevant answer to these questions is found in an article in the periodical *Science* (June 7, 1996) where the authors state that estrogenic chemicals become more potent and bioactive when they are exposed to each other. Scientists at Tulane University specifically studied pesticides that are estrogenic in nature and found the following to be evident:

> Using relatively weak environmental estrogens such as dieldrin, endosulfan, or toxaphene, the estrogenic potencies of chemical combinations were screened in a simple yeast estrogen system containing human estrogen receptor (hER). Combinations of the environmental estrogens in pairs "were 1,000 times as potent... as any chemical alone," the researchers report.[36]

From a physiological point of view, our estrogen receptors don't distinguish between the source of the estrogen molecule, be it bioidentical or synthetic. In our tissues, these multiple sources now act in combination with other exposures to estrogens that we can't avoid or eliminate. Needless to say, supplementing with the so-called safe estrogen (estriol) cannot prevent its effect on our cells. Neither can it perform the many necessary physiological and vital functions that are inherent with the use of natural progesterone.

Estriol is most dominant in a woman during pregnancy when very large quantities are produced in the body, along with very low levels of the other two common estrogens. However, we need to remember that the placenta is producing copious amounts of progesterone (300 to 400 mgs/day in the third trimester) to keep the increased level of estriol in check. In contrast, most women taking HRT are not using anywhere near this quantity of natural progesterone, if any at all. Dr. Lee reports that a study of women with breast cancer found they had 30 to 60 percent less estriol in their urine than did a control group of women without cancer. Although this phenomenon could be related to the reduced liver function of most cancer patients and not to any cause-and-effect relationship, it has been surmised that supplements of estriol might block the carcinogenic effect of excess estradiol and estrone and act, in effect, as a cancer-preventive (or anticancer) agent.[37] Unfortunately, the lack of agreement among scientists on this theory stems from the scarcity of research data.

The situation with endometrial cancer is similar. A study reported by the *Journal of the American Medical Association* showed estrone to be the principal component in the induction of endometrial carcinoma.[38] And a respected researcher tells us that the only known cause of such cancer is the presence in the body of excessive quantities of certain estrogens (in particular estrone and estradiol), accompanied by low levels of estriol and unopposed by the counteraction of adequate progesterone.[39, 40] Dr. Peat cautions, however, that there is evidence that estriol and other phytoestrogens can add dangerously to the body's total estrogen load.[41] An example is a Dutch study in 1988 in which estriol was shown to metabolize into a form of estrone in the uterine tissue of postmenopausal women.[42]

Since the last edition of the book we have discovered more information concerning the dangers of what we thought to be a safe estrogen (estriol). These studies that have cast some doubt on the safety of estriol for some women include the 1977 work of Lippmann et al., which showed estriol to *stimulate* the growth of human breast cancer cells.[43, 44] The National Toxicology Program advisory committee evaluated the use of birth control pills in treating postmenopausal women and voted 8-1 that steroidal estrogen use was associated with endometrial and breast cancer.[45]

The *JAMA* studies also show the risk of breast cancer to increase with the use of oral contraceptives, especially in women with a family history of cancer.[46] Furthermore, we have found that the majority of women who had breast cancer never had any genetic tendencies or family members with the disease. Personally, we feel that blaming the cause of a disease on "our genes" is too often an excuse so we (or our doctors) don't have to take on responsibility for our health and well-being. And today, with all the research available, we can all become more knowledgeable in understanding what our *body really needs*. This empowerment and freedom of choice is now at our fingertips.

Some important in-vitro studies were conducted recently at the University of California, Santa Barbara. They demonstrated that test tube cancers of both the male and female reproductive systems were stimulated on a genetic level by the addition of estrogen. Specifically, the addition of estrogen "turned on" the gene known as Bcl-2, which has a stimulatory effect on cell growth, and caused these cancers to grow. On the other hand, progesterone was found to inhibit growth—via the gene p53, which when activated results in a remarkable reversal of excessive cell growth such as that found in reproductive system cancers in both men and women.[47]

A 1995 research review published in the *American Journal of Epidemiology* examined a large eight-year study at Emory University that demonstrated "the risk ratio of fatal ovarian cancer to be 72 percent greater in women who were using unopposed estrogen replacement therapy (HRT) for six years or more." It concluded that women whose own (endogenous) estrogen levels were higher than their progesterone levels would also be at risk,[48] another reminder that estrogen overload can come from many sources—all of which can potentially contribute to the body's total saturation level of estrogen. For more information on the causes of and remedies for cancer, please see appendices D, E, and G.

It's a sad fact that the approved and medically preferred estrogens prescribed orally to women are combinations of estrone and estradiol, or estradiol by itself;[49] and these are the very forms traditionally used as supplements to combat osteoporosis.[50] The grim consequences of these hormones also befall menopausal women who are on short-term supplementation during the usual five-year period of menopause. Such estrogen supplements have been shown to increase the risk of hormonal-driven cancers sixfold—with longer-term use multiplying the risk by as much as fifteen times that of non-users. A study in Sweden also showed that women using high doses of the synthetic estrogen known as ethinylestradiol (used in lower doses in the birth control pill in the United States) had an increase in breast cancer.

Because of the known risks of the synthetic products, many doctors open to natural alternatives now believe that supplemental estrogen is not necessary as long as a woman is receiving natural progesterone. Since progesterone is a substance from which estrogen is formed—that is, a precursor of it and other hormones (cortisone, testosterone, and aldosterone)[51]—under normal conditions it will stimulate production of one's own estrogen.

Why, then, are the medical doctors continuing to give us synthetic estrogens or even natural bioidentical estrogens? Why do so few physicians prescribe the wiser choice of natural progesterone instead of synthetic progestins? And how do we, the recipients of such drug treatments, make sense of this baffling approach?

I can say from my own research and experience that for those who have been through menopause or have had their uterus or ovaries removed, the need for a careful approach to estrogen supplementation seems glaringly obvious. The case seems pretty clear: breast and endometrial cancer are caused to a great extent by excessive, unopposed levels of estrogens, which we acquire from a variety of sources. Therefore the addition of progesterone would be an important factor in cancer prevention because it has been shown to stop cells from multiplying.[52]

Is There a Safe Estrogen?

When I read in an article that was buried in a 1978 issue of the *Journal of the American Medical Association* that diethylstilbestrol, the hormone mainly prescribed for advanced cancer, "is not a steroid but is a chemical complex that acts like estrogen and is as carcinogenic as estrone,"[53] I wondered why most gynecologists or other medical specialists never mention these things. As we try to understand whether or not we need more estrogen than what is already produced in our body, even during menopause, let's hear what a prominent authority on this subject says: "One of estrogen's relatively normal effects is to shift metabolism toward the production of more lactic acid. . . ." The mere presence of lactic acid in the blood displaces carbon dioxide, with many harmful consequences (all of which are seen in the estrogen dominant state). Carbon dioxide is in effect our basic protection against free radical damage.[54] Pretty grim prospect to think that excess estrogen can lead to free radical hypoxia (oxygen deprivation to cells).

Nevertheless, Dr. John Lee's work on NHRT does give women this information to add to our treasury of knowledge:

> The addition of progesterone enhances the receptors of estrogen, and thus [a woman's] "need" for estrogen may not exist. If neither vaginal dryness nor hot flushes are present after three months of progesterone therapy, it is unlikely that estrogen supplements are needed. . . . Once progesterone levels are raised, estrogen receptors in these areas become more sensitive, and hot flushes [flashes] usually subside. The validity of the mechanism can be tested by measuring FSH [follicle-stimulating

hormone] and LH [luteinizing hormone] levels before and after adequate progesterone supplementation.[55]

Finding all this information was enlightening. However, first I had to experiment on myself. A pragmatist by nature, I then saw my goal become clear. After I had read books, articles, abstracts, reports, and studies to find what was available on the subject and contacted Emory University, pharmacies, medical centers, and reference libraries for pertinent documentation, I started on NHRT.

During and after the six months of my experiment, I felt better than ever before, so my second goal became obvious. I wanted to reach as many other women as possible to encourage them to take action on behalf of their own health and well-being, to consider any as-yet unknown long-term effects, and to evaluate and monitor their bodies' reponses to the treatment of their choice. In this way, they could perhaps gain as much as I, relieving not only their fears and frustrations but their mental and physical disorders as well.

Synthetic Hormones Create Imbalance

Wallace Simons, R.Ph., of Women's International Pharmacy told me that when progestins occupy the sites of progesterone receptors in target cells throughout the body it is as if these synthetic components are blocking the progesterone sites. As Dr. John Lee describes it, the body perceives that since the progesterone sites are all occupied, its own natural progesterone (assuming the woman is still ovulating) cannot be utilized, and therefore production is cut back.

Without the adequate opposition of progesterone, estrogen then becomes dominant and runs rampant. This in turn causes the body's feedback mechanism to recognize that something is still needed in the body's many progesterone receptors (as discussed in chapter 4). A message is sent to the ovaries to increase their own progesterone output to fill the receptors. But because these sites are unavailable, this additional progesterone cannot be used properly. The woman plunges into bodily chaos, which affects her emotions, memory, sex drive, body temperature, and other physiological functions that mirror hormonal decline.

Excessive environmental estrogens and the prescription of additional synthetic estrogens and progestins may play an underlying role in the stimulation and rapid multiplication of cells (often in breast or cervical tissues) and lead to hormone-fed cancers. Dr. Ray Peat explains another reason this happens: "The thymus gland is the main regulator of the immune system.

Estrogen causes it to shrink, while progesterone protects it." Furthermore, he says that estrogen excess actually obstructs oxygenation of the blood.[56] This is significant in view of Dr. Otto Warburg's finding that "normal cells use oxygen-based reactions as their source of energy, but cancer cells can form from cells not receiving adequate oxygen."[57] The body becomes overwhelmed and run down by the resulting imbalance, and the immune and circulatory systems are weakened.

In an important study reported by Johns Hopkins University in the *American Journal of Epidemiology*, women were first measured for their estrogen and progesterone levels and then placed in two separate groups to monitor their susceptibility to cancers. The findings proved quite interesting:

> A test was run for 40 years. They found when the "low progesterone" group was compared to the "normal progesterone" group, the women in the low progesterone group had [approximately] 5½ times the risk of breast cancer.[58]

A further conclusion was that the "low progesterone" participants encountered a tenfold increase in deaths from *all* types of cancer, compared with the "normal progesterone" participants. This should be headline news! However, according to Dr. John Lee, these important test results were not distributed or further publicized. Why? Can you imagine the thousands of women who might have avoided the dreaded disease of cancer, and even the difficulties of menopause, through natural prevention? Instead, women were given little hope—or choice—by their doctors except the radical methods of radiation, chemotherapy, and/or surgery.

There is a much simpler and saner way: balance the hormones so the body's own defense system kicks in, stopping disease in its tracks before it gets started. Indeed, progesterone alone seems to be the hormone of choice for most conditions. If, however, estrogen supplementation seems unavoidable, some women have found that several specific botanical sources have come to their aid. Among them are adaptagenic herbs, which exert a balancing action on hormone metabolism—lowering levels if too high and raising them if too low. They contain progestagenic and/or estrogenic substances. This information can be found in chapter 6. These are listed in a chart, along with other herbs that have been traditionally used to address hot flashes and night sweats during the transition of menopause. These, of course, are most effective in harmony with natural progesterone cream in helping to neutralize any excess or correct a deficiency of some of our other hormones.[59–61]

BREAST CANCER

Is it any great mystery that more and more women are succumbing to cancer at such a rapid rate? Just look at the statistics, which speak for themselves: Breast cancer is the leading cause of cancer death in women in the United States. According to *Morbidity and Mortality*, the report published by the Centers for Disease Control, the incidence of breast cancer increased 52 percent between 1950 and 1990.[62] Ninety thousand new cases are diagnosed annually, and 37,000 women per year will die of it.[63]

If natural progesterone therapy were given as much commercial time as is mammography for preventing breast cancer, women would certainly have a greater opportunity to learn the true meaning of prevention of disease. And when it comes to progesterone, it seems reasonable that what's good for the development and health of the embryo (progesterone being the dominant hormone) would also be a good equalizer for women going through the many changes and stresses in their lives. To understand why this is, take a look at Dr. Lee's response to a question asked of him during an interview by Ruth Sackman, president of F.A.C.T. (Foundation for Advancement in Cancer Therapy):

> We know that a woman is protected from having breast cancer if she has multiple pregnancies. In multiple pregnancies you have long periods of time where progesterone is the dominant hormone. In breast-feeding the ovaries do not start raising estrogen. So if a woman combines pregnancies with some time of breast-feeding, her breasts will be much protected against the estrogen effects.[64]

Dr. Lee's work with cancer patients who at the same time were suffering from osteoporosis has laid the foundation for a transformation in how today's women will approach menopause. The lesser-known hormones have been quietly written about for years. But women at large, who don't have ready access to medical journals, have not been made aware of the implications. Fortunately, however, Dr. Lee discovered the importance of natural hormones as far back as 1981. For more than fourteen years he observed the results of progesterone therapy in his patients and saw absolutely no return of their cancers. By making known to us his lifesaving findings, Dr. Lee has given women worldwide the benefit of his efforts.

Barbara Joseph, M.D., not only a survivor of breast cancer but also an obstetrician/gynecologist, relates some astonishing facts that are worth noting. In seeking the truth, she found, as many of us know, that the helpful information needed to fight this deadly disease is not accessible to most women. It is out there if we search for it but, as she says, "has been either downplayed or ignored by the medical profession."[65]

Approximately 80 percent of the women who get breast cancer have no inherited tendencies. Studies show that the woman who gives birth to children, breast-feeds, and also has been breast fed as a child "decreases her risk of breast cancer."[66] Also, abortions that take place during the first-trimester of pregnancy will "increase breast cancer risk by an overall odds ratio of 1:3."[67–71] Increasingly we are learning that diet, environment, and hormonal imbalance can bring about abnormalities in our cells.[72] What we eat, drink, and breathe, as well as our exposure to radiation and toxic chemicals in household products and personal care items, can affect our genes. Dr. Joseph says with conviction that radiation "is a risk factor for developing breast cancer. . . . The younger you are at the time of radiation the more likely it is that radiation, itself, will cause another cancer."[73] There is plenty of medical documentation to substantiate that an accumulation of radiation over the years (such as from routine X-rays of the teeth, chest, breast, and spine) can be linked to breast cancer, as well as to thyroid disorders and other potential diseases.[74, 75] (See also appendix D, which discusses mammography and breast cancer.)

PROGESTERONE RECEPTORS AND BREAST CANCER

This may be the time to bring up a very important point. Many readers who have had breast cancer, and who have educated themselves and now want to use natural progesterone with their doctors' blessing, are going to run into a very common brick wall. If a cancer patient has undergone breast biopsy, more than likely she has also had the standard estrogen and progesterone receptor assay. This test is used to measure the quantity of hormone receptors on the tumor cells and then, theoretically, to serve as a guide to the advisability of hormone treatment of any kind. If the results show that the number of progesterone receptors is high, most doctors will not prescribe progesterone. They're unsure of how to interpret the test results.

After getting this same response from several doctors, even the more open-minded ones, one patient took matters into her own hands and wrote to the company in California that had run her tests, asking for the medical abstracts on which the evaluation was based. The only articles available turned out to be over a decade old and seemed to conclude that more study was definitely needed.[76–78] The laboratory did, however, admit that the assays are performed using *synthetic* progestins—leading one to wonder just how much value they hold! The woman's gynecologist was also very surprised to learn this.

Obviously she is not alone, because Dr. John Lee is asked about this dilemma all the time. He wrote to her, "Like many other things in life, we are forced to make decisions despite incomplete knowledge. . . . The available knowledge concerning the significance of hormone receptor status is still a bit murky, [and] the testing procedure itself involves some uncertainties." First of all, he pointed out, "One cannot assume that tumor cells are all alike."

Dr. Lee, in his explanation to the frustrated woman, said that progesterone receptors (PgRs) "do not develop in breast cells (or tumor cells) unless estrogen is present in good quantities. The very presence of a high number of ERs [estrogen receptors] and PgRs is a good sign, in the sense that the tumor cells are more like fully differentiated normal cells."

Estrogen acts to increase cell proliferation. Progesterone, on the other hand, acts to induce cell maturation and differentiation. Therefore, said Dr. Lee, "the presence of PgRs allows the hypothesis that the addition of progesterone makes the tumor cells more mature and more differentiated, creating a lower level of malignancy among them. The authors of the papers [on the ER/PgR assay] fail to consider the different actions of the hormones involved."

So his advice to the doctor of the breast cancer surgery patient is this: "From all the evidence I've seen, even if . . . the receptor sites are there for progesterone, the patient is a perfect candidate to use progesterone. . . . That's the only way the progesterone could ever work. Whereas if it's estrogen-site positive, then she should not have estrogen because it causes the cell to multiply. What does progesterone do? It causes [the cell] to stop multiplying."[79]

According to Dr. Lee, "My long experience in using natural progesterone in patients with a past history of breast cancer treated by surgery alone, and the finding that none of them have shown late metastases or recurrences, leads me to believe that natural progesterone poses no increased risk to such patients . . . [and is] quite probably a benefit." He concluded, "If the PgR test is negative, the cell will be unaffected by progesterone. If [it] shows a good quantity of PgRs, supplemental progesterone may make the tumor cells less malignant."

And now, let's take a look at some risky practices associated with either the cause or the treatment of hormone-related cancers, and the forces that are at play. On the one hand we have the environmental, synthetic estrogens and the bad estrogens that could dominate the body (in Dr. Lee's conviction these are the estrogens that are "the sole cause of fibrocystic breast disease [and] the only known cause of cancer of the uterus"[80]). But on the other hand, to bring about balance, we have plant-derived progesterone and what may or may not turn out to be "good" estrogens—such as estriol and other forms that come from plants. What follows, however, is what we're up against if *not* given the choice of natural hormone replacement therapy.

AVOIDABLE HYSTERECTOMIES AND THEIR AFTERMATH

Hormone deficiency is a fact of life that we must address in order to understand the problems that may begin at childbearing age. The slow decline of progesterone, such an essential hormone, is overwhelming enough; but when there is a sudden halt, it can be devastating. A complete hysterectomy, in which the ovaries are removed, can create numerous problems, such as adrenal and pancreatic disorders (e.g., diabetes) and other side effects, including vaginal dryness and sudden hot flashes.[81]

Estrogen is traditionally prescribed at this time, but as Dr. Lita Lee comments, "This seems such a dichotomy to me, since estrogen excess and/or progesterone depletion is one of the primary causes of problems leading to hysterectomy (excessive bleeding, fibroids, endometriosis, and cancer). The more research I read, the less inclined I am to think that women need supplemental estrogen even after menopause."[82]

If the doctor prescribes synthetic estrogen, it won't be long before one or more of the following conditions inevitably arises: abdominal cramps, interruption of periods, bloating, breast tenderness and enlargement, cystitis, high blood pressure, endometriosis, gallbladder disorders, hair loss, elevated blood fats, jaundice, depression, nausea and vomiting, sustained vaginal bleeding, decreased carbohydrate tolerance, skin outbreaks, blood clots in the legs, unwanted weight loss or gain, or vaginal yeast infections.[83]

Any woman who develops these problems has really been mistreated fourfold by the doctor prescribing the estrogen: (1) It is unopposed by natural progesterone, (2) synthetic estrogen can in the long run cause problems worse than the original complaints, (3) Provera and other imitations of progesterone, if prescribed, exaggerate the symptoms even further still, and (4) all of the above conditions not only accelerate the aging process but open up an environment favorable to cancer.

When such symptoms appear, some action may be necessary before a more severe stage of development, such as a tumor, occurs. We need to watch and listen for "signals," be armed with proper information, and be prepared to make changes before it's too late. Research shows that postmenopausal women with either benign or malignant ovarian tumors register low progesterone levels prior to surgery.[84] What do all these studies tell us? It seems that the use of progesterone before and after surgery may prepare us for dealing with stress and promote more efficient healing.

CONTEMPORARY SYNTHETIC HORMONES

Women of all ages, from premenopause to postmenopause, are now under pressure to use designer drugs to prevent breast cancer, and recently we have heard much about a drug called Tamoxifen. This is a synthetic hormone, a "nonsteroidal antiestrogen," and is related to the carcinogenic hormone DES. It has been used since 1977 to treat advanced breast cancer but is now believed to have many harmful side effects, some of which are similar to those of estrogen, which can promote more tumors. Nevertheless, doctors are prescribing Tamoxifen for use in hormone replacement therapy. In one study almost half of the Tamoxifen recipients "complained of 'persistent vasomotor, gynecologic, or other major side effects.' "[85]

The women enrolled as volunteers in the clinical trials of Tamoxifen as a breast cancer deterrent were apparently informed of a statistically known increased risk of endometrial cancer.[86] In February 1996, a review by the International Agency for Research on Cancer—based in Lyon, France, and composed of scientists from various countries—concluded definitely "that there is sufficient evidence to regard Tamoxifen as a human carcinogen that increases a woman's risk of developing . . . cancer of the endometrium, the inner lining of the uterus."[87]

Is it any wonder that author Sherrill Sellman's research explains Tamoxifen to be a "Major Medical Mistake,"[88] and shows that by taking Tamoxifen as prescribed, women are at further risk for developing cancer.[89-91] Several studies show that Tamoxifen, anti-depressants, certain antibiotics, and cardiac medications can all cause risk of arrhythmia and even cardiac death.[92, 93] In May 1995, the California State's Carcinogen Identification Committee voted unanimously to add Tamoxifen to its list.[94]

A study that is not readily available to the public (Veronesi, 1998) shows that tamoxifen is causing blood clots, strokes, and high triglyceride levels.[95] In another study (Powles, 1998), "four cases of endometrial cancer occurred in the tamoxifen group compared to one in the placebo group."[96] The British journal *The Lancet* has reported two recent three- to four-year studies that demonstrated no evidence of any difference in breast cancer rates from the control group versus those women using tamoxifen.[97, 98] This overlooked information seems to contradict the shorter (only two-year) U.S. study. Women need to realize that the shorter the study time, the less reliable the conclusion. Dr. John Lee confirms that Tamoxifen increases "the risk of endometrial cancer and blood clots, including fatal blood clots in the lung."[99] Other researchers confirm these same dangers[100–102] and even show it to create a slightly higher risk for ocular disorders as well as uterine cancer.[103, 104]

Tamoxifen has also been linked to liver cancer, eye disease, and depression. "Despite that," says Dr. Marcus Laux, "there's talk of selling this to millions of women at high risk as a 'preventive'!"[105] No wonder Dr. Lee says that other countries view our giving tamoxifen to postmenopausal women as "another American joke."[106]

Of course, it's impossible to keep up with all the new synthetic hormones and drugs that continue to be approved for today's market. Appendix B, for example, lists some of the numerous terms that apply to synthetic estrogens and progestins. Certainly, great caution should be used when taking synthetic or conjugated estrogens. As one of the most often prescribed, Premarin, is described this way in the physician information sheet: "Premarin is a mixture of estrogensulfates blended to represent the average composition of material derived from pregnant mare's urine (Pre-mar-in). It contains estrone, equilin, 17a-estradiol, equilenin, and 17a-dihydroequilenin."[107] In fact, says Dr. Marcus Laux, "Premarin is the number-one best-selling drug in the country,"[108] and contains synthetic additives and "foreign estrogenic elements . . . that we believe [are] dangerous and potentially cancer producing."[109]

So how can some doctors and pharmacists honestly say that Premarin is natural? The authors of *Women on Menopause* write that Premarin "cannot be natural to humans, although it is to horses."[110] As it is not bioidentical to our human estrogen, we shouldn't be too surprised that we eventually see side effects and even tumor growth as a result of the synthetic components of this drug, not to mention its inevitable contribution to estrogen overload.

Maggie Fox, health and science correspondent, states in Reuters (January 22, 1998) that the breakdown of the synthetic version of Premarin can react in an unusual way with DNA and that such damage to DNA can cause cancer. "If this reaction were to occur with DNA in breast cells, and that damage is not repaired, mutations could result, leading to the initiation of the carcinogenic process in the breast." Dr. Peat explains this occurrence in another way, as he tells us that estrogen increases the formation of a nitric oxide free radical. This has numerous harmful effects ranging from damaging DNA to damaging the mitochondria.[111]

Studies continue to prove that the "prolonged, uninterrupted action of estrogen . . . is profoundly harmful . . . [as it's] . . . the prolonged shock-like state that contributes to the degenerative diseases, which typically begin with a sort of diabetes, an inability to use glucose for energy because of the accumulation of too much of the wrong kind of fat"[112] stimulated by the storage of our excess estrogenic molecules in these very fat cells.

And then there are the imitation progesterones, such as the commonly prescribed Provera (methoxyprogesterone acetate). Majid Ali, M.D., calls this progestin a "synthetic molecule that does not fit well with the natural order of hormonal rhythms."[113] Thus, introducing it along with Premarin seems like adding fuel to an already hazardous fire. In fact, in a seminar presentation Norman Shealy, M.D., cautioned that Provera and all the other progestins actually lower DHEA levels, as does Premarin.

When a patient reacts badly to one of these compounds, the drug is put aside and one of the many other synthetic substitutes is prescribed instead. Whenever you have a prescription filled, ask your pharmacist for a copy of the package insert that is prepared for the doctor and the patient. The warnings and contraindications concerning the new drug assigned to you will be clearly stated. See appendix B or refer to the *Physicians' Desk Reference* (PDR) and other books available at your library or bookstores to confirm whatever side effects you should be aware of from any medications you are taking.

THE WARNINGS ABOUT SYNTHETIC HORMONES

Women are now paying more attention to the cautions about dangerous side effects. Concerned about their own possible reactions to these drugs, they are looking around for alternatives.

Synthetic estrogen, to begin with, is prescribed by doctors for many situations, such as cramps, acne, irregular periods, birth control, infertility, menopause, postmenopause, and osteoporosis. Precautions come with all drugs, but with the typical estrogen package, the warnings on the inserts are so small that it's easy for your vision to fade following the first few sentences. However, it's essential to read on. Here is an example from the literature for the synthetic hormone Premarin:

> **Endometrial Cancer.** There are reports that if estrogens are used in the postmenopausal period for more than a year, there is increased risk of endometrial cancer (cancer of the lining of the uterus). Women taking estrogens have roughly 5 to 10 times as great a chance of getting this

cancer as women who take no estrogens. . . . Estrogens can cause development of other tumors in animals, such as tumors of the breast, cervix, vagina, or liver, when given for a long time.[114]

Estrogen incites cell multiplication, and at high levels it starts activating the formation of cysts and tumors. With regard to the synthetic Premarin, *The People's Pharmacy* tells us that five out of fourteen of the women who are prescribed it for menopausal problems are increasing their risk of cancer of the uterine lining (endometrial carcinoma).[115] And of course, the longer we take estrogen, the higher is our risk for acquiring such cancer.

Progestin therapy together with estrogen is often recommended by your medical doctor, but even so, as the "Information for the Patient" by Mead Johnson Laboratories says:

> The possible risks include unhealthy effects on blood fats (especially a lowering of HDL cholesterol, the "good" blood fat which protects against heart disease risk), unhealthy effects on blood sugar (which might worsen a diabetic condition), and a possible further increase in the breast cancer risk which may be associated with long-term estrogen use.[116]

Even if we do everything right in the way of avoiding harmful radiation and synthetic hormones, the picture is not complete and we are unlikely to succeed in our effort to avoid "diseases of civilization" such as cancer unless we adopt an otherwise healthy lifestyle. In *My Healing from Breast Cancer* Dr. Barbara Joseph urges, "We need to buy and eat organic food whenever possible. This nourishes us, keeps carcinogenic chemicals out of the body and at the same time makes a powerful political and economic statement. Health is not achieved by going for yearly checkups, getting Pap tests or scheduling mammograms."[117] (See appendix D.)

How true! Only when our bodies are provided proper nutritional support can substances such as progesterone achieve their full impact on the system. Any approach to cancer prevention or control must embrace the entire person—mind, body, and spirit. We should choose health care providers who will try to help us reestablish internal balance at deeper levels so that the body can heal itself as it is programmed to do.

A more complete discussion of cancer, mammography, nutrition, and other aspects of natural cancer therapy is beyond the scope of this book. However, it is vitally important that we become aware of the dangers of blindly following standard allopathic procedures, especially mammograms. It is suggested that the reader refer to the selection of books in appendix D. In particular, Dr. Ralph Moss's book *Cancer Therapy: The Independent Consumer's Guide to Non-Toxic Treatment and Prevention* covers many of these subjects in greater detail.

IMPORTANT TESTS YOU SHOULD KNOW ABOUT

AMAS (Anti-Malignin Antibody in Serum) Test

This revolutionary test has been found to be 95 percent accurate on the first administration and 99 percent accurate on repeat analysis for identifying cancer anywhere in the body. Dr. Samuel Bogoch, M.D., Ph.D., discovered this diagnostic technique in 1974. Frank D. Wiewell, the executive director of People Against Cancer, tells us that this simple blood test is a breakthrough in that it works for all types of cancer cells and does so up to nineteen months, in some cases, before they are detected by any other method.

Dr. Marcus Laux points out that 90 percent of breast lumps are found by self-examination. Because of this fact, he recommends that you insist on an AMAS (Anti-Malignin Antibody in Serum) test before agreeing to any kind of X-ray or invasive procedure such as needle biopsy or aspiration.[118] This diagnostic method is superior to other tests, such as mammograms or diagnostic ultrasound, in that it can detect malignancy anywhere in the body (except for last-stage terminal cancer) almost two years earlier[119] than more conventional assessments. It can be given as part of an annual check-up and provides "early detection, particularly with breast and ovarian cancers, which can be difficult to detect until they are advanced,"[120] says Dr. John Lee.

With an accuracy rate of 95 to 99 percent, the AMAS test has been used to monitor large numbers of breast cancer patients. Unfortunately this test is still not known or used by many doctors despite decades of research, published peer-reviewed scientific literature, and thousands of positive double-blind clinical experiments by researchers. This is pretty sad considering that the test was already approved for marketing by the FDA in 1977 and is covered by many insurance carriers, including Blue Cross/Blue Shield and Medicare. This is yet another reason why we must courageously demand that this test be made widely known and available before inferior or risky tests are administered.

You or your doctor can call Oncolab, one of the laboratories that will perform this assay, at (800) 922-8378. This organization can provide literature and special test kits. The cost is approximately $135. Due to the thousands of people who have saved their lives through this early testing, Dr. Bogoch will probably receive the Nobel Prize for his incredible discovery that has the potential for saving many more lives in the future.

A friend of mine decided to pursue the results from a CAT scan as well as the AMAS. She had the CAT scan done for her own peace of mind—as another source of information to either confirm or deny the AMAS blood test results. She was happy to find that there were no indications of the cancer having spread to other organs. The CAT scan will report on whether the primary tumor disappeared as it shows the physical structure, size, shape, etc. It is always comforting to be knowledgeable about what is going on in your body, and sometimes this means that we should look at the range of tests available in order to determine if they are all in agreement with each other or not.

Early detection is important because it provides the patient more time to seek out, study, and then utilize their choice(s) of natural alternatives in fighting cancer and keeping it in remission. Natural therapies for preventing and combating cancer are numerous and we have listed them under different categories in appendix D. These essential health care approaches can range from improving dietary lifestyles to addressing hormonal, neurological, and nutritional deficiencies.

We all need to pass the word on to friends and family members about this information. In the end we will be the ones who are playing the active role in the revolution in the war against cancer. We can't count on the powerful organizations that have a vested interest in drugs and medical technology to turn the tide.

Tumor Marker CA-125

You may have also heard about the tumor marker CA-125. This simple blood test is considered a good indicator of ovarian cancer (stage II through IV).[121] Unfortunately, it produces 95 percent false negatives for early stage I ovarian cancer. Nevertheless, another friend, Carolyn Benivegna, insisted upon it when the medication her doctor prescribed for a diagnosis of "irritable bowel syndrome" had no effect on her distended abdomen.

When she was subsequently hospitalized to have five pounds of fluid extracted, cancer cells were discovered. At this point, she asked for this inexpensive blood test (the CA-125), which ultimately identified her cancer as "essentially ovarian cancer." This news was shocking to Carolyn, as she had undergone a hysterectomy several years before. After having had this procedure, she states, "I thought I did not have to worry about getting any of the female reproductive cancers since I no longer have my ovaries or uterus!"

While the CA-125 correctly diagnosed Carolyn's disease, John Bernard Henry, M.D., in *Clinical Diagnosis & Management* cautions that sometimes CA-125 levels can become significantly elevated during the menstrual period and in patients with acute pelvic inflammatory disease or endometriosis.[122] Nevertheless, this test is often used to help identify ovarian cancer and as a follow-up after ovarian cancer surgery. Again, it can't be emphasized enough that as a basic screen Dr. Lee suggests a yearly blood test to include the AMAS (anti-malignin antibody in serum) test as a check for the presence of malignant cancers.[123]

HORMONE TREATMENT FOR MEN

Hearing the personal stories of the "incurable" helps us to see clearly the merits of prevention and to understand that the whole truth concerning health is made up of a variety of natural choices. However, it seems evident from diverse studies that more research should be done, not only for women but also for men. To illustrate, *Choices in Healing* describes a case history in which a man with prostate cancer was given all the best conventional procedures, including chemotherapy. Nothing seemed to help, and he became quite weak. However, his doctor prescribed specialized hormone therapy, by means of which he recovered.[124]

This story was interesting but did not leave much of an impression on me until one day when I was having a casual conversation with the owner of our neighborhood health food store concerning the many benefits of natural hormone supplementation for women. During our discussion, a man in the store overheard us and asked, "Can natural progesterone help with male as well as female problems?"

The question does need a response, especially in light of the published statistics we have listed in appendices D, E, F, and G.

Author Sandra Coney surmises that the sea of environmental estrogens in which we find ourselves might explain "the rise in male prostate cancer paralleling the rise in female breast cancer."[125]

Furthermore, Al Sears, M.D., explains: "As a man ages, his testosterone decreases while his estrogen increases, partly due to a conversion of testosterone to estrogen. One recent study found that estrogen levels in an average 54-year-old man are higher than those of an average 59-year-old woman! And the problem compounds itself. Lower levels of testosterone make it more likely that you'll be overweight. And studies show that fat cells generate the aromatase enzyme that converts testosterone to estrogen. It's a vicious cycle of decreasing testosterone and increasing estrogen."[126] More information can be found on this subject in a popular guidebook entitled *Alternative Medicine: The Definitive Guide,* with chapters written by 350 leading health care professionals and scientists. The book presents a wealth of effective treatment options. One of the personal accounts, written by a medical doctor, would certainly be of interest to the man who asked the question about men and progesterone:

> Topical application of natural progesterone may prove beneficial in the treatment of prostate conditions. The doctor reports working with twelve men, all in their late seventies, who were suffering from osteoporosis. As it has been well established that natural progesterone, applied topically, can relieve osteoporosis, the physician suggested that the men systematically massage it into their skin on a daily basis. All of them began to experience relief from their condition, and later called to tell [the doctor] that, after three months, . . . they were also experiencing an improved urine flow, with less pressure on their prostate glands and noticeable decrease in nightly urination.[127]

The physician who treated these men did not choose to have his name publicized. He preferred to remain anonymous rather than be associated with natural alternatives in healing and then be ridiculed by those of his peers who focus on orthodox medical standards and who use only prescription drugs to treat their patients. Sadly, this attitude is what creates the greatest obstacle for the many patients who desperately wish to obtain natural products from their medical doctors.

Perhaps when this doctor retires and no longer fears being discriminated against, he will write a book for the large numbers of men who suffer from prostate enlargement and its unpleasant symptoms. The good news that natural progesterone and herbal remedies can actually reverse many prostatic disorders would certainly be a relief to the ten million men in the United States who are afflicted with impotence (often a side effect of an enlarged prostate), of whom only 200,000 actually seek medical help.[128, 129]

Dr. C. Norman Shealy, noting that women after the age of about fifty are not deficient in estrogen but in progesterone, theorized that this hormone must also decline in men as they age. Studies confirm this. Dr. John Lee's investigation found that in older men not only do progesterone levels decline, but their testosterone converts into dihydrotestosterone (DHT), which can stimulate the prostate gland to grow.[130] He says that levels of estradiol in aging males are the same or higher than those in postmenopausal females because of the decline in testosterone and its conversion to DHT. Fortunately, "progesterone inhibits the conversion of testosterone to DHT"[131] This is especially important in consideration of the fact that "DHT is a far more potent stimulant of prostate cell growth than testosterone."[132]

Dr. Lee advocates that "whatever we can do to avoid or oppose those estrogens will help us prevent prostate disease. . . . Men synthesize progesterone in smaller amounts than women do, but it is still vital. And yes, I believe it may be important in the prevention and/or treatment of enlarged prostate (BPH) and prostate cancer."[133] A question we often get during our lectures concerns whether men benefit from natural progesterone? Progesterone is not just a hormone produced by women. Men also produce it. However, it doesn't decline as readily in men as it does in women. Estrogen dominance is induced in men also if they work around environmental toxins or if their diet is highly estrogenic (consuming soy products or meats not free of hormones additives and antibiotics). In an article by James South, M.A., on progesterone for prostate health we are given more crucial documentation on this subject.[134] For instance, M. Krieg, along with his researchers, reports that estrogen creates a cellular response in the prostate gland on a biochemical level.[135] Another study goes on to implicate the negative impact of estrogen overload in men as contributing to conditions such as benign prostatic hypertrophy (BPH), better known as prostate enlargement, with all of its complications.[136] S. Boehm and coworkers are investigating the value of estrogen suppression as a therapeutic strategy in the treatment of BPH.[137]

On this subject, let me share a little anecdote. I was asked to speak about *The Estrogen Alternative* to a homeopathic group who meet regularly in Philadelphia. There was an ex-Marine sitting in the front row. It didn't faze him at all that he was the only man in a room full of women. I later learned that he had tried everything for his prostate cancer. When his wife began using progesterone cream to keep her cancer in remission, he also began to use it. He found it was the only therapy that brought his PSA levels back to normal and that it was also keeping his cancer in remission.

Supplementing with a natural transdermal progesterone cream seems a safer and more natural approach when seeking preventive care. Some advocate the use of natural testosterone cream, but this may then unfortunately convert into dehydrotestosterone, which could only aggravate any problems. Dr. Raymond Peat also reports that not only has progesterone been used successfully to treat benign prostatic enlargement, but "in cases of specific progesterone deficiency in men, small doses can cure impotence."[138] As we have previously mentioned, progesterone is not just a "female hormone," a healthy man will also produce progesterone in his testicular tissue as well as his adrenals.[139]

Concerning men who suffer impotence after undergoing a vasectomy, Dr. Peat speaks out on how small doses of progesterone can possibly restore normal potency. "This is because damage to the vas deferens can specifically, but temporarily, suppress progesterone production." Dr. Peat not only recommends supplementing progesterone for this situation but for other disorders ranging from circulatory problems such as migraines and strokes to arthritis, epilepsy, dementia, and cancer.[140]

Years ago when Dr. Shealy could not find any progesterone studies in men he started using natural progesterone on his older male patients. The progesterone apparently caused one patient's DHEA hormone level to double. His libido soared, and he felt better than he had in years. In fact, Dr. Shealy discovered that the majority of men who used the natural progesterone cream showed a marked increase (60 to 100 percent) in their DHEA.[141] This is important news, since DHEA seems to spark the metabolism of both men and women and helps balance the entire glandular system. More research on the connection between these two hormones is definitely in order.

But one more point before we leave the subject of hormone imbalance in men. A story from Dr. Peat's *From PMS to Menopause: Female Hormones in Context* tells about a sizable settlement awarded to a widow because her husband had mistakenly been given "a female sex hormone" and suffered several strokes and died.[142] It's ironic that the newspaper story he quoted would focus on the woman's monetary settlement rather than the real issue—the dangers of estrogen therapy. Regardless of our gender, Dr. Peat makes clear that an overload of estrogen can lead to heart disease, strokes, and a host of other serious conditions.[143]

The possibility that estrogen dominance will precipitate strokes is often subtly downplayed in this world of overmedication. The important lesson to be learned here, however, is that this story authenticates the studies that clearly show synthetic hormones (estrogen and progestins) to be a cause of many cardiovascular disorders.[144–146] Telling the public anything different is, quite frankly, playing a game of Russian roulette with people's health, and quite possibly their lives.

In appendix D you will find an extensive list of specific minerals, vitamins, herbs, and other plant sources that have been proven to be effective as natural cancer therapies. Studies also stress that a low-fat, high-fiber diet aids in fighting prostate cancer. Men with this disorder normally have low testosterone levels along with high estrogen levels. The typical American high-fat (omega 6 fatty acids), low-fiber diet is causing this dangerous ratio of high estrogen relative to low levels of testosterone and progesterone, which in turn is promoting prostate cancer.[147] On the other hand, biological studies stress that omega 3 fatty acids can inhibit growth in the prostate gland.[148] For documentation that proves how the low-fiber/high-fat diet is becoming a major cause of prostate disease, take a look at the incredible number of studies listed in appendix F.

MELATONIN AND BREAST CANCER

Speaking of hormones, we should mention one that has become a popular item in the newspapers, magazines, talk shows, health stores, and drugstores. Melatonin, a hormone secreted by the pineal gland, has been reported to inhibit cell division and "block the growth of breast tumors in laboratory animals."[149] It is suspected that one's level of melatonin may be an early predictor of some types of cancers, "since women with ER [estrogen-receptor]-positive breast cancer and men with testosterone-dependent prostate cancer have lower levels of melatonin than those without the disease."[150]

Mice given melatonin in their water at night never developed terminal cancer, which often affects the particular breed studied. The mice that didn't get the melatonin lost neuromuscular coordination, their immune and thyroid functions declined, and they died of cancer.[151]

If you do decide that melatonin is a supplement you would like to try, be aware of possible side effects. These appear to be related to the timing of its use as when it is ingested seems to be a key factor in preventing estrogen from becoming dangerously high.[152] Researchers have found melatonin injections in the morning to be risky because given at that time they stimulated tumor growth. However, when given in the evening they retarded cell proliferation.[153]

THE POWER OF NATURAL ALTERNATIVES

When I began looking into natural means of ridding poisons from my body and countering the toxic surroundings that are increasingly difficult to avoid, it was a comfort to become acquainted with like-minded medical doctors who are getting off the track of medicating the *symptoms* of disease and getting on the track of preventing the *cause* of disease. My hat goes off to them for thinking of the patient's needs first.

Stuart Berger, M.D., advises that when we choose a medical doctor, we should "avoid powerful ways that our medical system and its illness-centered view of medicine keep us unhealthy . . . and actually raises our risk of medical problems."[154] Medical doctors, like everyone else in this world, should be held accountable for their actions. However, we also need to be personally accountable by keeping in tune with our bodies and learning about natural substitutes for medication. A drug may be essential in cases of acute disease, but prolonged use of a prescription drug often covers up the underlying cause.

Dr. Lorraine Day faults medical science for attempting to blame cancer and other diseases on genes, thus taking away our personal responsibility. She states—and I can vouch for this from personal experience—that often doctors will tell their patients it's O.K. to eat anything they want![155] She points out that they may know little about nontoxic therapies because they offer less profit potential and do not receive funding for the hugely expensive studies required for approval by the FDA.[156]

Let's reflect for a moment on the divergent philosophies. Our distinctive choices in health care may produce entirely different conclusions: (1) Masking the symptoms (temporarily avoiding disease and/or surgery through medication) is focusing on the *disease*. The cause of the illness is still festering—but since medication may slow down the need for immediate surgery, the medical field calls this prevention. (2) Aiding the body to avoid disease or to heal itself through good nutrition and natural therapies is focusing on health.

We should recognize abuses. If some of our gynecologists could have a taste of their own medicine (unnecessary needle biopsies, hysterectomies, mammograms, toxic synthetic estrogens or progestins, Tamoxifen, Evista, etc.), they might be more inclined to respect their patients' rights to natural choices and would give higher priority to knowing what will harm the body and what will heal. It could be that we who have to live with illnesses and the side effects of drug treatment need to be the ones to make a change: to become fit in order to be survivors. It is up to us to reshape the public's attitude toward health and disease.

With a little curiosity and effort we, too, can learn not only how to avoid the hazards of certain modern technology but also how to counter the depletion of our energy by the continual use of toxic drugs. The suffering that results today from the many drug-driven diseases is often unnecessary. We deserve more than this and so do our families.

A phenomenal healing potential exists within the human body. Once released, the life force can manifest itself in a degree of wellness that many of us don't even realize is possible. Admittedly, learning how to harness this on our own can be time-consuming and trying. But once we find the right professional to work with us, we'll discover that *implementing what we instinctively know to be true is truly living.* By striving to achieve a harmonious synchronization of the body's systems, we'll enable the many parts to work together to create a healthier, disease-defying whole.

For specific advice on natural hormone replacement therapy, please see chapter 7. It tells you how to make wise choices, understand the doctor–patient relationship, and confidently communicate your needs. Self-help advice and valuable resources, including names of recommended books, pharmacies, and manufacturers, are found in appendix F (Clinical Studies and Research Reports) and appendix G (Sources of Natural Progesterone).

PART III

Making Assertive Lifestyle Changes

SIX

Hormonal Support from Our Foods

A person should take every care of his body . . . not for the sake of the body, but in order that the soul in a sound body may act . . . rightly, and may have the body as an organ perfectly obedient to it.
                                                            Emanuel Swedenborg [1]

To use natural healing methods effectively requires modifying our habits and developing a good deal of discipline. At one time I had trouble making such a transition in my own health regimen. Instead of getting involved with prevention, I tried to tell myself that I was not going to have menopausal problems. If I didn't think about it and just kept busy, I hoped to bypass "the change." So instead of facing it and looking for alternative solutions, I allowed my symptoms to grow worse. The stress and the aging process simply accelerated. Not in control of my life, and skeptical of natural remedies, I was paying very dearly for my reluctance to deal with the transition. It was from this low point that I gradually became more aware of prevention and the necessity of a healthy lifestyle.

Women suffering from intense loss of energy or drive during PMS will be interested in Dr. Katharina Dalton's recommendation that they snack on a complex carbohydrate food every three hours. In fact, many nutritionists "encourage sufferers to be 'grazers,' eating at frequent intervals, and not 'gorgers,' only eating three times a day," and point out that starchy foods such as rice, oats, potato, rye, or corn prevent "adrenaline release from low blood glucose."[2,*]

---

* This would not apply to those concerned about a tendency to diabetes. Raymond Peat, Ph.D., recommends a *low*-starch diet to avoid elevated blood sugar, insulin and fat over-production, cell death, and allergies.[3]

It's quite interesting that some of these same foods are discussed in *Modern Pharmacognosy* as sources of progesterone: "Small amounts are . . . found in plants, e.g., yeast, rice, wheat, cabbage, and potato."[4] Dr. John Lee says that in "cultures whose diets are rich in fresh vegetables of all sorts, progesterone deficiency does not exist. . . . Many (over 5,000 known) plants make sterols that are progestogenic."[5] As for estrogen activity, it is associated with soy products, such as tofu, soybeans, and soy milk, as well as alfalfa, pomegranates, and boiled beans.[6, 7] Those wishing to limit their total estrogen intake may find such information helpful. Fermented soy items such as miso, tempeh, and tamari are considered to be safe and they also provide less potent levels of estrogen.

We might want to reconsider the widespread assumption that estrogens derived from plant sources (phytoestrogens) can automatically provide viable health benefits. Shocking news is surfacing specifically about the estrogenic effects of soybean consumption resulting in numerous health problems.[8] Investigations made by toxicologist Mike Fitzpatrick, Ph.D., confirm the facts that soy has been linked to thyroid disorders, infertility, and even leukemia. His studies on the dangers of soy isoflavones have been submitted to the U.S. Food and Drug Administration (FDA).[9] Many testimonials tell of the unhealthy effects of soy. For instance, Joyce Gross, M.A., R.D., L.D.N., was educating women as to what she thought were the beneficial effects of soy. As she says,

> In March of 2001, I was promoting the beneficial effects of soy along with a majority of the medical profession. I was consuming a soy shake supplement that was, and is still, being marketed for its phytoestrogen effect to alleviate menopausal symptoms. I was duped like so many other non-suspecting consumers.
>
> After taking the supplement for about two months, I developed symptoms that included severe joint pain, especially in my hands, "trigger finger(s)," carpal tunnel syndrome, chronic fatigue syndrome, a "brain fog," depression, and excessive weight gain. Later on, I also developed ulcerative colitis and rheumatoid arthritis.
>
> Prior to seeking medical advice, I developed a "hyper" active state where my resting pulse rate was 125, and I was having hundreds of heart palpitations a day. I saw a cardiologist who did a myriad of tests and was told, "There's nothing wrong with you. Go home and take your estrogen and you'll feel better." Well, I won't tell you how angry that made me. I insisted that there was something wrong with me and told the doctor that I would look for another doctor to help me.
>
> The only thing that was different in my diet was the soy supplement.

I did some research online and found out that soy is an endocrine disruptor and can [actually] cause hypothyroidism. Of course this didn't make sense to me at first since I had a resting pulse rate of 125! But as I delved further into my research, I found that this is quite common in women who have Hashimoto's Thyroiditis, which is what I was eventually diagnosed with.

I learned that my symptoms of the "hyper" state are sometimes quite common and many women wind up in the emergency room as a result. Apparently, in Hashimoto's disease, just before your thyroid stops working completely, it can go "haywire" and put you into an alternating hyper and hypo state.

It took eight months for Joyce Gross to start feeling better once she stopped the soy shakes.

Whether we want to consume soy in any of its many forms or not, we have little choice as it has become a manufacturer's food fad and is included as an additive in almost all packaged products we buy. Unbeknownst to us, and whether we want it or not, it has become a dominant food in our daily diet. It's hard to keep up with these denatured ingredients, which are foreign to the cells in our body and which build up in the tissues with a variety of toxic and even carcinogenic effects. With the consumption of processed, sugar-free ingredients from chemical sweetners such as Splenda (brand name for sucralose)* and Nutra Sweet (Aspartame)[10] to the harmful fats, such as olestra, which deplete us of essential minerals,[11] is it any wonder we eventually develop stress leading to hormonal imbalance and eventually suffer from disorders such as fibromyalgia and arthritis due to the toxins that sooner or later settle in our muscles and joints?[12]

ARE SOY FOODS UNHEALTHY?

Current health news and the media focus on soy products protecting against breast cancer notwithstanding, we should look carefully at the studies that give another perspective. David Zava, Ph.D., a biochemist and breast cancer researcher, tells us that his extensive research on the subject shows differently, and that "soy protein isolates increased the proliferation of normal breast cells in intact humans [and that] genistein [from soy] acts like a pro-estrogen, not

---

* According to the Sucralose Toxicity Information Center, research demonstrated that years of sucralose use might lead to immune system and neurological disorders. Sucralose users are essentially venturing into the unknown.

an anti-estrogen."[13] Experiments with soy-derived coumestrol, another phytoestrogen, have demonstrated the same thing.[14, 15] Researchers found that consumption of phytoestrogens from soy for even a relatively short interval can significantly elevate estrogen levels in the brain. It can also interfere with the calcium-binding proteins in the brain.[16] Studies show how the genistein (isoflavones) from soy foods causes an estrogenic effect on the brain, breasts, and reproductive system.[17] Furthermore, according to *Cancer Research* "Genistein . . . is more carcinogenic than DES."[18]

And yes, DES is the drug that caused death and disfigurement for countless women and their newborn infants. We are alerted through numerous studies that soy products should not be eaten due to their toxic effects to our thyroid, liver, and endocrine glands.[19] A 1996 study reported that women who consumed soy protein isolates had a greater risk of experiencing abnormally excessive cell growth (described by our doctors as cervical or endometrial "hyperplasia"), a symptom that can be a forerunner to malignancies.[20] Studies being conducted by researchers are finding that women should not consume soy products thinking that they are preventing breast cancer, because the genistein in soy food is found to actually stimulate breast cell growth.[21, 22]

But the powerful influences from the media and food manufacturers convince the public otherwise, saying that soy foods stop tumor growth, protect against cancer, and should be used as a protein substitute for meat. But today we are finding more studies confirming that a high rate of thyroid disorders and cancer risks are linked directly to soy consumption.[23–26] Nevertheless, many women (and their well-intentioned doctors) have embraced the soy fad (or mania?), and they don't understand why they are still estrogen-dominant and in many cases very allergic. A typical story comes from Heather Campbell:

> After about a month of taking a vitamin E product that was mixed in soy oil, my menstrual cycle was thrown way off. I also experienced extreme breast tenderness as part of PMS. Normally my periods were quite regular and pain-free, but this product made my period come 10 days early. After discontinuing the product my periods went back to normal, but it took several cycles for the PMS breast tenderness to disappear.

Such stories are dramatic reminders that we need to become more informed about the foods we buy and consume. As we try to live normal healthy lives, we also need to arm ourselves with information, not gleaned from commercials, but from bona fide evidence-based clinical studies done by researchers and doctors who put the health of their patients first and foremost. We must ask ourselves, "Who is providing the enormous financial backing for this commercialized data? Is it from one of the powerful agricultural lobbies or the pharmaceutical companies promoting their own interests?"

If we would like to use soy as our principle source of protein, perhaps the *Cancer Forum* will give us some insights on such an option. As far back as 1996, warnings were issued that soy can interfere with the functioning of our digestive enzymes, "which is a serious handicap for good metabolism."[27] Substituting soy for milk, cheese, and meat can block the absorption of important nutrients.

As individuals with varying needs, we need to be able to make educated decisions regarding health and diet. An excellent treatise on the subject of soy as a food source appeared in *Health Freedom News*. Its argument is that only *fermented* soy products such as miso, tempeh, natto, and soy or tamari sauce are digestible or safe, because fermentation, to some degree, reduces soybeans' powerful enzyme inhibitors (which interfere with protein digestion), clot-promoting agents, and phytic acid. Unfortunately the phytate content of soybeans, as well as the trypsin inhibitors, interfere with many vital enzymes and amino acids.[28, 29] Phytates also block the intestinal uptake of essential minerals, especially zinc. This destruction of such minerals by phytic acid occurs with unfermented soy products more than any other grain or legume. Also we are told that soybeans are high in protein, but what we are not told is that soybeans actually block the action of enzymes and minerals that are essential in the digestion of protein. "Precipitated" soy products such as tofu especially have this effect if they are not accompanied by a little fish or meat protein.[30] Asian and Western children who do not get enough meat and fish products to counteract the effects of a high phytate diet are subject to rickets and other growth problems.[31] Contrary to accepted opinion concerning the healthy effect that consuming soy has on Asians, a *New York Times* article (June 6, 1996) has cited that more than 100 million cases of "goiter" are presently reported in China.

Decades ago soybeans were not utilized as food; they were used—more appropriately—in crop rotation. Unfortunately, however, the soybean industry cleverly thought of a way to process the bean for human consumption and at the same time generate a fine profit. As you will notice in your food pantry, soy has become an additive in almost all packaged products as hydrolyzed or texturized soy isolates.

HOW ARE SOY PROTEIN ISOLATES (S.P.I.) MADE?

Much of the difficulty with nonfermented soy foods comes from their processing. Textured vegetable protein, the result of high-temperature, high-pressure extrusion, has been shown to damage vital organs in animals. The fatty acids in soybeans are very susceptible to rancidity under high pressure and heat; and soybean oil cannot be extracted without dangerous solvents, some of which remain in the final product.[32] An alkaline solution is added to it in order to remove the fiber, which produces a toxin called lysinoalanine.[33] Another step involves adding an acid to separate the components. This is done in aluminum tanks, which leach high levels of aluminum into the final product. It is then spray-dried at high temperatures to make a protein powder. Additionally, nitrites (potent carcinogens) are formed during the spray drying. The use of additional high temperature and pressure produces textured soy protein.[34] Finally, even though much of the trypsin inhibitor content can be removed through high-temperature processing, it's not all removed during this processing. This remnant can vary as much as fivefold[35] and adds to the negative effects of soy isolates. This leftover anti-nutrient (a toxin) becomes more of a concern when MSG is added in order to mask the unpleasant taste of this texturized soy product. This additive can often create an allergic reaction as well as a need to increase intake of vitamins E, K, D, B_{12}, calcium, magnesium, manganese, molybdenum, copper, iron, and, of course, zinc.[36] The effect of such mineral-blocking enzyme inhibitors in soy can result in any number of conditions, including endocrine disruption, goiters, reproductive disorders, and allergic reactions.[37]

THYROID DYSFUNCTION LINKED TO SOY

Soybeans are also listed in *Nutrition for Women* as one of the foods that inhibit thyroid function.[38] The National Center for Toxicological Research reports that soy isoflavones (genistein and daidzein) "inhibit thyroid peroxidase-catalyzed reactions essential to thyroid hormone synthesis."[39] Japanese researchers studied the effects of consuming as little as two tablespoons of soybeans a day. Even when healthy people were put on this diet for a short period of time, it was found to suppress thyroid function with development of goiters in "especially elderly subjects."[40] (See page 169 where we discuss how doctors recommend supplementing with maca root, as it is rich in iodine and is often able to restore thyroid function.)

Additionally, it only takes a mere 45 mg of isoflavones daily in premenopausal women to create a biological effect that can cause a reduction in the amount of hormones needed for proper thyroid activity. Numerous women are on thyroid medication, yet at the same time they are increasing their soy intake. The two seem to be at cross-purposes. Women as well as men who believed that soy foods were healthy are now feeling compelled to tell their stories. For instance, Debbie Compton says, "I believe that consumption of soy-based protein powders and low-carbohydrate diet bars containing soy products may have taken my hypothyroidism to all new heights." Is it any wonder Debbie had problems?

Research clearly points out that dietary soy damages the enzymes that manufacture thyroid hormones—enzymes so essential to thyroid functioning.[41, 42] Besides this bad news, scientists have known for years that isoflavones in soy products can cause enlarged thyroid glands. Test animals fed soy protein isolates (SPI) develop enlarged thyroid as well as enlargement of other glands, most particularly the pancreas. Their diets, which were high in trypsin inhibitors led to the development of pathological conditions of the pancreas, including cancer.[43] A biochemical pharmacology study confirms that fatigue, as well as goiter problems, are associated with consuming soy foods.[44]

The soybean industry is a multibillion-dollar business in this country. No wonder we are not able to purchase foods that do NOT contain soy in the list of ingredients on the product. Perhaps this fact alone will give us some insight as to why we need to take a look at package labeling and acquire a bit more knowledge about what is healthy in our diet.

For more information see appendix D where we list studies and Web sites that will direct you to the documentation that deals with adverse effects of soy on thyroid function as well as other endocrine disorders. Also look at the Web sites www.soyonlineservice.co.nz and www.westonaprice.org/women/wise_references.html. To reinforce our understanding regarding the debilitating effects of soy, we have found numerous testimonials to show what can happen to our bodies when we are not informed about what we should and should not be consuming in order to remain in good health.

> An article about the dangers of soy for thyroid patients opened my eyes to the fact that I had been poisoning myself for 3 years with a food I didn't even like. Within a month after throwing out all the soy products in the house and vowing never to touch them again, the hypothyroid symptoms began to melt away. I'm walking the road to health once again.
>
> Leslie Blumenberg

> I personally have suffered from consuming soy protein shakes once a day for breakfast for a period of 2–3 years. There are no warning labels on these products! I have been hypothyroid for many years and was taking Synthroid at the time, in spite of the medication I became ill from the effect that soy had on my thyroid.
>
> Colleen Witzel

I have moved and changed careers and have almost completed my first year in medical school in D.C. But what I wanted to say is this. Ever since I quit Isolated Soy Proteins (ISP) my T$_3$ levels went off the roof and my thyroid replacement hormone had to be cut drastically . . . like my doctor put it, seems as if my thyroid's kicking back in. Sure enough, I'm almost finishing my second year in med school, and my thyroid meds had to be decreased by 75 percent.

Franklin Westhout

Soy milk can be highly allergenic in itself, lacking in needed natural vitamins and cholesterol. Its production creates an incomplete, denatured protein with possible chemical contamination. Athletes should be aware that the "soy protein" drinks they are consuming in order to build muscle tissue may actually cause muscle protein breakdown.[45] *The British Journal of Nutrition* informs weight-training athletes that diets consisting of soy protein may increase protein breakdown in skeletal muscle.[46] And speaking of musculoskeletal weakness, author Elaine Hollingsworth's research shows "all soya bean products, especially soya milk, leach calcium from bones, depress the thyroid gland, and create havoc in the body."[47] In addition, soy baby formula contains many additives,[48] and some researchers stress the need to study the question of feeding infants and children, sometimes for years, a substance known to have estrogenic properties.[49] The most natural solution? Breast-feeding, enhanced by progesterone therapy. However, if this is not possible, homemade formulas can be prepared with a base of broth or raw, organic whole milk (see appendix C).

FRIENDLY HERBS FOR HORMONAL SUPPORT

The plant world provides us both food and medicine. Herbs come in many forms, from teas to capsules and everything in between, and can be used for almost every condition and symptom. Many books have been written informing us how much to take and for which illness. We will very briefly review some of those herbs that are for menopausal problems. It is important to remember, however, that herbs are powerful and some can be dangerous if combined with certain prescription drugs or taken in excess. Always consult a reputable herbalist before deciding which herbs are right for you.

Some dear friends gave me an herb book that notes the natural estrogenic qualities of damiana for relief of hot flashes, and blessed thistle and saw palmetto for other female disorders.[50] Marcus Laux, N.D., expands the list of plants with estrogen-receptor activity: dong quai, alfalfa, black cohosh, fennel, anise, flaxseed, yellow dock, hops, sesame, garlic, many kinds of fresh and dried beans, cabbage, and olives.[51]

The Herb Lady's Notebook stresses that progesterone is the most important hormone for balancing the thyroid and entire glandular system.[52] Especially affected is adrenal activity.[53] Herbal progesterone-like qualities are found in sarsaparilla, ginseng, licorice root, bloodroot, red clover, mandrake, nettle leaf, nutmeg, damiana, turmeric, sage, oregano, thyme, and unicorn root.[54] Dr. John Lee points out that dong quai and fennel have active progestogenic as well as estrogenic substances.[55]

HERBS FOR HORMONAL SUPPORT

Herbs with Phyto-Estrogen Qualities	Herbs with Phyto-Progesterone Qualities	Adaptogens
Alfalfa	Bloodroot	(Exerting alternative action
Anise	Chasteberry*	on hormone metabolism.
Black cohosh*	Fenugreek	They contain progestogenic
Blue vervain	Sarsaparilla	as well as estrogenic substances.)
Cranesbill*	Mandrake	
Damiana	Mistletoe	Dong quai
Dandelion root	Nettle leaf	Fennel
Flaxseed	Nutmeg	Ginseng
Hops	Turmeric	Licorice root
Red clover tops	Oregano	
Sage*	Thyme	
Sesame	Vitex	
Strawberry leaf*	Yarrow	
St. John's wort buds		
Wild oats		
Sage leaf		
Yellow dock		
Yorkum*		

* Herb traditionally used to address hot flashes and night sweats during the transition of menopause. Most effective when used in conjunction with natural progesterone cream to establish hormone balance.

Dr. Julian Whitaker adds that motherwort, chamomile, and chasteberry are good for relaxing the nervous system and reducing hot flashes, night sweats, and heart palpitations. In addition, oat straw and blue and black cohosh are good for muscular toning and as uterine tonics. For muscular spasms or cramps, lack of energy, or mild depression, skullcap is recommended. For endometrial pain, some excellent herbal tonics are discussed in detail in *The Women's Book of Healing Herbs* by Sari Harrar and Sara Altshul O'Donnell.[56] To relieve vaginal dryness you could include licorice, wild yam, and goldenseal. There are also topical lubricants, which include calendula (marigold), slippery elm, aloe vera gel, and vitamin E.[57]

Supplementing one or more of the adaptogenic herbs listed above can be quite helpful in our desire to achieve hormonal balance. For instance, if you think you need herbal estrogen, I have found the use of licorice root *(Glycyrrhiza glabra)* to be an excellent choice in that it is an invaluable aid for maintaining a healthy immune system.[58] "Licorice is believed to exert an alternative action on estrogen metabolism," according to *The Healing Power of Herbs.* "When estrogen levels are too high, it will inhibit estrogen action, and when estrogen levels are too low, it will potentiate estrogen action. . . ."[59] In other words, it may act on the body as an adaptogen.

Let's talk a minute about stress and the adrenal glands. These triangular glands are located above the kidneys and "share a close common ancestry with both the ovaries and the testicles. . . . Although Western medicine only acknowledges the most extreme cases of adrenal failure as a problem, adrenal exhaustion is epidemic. . . . Adaptogens include well-known herbs such as panax ginseng, Siberian ginseng, and astragalus . . . Licorice root is a specific for low adrenal function and contains substances very similar to some adrenal hormones."[60]

However, the use of natural progesterone is essential in the treatment of adrenal exhaustion due to its role as the precursor hormone in production of the adrenal steroids. In fact, without inclusion of natural progesterone, adrenal recovery is greatly impaired. Because adrenal health is so important during menopause, I have found herbs with adaptogenic qualities to be effective when suffering from low adrenal function. Keep in mind that they should always be used in combination with regular application of transdermal or sublingual progesterone.

Black cohosh *(Cimicifuga racemosa)* functions in a similar way to human estriol. This herb is also thought by some to be able to balance one's own estrogen. However, many herbs have the potential for unintended side effects if used in excess.[61, 62] Being observant of any obvious physiological changes—favorable or otherwise—can help in making a reasonable decision whether to use more, less, or none at all.

Jesse Hanley, M.D., notes that because women are not getting the help they want from mainstream medicine, they are experimenting with self-help treatment through herbs. Dr. Hanley warns that although certain estrogenic herbs might relieve your symptoms, they could also increase the risk of fibroids, tumors, and cancers, and therefore advises us, "Make sure your formulas contain progesterone-precursor herbs, such as sarsaparilla and chaste berry *(Vitex agnus castus)*."[63] (Sarsaparilla, incidentally, also has been found to be a precursor of testosterone.) James Jamieson, pharmacologist, also emphasizes the importance of balancing the estrogenic herbs with a natural progesterone source.

A NOTE ABOUT PHYTOESTROGENS

We are going to be hearing about the plant estrogens for some time to come, as this field of research expands. We know that a single plant may contain numerous estrogenic substances that work in different ways. Perhaps we should heed statements such as these from journal articles published in the mid-1990s which "make it clear that phytoestrogens have some of the same capabilities to induce developmental toxicity as do other estrogens. . . . There is a clear need to carry out detailed pharmacological studies to define relative [estrogen] agonist and antagonist activities in different tissues. . . ."[64]

Furthermore, "few studies have actually demonstrated that isoflavonoids [a class of phytoestrogens] are estrogen inhibitors;" and the findings of more than one study "contradict the assumption that all phytoestrogens are necessarily antiproliferative [cancer-protective] agents."[65] An article in the *Journal of Nutrition* "argues for the importance of fully characterizing each [dietary] phytoestrogen in terms of its properties, natural potency, and short-term and long-term effects."[66]

In an article in *In Vivo*, "Estrogen-Induced Cancer: Estrogen's Role in Cancer," Susan Conova writes that the allegedly "safe" estrogens that are promoted as "replacements for the estrogens in hormone replacement therapy may not be so safe after all."[67] Dr. Hari Bhat, assistant professor of environmental health sciences suggests "even non-carcinogenic estrogens can cause cancer given the right conditions." This research was published in the April 1, 2003, Proceedings of the National Academy of Sciences and was supported by the NIH and the Jean Sindab/AVON Breast Cancer Foundations. Dr. Bhat says, "If we have oxidative stress in cells from other chemicals, then women are at risk for cancer even with estrogens that are considered non-carcinogenic. . . . The therapy may be safer if taken with antioxidants, but more research is needed to make safe and more effective antioxidants."[68]

We need to understand that since estrogens of various kinds often act by mechanisms or pathways other than by binding to the estrogen receptors, the focus only on receptor-binding may not tell the whole story. Also keep this in mind before turning to the latest antiestrogen designer drugs known as "selective estrogen receptor modulators," such as Evista (see chapter 4 for more information). As it is vital that we obtain hormonal support from our foods, it seems appropriate to provide more facts about a plant source that provides health benefits in this area.

MACA ROOT *(Leoidium meyenii)*

We have now seen through research, documentation, and testimonials how rebalancing our hormone levels with natural progesterone will aid in relieving women of many uncomfortable PMS and menopausal symptoms. However, if hot flashes or vaginal dryness persist, the use of maca root supplements, rather than the use of those of an estrogenic nature, often provides a valuable partner to progesterone. This phytonutrient is particularly helpful when a woman begins to gradually taper off her synthetic HRT. The health-promoting effects of this root are far superior to any phytoestrogen, says anthropologist Dr. Viana Muller.[69] In fact this root medicine has been used for more than 10,000 years with few, if any, known adverse effects.

Hugo Malaspina, M.D., a cardiologist in Lima, Peru, explains that maca aids in normalizing the hormonal secretions of the pituitary, pancreas, and adrenals. He finds in his practice that it has been especially beneficial following a hysterectomy.[70] The root portion of this plant helps the endocrine system (e.g., thyroid, testes, ovaries, and pancreas) to stay in balance.[71] Chris Kilham, a medicinal plant researcher at the University of Massachusetts, writes how maca is commonly used to enhance energy and endurance.[72] Henry Campanile, M.D., practicing in St. Petersburg, Florida, recommends maca root to his patients to balance and nourish the adrenal glands. He personally found that supplementing with maca has given him much more energy.

Doctors often recommend maca in their practice because it is rich in iodine and is often able to help restore thyroid function. Researcher and author Elaine Hollingsworth tells us that many symptoms relating to thyroid disorders (e.g., low energy, depression, memory loss, low body temperature) have been "banished with the use of maca."[73] In her book *Take Control of Your Health and Escape the Sickness Industry* she provides numerous testimonials from doctors and patients alike who have benefited from this medicinal tuber. On a personal note, I use maca root because I have always had low thyroid. In my case, ongoing use of supplemental progesterone, with intermittent or occasional addition of maca, proved to be quite helpful when I've been under more stress than usual.

We can see why this tuber is valued for its medicinal qualities, as it contains amino acid proteins and is an excellent source of complex carbohydrates. It also contains fatty acids (linolenic, palmitic, oleic), and polysaccharides. Philip N. Steinberg, a certified nutritional consultant tells us that many B vitamins and steroidal glycosides are present in Peruvian maca. Vitamins C and E as well as numerous alkaloid minerals have been found in the root portion of this plant. It's no wonder so many doctors are now speaking out about its benefits.

Richard Brown, M.D., in his book *Stop Depression Now* speaks about using maca for the treatment of depression for both men and women. Hugo Malaspina, M.D., Viana Muller, M.D., Gloria Chacon de Popivici, Ph.D., Garry Gordon, and Burton Goldberg (president of Alternative Medicine Publishing) tell us to forget dangerous and expensive drugs such as Viagra. An article called "Move Over Viagra" printed in *Nutraceuticals World* (June 2002) explains how maca can help fertility enhancement. Biologist Gloria Chacon de Popivici informs us that maca is not a hormone replacement, but it does aid in supporting the function of the hypothalamus and pituitary.

With all these benefits we have to wonder why haven't we heard more about this cruciferous vegetable, which has been used for more than 10,000 years to boost the immune system? One reason is because of the lack of education concerning natural remedies in today's world of "organized medicine." Fortunately, we can once again learn from the Peruvians, who have used this ancient food remedy for thousands of years on a daily basis to keep the body in nutritional and hormonal balance.

However, as for the possibility of any contraindications, Stephanie Sulger-Smith, RN, MS, says, there may be a few individuals who could perhaps develop an allergic reaction.[74] Should you want to supplement with this root, or any herb for that matter, be observant to any physiological changes in your body.

THE B-COMPLEX VITAMINS

The significance of the B vitamins became clear to me when I read Dr. Carlton Fredericks' findings that B-complex vitamins will help to convert estrogens, such as estradiol, to estriol for excretion from the body. We can assist the Bs in this process by keeping the colon clean and allowing the liver to do its work.

Among the liver's many important functions are the conversion of various hormones, especially the estrogens, for elimination. Eating frequent small meals and healthy snacks rather than a few large meals helps stabilize the blood sugar and provides a steady source of energy to the liver, without overloading it and making it sluggish. This may be an especially important issue for women who are considered at risk for breast cancer. As Dr. Richard Passwater tells us, "Breast cancer patients have lower levels of estriol than normal" (see chapter 5). Therefore, including B-complex on a daily basis from adolescence on may actively assist in the liver's conversion of estrogen.[75]

This was confirmed by Dr. Fredericks, who found that cancer is linked to deficiencies in B-complex (especially folic acid) along with vitamins C, E, and A. "B-complex vitamins help the liver regulate the estrogen level," says Dr. Fredericks.[76] He goes on to advise that the "control of estrogen is a nutritional process. . . . It is not properly achieved by prescribing more estrogen."[77] He says that "vitamin B complex cuts down excess activity of estrogen, whether prescribed for menopause or birth control or produced by the woman's own ovaries. . . . [It] helps to counteract the effects of high levels of estrogen which has not been detoxified by the liver."[78] Studies are also underway to explore how certain types of dietary fiber, such as wheat bran, may moderately speed up intestinal transit time. This may relieve or prevent congestion in the colon and lower the concentration of estrogen in the blood.[79]

When taking a B vitamin, remember that they all work together, each one needing the other. In general, almost all of us need a B-complex supplement because these vitamins are often lost in the processing of foods. Dr. Fredericks states in his book *Guide to Women's Nutrition: Dietary Advice for Women of All Ages* that progesterone can be stimulated by vitamin B₆, which can be useful *in moderate amounts* for women who suffer from bloating and water retention. He says that if "a woman takes the birth control pill, she develops vitamin B₆ deficiency and then folic acid deficiency,"[80] along with the obvious progesterone deficiency. Thus, he says, B₆ may help to counter "the negative effects of the birth control pill. . . . Vitamin B₆ has also been helpful for women in offsetting the tendency to store water, particularly in the premenstrual week, and helps clear up premenstrual acne."[81] He also states that you can encourage "safe progesterone production with vitamin B₆—a critical factor in controlling estrogen."

Furthermore, according to Gail Sheehy in *The Silent Passage*, taking progesterone with B₆ may be helpful for women suffering from exhaustion.[82] As for some of the foods that contain B₆, Dr. Fredericks lists "beef liver, kidney, fresh fish, bananas, cabbage, avocados, peanuts, walnuts, raisins, prunes, and cereal grains."[83]

A NATURAL APPROACH TO DEALING WITH ANEMIA

In some situations, iron pills may intensify anemia "or even be the cause of it," warns Dr. Ray Peat. He points out also that it "would seem reasonable to consider the role of vitamin E in anemia, before giving a woman iron pills."[84]

Concentrating on one's diet is safer than taking iron salts, which have a destructive effect on vitamin E. Iron accumulation can lead to inflammation, calcification, cancer, and suppression of progesterone synthesis.[85, 86] Should you have a deficiency, natural sources of iron include red meat, liver, eggs, wheat bran, wheat germ, oatmeal, brown rice, raisins, dried apricots, prunes, dates, apples, bananas, cherries, grapes, oranges, parsley, carrots, celery, onions, and blackstrap molasses.

Dr. Peat also makes the interesting observation that more often than not, anemia is a thyroid/estrogen problem, related directly to the temperature of the long bones of the arms and legs, where red blood cells are formed in the bone marrow. Thus, in addition to warm clothing, an answer may be support for the thyroid, which is instrumental in body temperature regulation.

Speaking of the thyroid, many women who consistently use the maca root may want to also add homeopathic support to their regime: Thyroidinum (thyroid gland) 6x, 12x, 30x and Lactose. Putting to use a combination of a variety of natural therapies can make a vast improvement in one's energy, mood, and metabolism.

VITAMINS A AND E AND PROGESTERONE: A DYNAMIC TRIO

Dr. Fredericks' *Guide to Women's Nutrition* gives some information that you can relay to your medical doctor, should he or she be skeptical about the use of vitamin E for PMS problems. Tell him or her that the *Journal of the American Medical Association* (which, as Dr. Fredericks says, "the orthodox physician is likely to regard with some awe if not trepidation")[87] states that vitamin E in doses ranging from 150 to 600 units daily decreases menstrual flareups, anxiety, moodiness, irritability, headaches, fatigue, pounding of the heart, and dizziness.[88]

If natural progesterone is not readily available in an emergency, there are vitamins we can temporarily use that also help to balance estrogen levels, especially vitamins A and E. In fact, Dr. Ray Peat says that vitamin A and pantothenic acid (B5) "promote natural progesterone synthesis,"[89] adding that both vitamin E and progesterone increase the amount of oxygen in the uterus.[90, 91]

Vitamin E has relieved some women of a variety of menopausal conditions, such as hot flashes and emotional problems.[92] In the book *Cancer and Its Nutritional Therapies*, Dr. Richard Passwater informs us that "vitamin E has been used successfully by many physicians to make fibrous cysts disappear."[93]

As for vitamin A, researchers recognized the relationship between vitamin

A deficiency and cancer as far back as 1925. *Cancer and Its Nutritional Therapies* refers to studies by Dr. Harold Manner of Loyola University in Chicago, wherein "vitamin A was a critical component of his protocol to *cure* breast cancer in mice." Dr. Manner also cites laboratory evidence that "cancers such as breast, lung, and skin tumors can be cured by treatment with vitamin A." This vitamin reversed "the effects of carcinogens in tissue cultures from the prostates of mice."[94] Dr. Ray Peat corroborates that "vitamin A protects some tissues, such as the breasts, against estrogen's effects, including cancer, and generally offers protection against estrogen by increasing progesterone."[95]

Vitamin E and riboflavin (B2 vitamin needed in red blood formation) will provide relief from hot flashes and severe PMS problems, says Dr. Fredricks; and a cream combining vitamins E and A has been successful for a large number of women with vaginal atrophy.[96]

PURE WATER: THE BEST MEDICINE

The importance of consuming plenty of water is emphasized in the book *Your Body's Many Cries for Water*. Its author, Dr. Batmanghelidj, scientifically explains why major diseases are often simply due to chronic, long-term dehydration. The water you drink will bring about cell volume balance in your body and result in more efficient cell activity.[97] When the body is in a hydrated state, proteins and enzymes become much more efficient. Dr. Batmanghelidj tells us, "The damage occurs at a level of persistent dehydration that does not necessarily demonstrate a 'dry mouth signal.'" Thus if we only drink when we are thirsty, our cells have already suffered.[98]

Of particular and critical interest to women is the role of chronic dehydration in the development of breast cancer. Dr. Batmanghelidj says the stress it creates "will increase the secretion of a hormone called prolactin, which can at times cause the breast to transform into cancerous tissue. . . . Also, the dehydration would alter the balance of amino acids, and allow more DNA errors during cell division."[99] Dr. Batmanghelidj says dehydration also suppresses the immune system by making one's natural killer cells less active.

He explains, "The breast is a water-secreting organ. . . . Whether you are having a child or not makes no difference. The breast must be ready to fulfill its predestined role. . . ." If a woman already has breast cancer, drinking plenty of water, he says, would assist with any therapy by flushing out toxins. "If you do not have breast cancer, or want to prevent a metastasis from occurring, it is urgent that you drink enough water. If you don't, your breast may suffer horribly because of its unique role in supplying fluids."[100]

The doctor makes the point that water "improves the uptake of hormones by the cells" by its action on the receptors at the cell membrane. He further stresses the necessity of avoiding caffeinated beverages or compensating for their diuretic action, and also the necessity of adequate salt intake in order to retain sufficient water in one's cells.[101]

It is sometimes recommended that we drink as close as we can to a gallon of water a day—or at least one-half ounce for every pound of body weight. But we need to remember, not just any water will do. In addition to the many contaminants found in tap water, many popular water filters create a breeding ground for bacteria and viruses. Because of the inorganic minerals contained in ordinary water, some authorities maintain that the best home drinking water is obtained from a distiller (using nature's water purification principle) or a reverse osmosis filtration system.[102–105]

THE SALT OF LIFE

Why should we insist on unrefined sea salt instead of ordinary table salt? Author Jacques de Langre, in *Seasalt's Hidden Powers,* tells us that when natural sea salt is processed and commercially treated with bleaching agents, valuable minerals are removed. Is it any wonder we hear that table salt, laden with additives, is not good for us and can cause water retention, back pain,[106] and even kidney problems?[107] That is because it interferes with the free movement of body fluids through cell membranes and blood vessel walls.[108]

Unprocessed sea salt, on the other hand, aids in metabolism and provides the body with a balanced array of many essential minerals.[109] Dr. de Langre, in fact, draws a vivid comparison to the salty, mineral-rich amniotic fluid that surrounds a baby in the womb.[110, *]

Fortifying our body with foods such as healthier forms of salt can often prevent deficiencies in iodine or iron.[111] These mineral deficiencies often bring about or aggravate thyroid problems. Balance is the key in anything, of course, as excess iodine may suppress thyroid function and could even create autoimmune thyroiditis (Hashimoto's disease). As discussed above, sea salt is a useful condiment for this purpose as it provides both iodine and iron in its natural form. However, consuming salt that contains the synthetic iodized form is not a wise choice.[112]

---

* A nutritious salt for your kitchen may be obtained from The Grain & Salt Society, 273 Fairway Drive, Asheville, NC 28805, (800) 867-7258.

SUGAR VS. STEVIA

It has been well documented that consumption of foods and beverages which are high in sugar content is associated with the prevalence of PMS,[113] as well as deteriorating bone health and other physiological disorders.[114–116] The fact of the matter is processed sugar is in almost everything. Like estrogen, it is ubiquitous, and because of its accumulative effect, it can promote diabetes and encourage growth of harmful bacteria, parasites, and yeast organisms such as candida.[117] When a food product is labeled "cholesterol free," the fat taken out is often replaced with processed sugar.[118]

Persistent ingesting of refined sugar is considered the #1 promoter of disease. Nancy Appleton, Ph.D., tells us in her book, *Lick the Sugar Habit,* that an excess of sugar in our body can "bind nonenzymatically with protein . . ." Sugar and protein are not supposed to bind together. If they do, "glycated protein" results and this can "permanently alter the molecular structure of the protein."[119] The protein becomes toxic, resulting in cells that do not function optimally.[120, 121] This excessive dietary sugar intake increases calcium excretion in the urine, upsetting the body's mineral balance,[122, 123] and most especially the calcium-phosphorous ratio, which in turn can cause joint degeneration[124, 125] and excessive calcium in the systemic circulation which becomes toxic and can cause such problems as bone spurs, arthritis, and kidney or gallstones.[126] High intake of refined sugar can also cause cataracts,[127] weakened eyesight,[128] hormone imbalance,[129] multiple sclerosis,[130] allergies,[131, 132] heart disease,[133] osteoporosis, and cancer in any of its many forms.[134–136] The list of disorders and studies are too numerous to list here. Eventually, the immune system becomes overwhelmed and exhausted.[137]

One healthy sweetener we speak about in greater detail in *Preventing & Reversing Arthritis Naturally* is an herbal sweetener called *stevia*. It is used as a natural nonfattening sugar substitute. Stevioside, the plant's sweetening agent, is 300 times as sweet as granulated table sugar. Steviosides actually normalize blood sugar levels, inhibit the growth of some types of bacteria and other unhealthy organisms, and are helpful in the treatment of hypoglycemia and diabetes.[138–140] Dr. Daniel B. Mowrey's investigation into herbal remedies has led him to write about their scientific validation.[141] It turns out that stevia not only sweetens our food but is also used for medicinal purposes in other parts of the world. In Paraguay, for instance, it is used to nourish the pancreas and to encourage its ability to function normally.[142] For more information about stevia's history, the FDA's involvement, and much more, go to www.stevia.net. For its long term use as a digestive and weight management aid and for strengthening the heart and vascular system, go to www.healthfree.com.[143]

For many health reasons I avoid processed sugar, hydrogenated vegetable oils, and other synthetic ingredients. This approach has caused me to resort to making my own healthy "gourmet" chocolates using the superior sugar substitute, stevia. The best part of this is that I don't feel guilty when I satisfy my chocolate craving following my evening meal.

NATURAL THYROID MEDICATION

Dietary approaches provide the optimal medicine for normalizing thyroid function. Joel Robbins, M.D., N.D., D.C., tells us that an imbalance in our alkaline/acid levels can be a large factor in maintaining health and avoiding the onset of a variety of diseases. His suggestion is that we should look to foods for healing, balance, and remedy, even in the case of thyroid disorders. Dr. Robbins suggests that approximately 80 percent of our diet should consist of alkaline foods. In other words we should eat more fruits, vegetables, almonds, and so forth.[144–146]

Avoid refined sugars, table salt, milk, white flour, processed foods, and all refined fat whenever possible. Also substitute organic (unrefined) coconut oil and unsalted organic butter for frying and baking foods, and use extra virgin olive oil when making salad dressings. Herbs that support the thyroid are gotu kola, bladderwrack, kelp (natural iodine), black walnut, cherry bark, nettles, Irish moss, tirazine, ginseng, parsley, and dong quai. Dr. Sherry Rogers' book *Tired or Toxic?* suggests detoxing with water containing pure ascorbic acid powder (directions are on the bottle) and supplementing with 300–600 mg of lipoic acid and 400–800 mg of glutathione. Make sure your daily supplements contain potassium, magnesium, and maca root (good for the hypothalamus), you eat plenty of green leafy vegetables, and your foods are rich in omega-3 fatty acids.

THE BODY'S NEED FOR GOOD CHOLESTEROL

Let's hear it for the good cholesterol that's in our bodies. This cholesterol (which Dr. John Lee says is of concern mainly when it is *oxidized*) is actually the precursor of progesterone, estrogen, DHEA, and other steroidal hormones. Wallace L. Simons, R.Ph., of Women's International Pharmacy, says that we've been sold a real bill of goods about cholesterol. As long as we consume plenty of antioxidants, we should not have a problem; arteriosclerosis is brought on in part when the "bad fats" are allowed to break down into free radicals.

We are told to stay away from many foods in order to avoid cholesterol problems; however, we may be mistakenly steered away from important foods in order to lower our dietary fat content. An example of this is seen in an interesting study from Denmark concerning the inclusion of eggs in our diet. Dr. Earl Mindell provides us with some vital facts: "When 21 healthy adults ranging in ages [from] 23 to 52 years old were given two boiled (not fried) eggs every day plus their ordinary diet, their *good* blood cholesterol went up 10 percent, while their total blood cholesterol only went up 4 percent after six weeks." It seems that moderate egg consumption may be quite beneficial where cholesterol problems are concerned.[147] Of great interest to us in this discussion of hormones is the statement by Dr. Ray Peat, in his book *Nutrition for Women,* that including eggs and liver in the diet will promote the formation of progesterone.[148]

We should also consider butter a preferred choice over margarine, an artificially engineered product whose partially hardened oils can be toxic and damaging to the arteries and the immune system. The vitamins A and D that butter contains "are essential to the proper absorption of calcium and hence necessary for strong bones and teeth."[149] Butter is also an excellent source of a highly absorbable form of iodine and assists the proper functioning of the thyroid gland.[150] Its lecithin helps to assimilate and metabolize fat constituents such as cholesterol,[151] and it is rich in antioxidants, including selenium and vitamins A and E. Even cholesterol is an antioxidant. Both the vitamin A and the short- and medium-chain fatty acids found in butter are valuable to the immune system, and its lipids protect gastrointestinal health. Because these fatty acids are burned for quick energy rather than stored in the fat tissue, *Health Freedom News* states that "the notion that butter causes weight gain is a sad misconception."[152]

HEALTHY OILS AND THEIR ROLE IN HORMONAL BALANCE

Clearly, the whole question of fats in our diet is one we need to approach cautiously. Fad follows upon fad, and we are at the mercy of public relations teams and pop journalists who often fail to delve into all the scientific facts. However, the subject is important, as it relates not only to weight control, heart disease, and cancer but also to the formation of all our steroid hormones, including progesterone. Fortunately, there are numerous interesting and ongoing studies currently under way regarding fats and oils and their effect on our health, which will help give us a new perspective regarding the good fat/bad fat dilemma.

Sorting out the confusion regarding fats/oils has been complicated by myths, misconceptions, and misinterpretation as to what is involved. The chemicalization of oils came about because food manufacturers and biochemists were anxious to produce "stable" products that would not turn rancid on the supermarket or kitchen shelves. In itself, that is a very viable and most necessary consideration for all of us to address. Unfortunately, liquid (poly- and monounsaturated) vegetable, nut, and seed oils turn rancid with exposure to heat, light, air, and pressure. This can happen long before they even get to the grocery shelves due to the combination of such environmental exposure during the manufacturing process.

In order to slow this process down, food chemists developed what they envisioned to be the perfect solution: partial or complete hydrogenation of liquid oils to a semi-solid or solid form. In so doing, hydrogen molecules are added to the unstable and unsaturated fatty acids as found in these oils. The fallacy in this course of action is that the developers of these artificial oils declared that if oil was partially hydrogenated, it must be "safe." What they didn't recognize was that in the very process of hydrogenation, they had created a new fatty acid, now known as a trans-fatty acid (TFA). These chemically altered fatty acids are foreign to our cellular processes and wreak havoc instead of health.

It is interesting to note that in May of 2003 a lawsuit was filed against Kraft Foods to discourage the consumption of trans-fatty acids via the marketing and sale of packaged foods (specifically Oreo cookies) to school age children. Currently the House Chairman of the Joint Committee on Health Care, Massachusetts State Representative Peter J. Koutoujian, is sponsoring legislation to "ban sales of soft drinks, candy bars, and fried foods in schools during school hours." Unfortunately, these "foods" are all laden with TFAs. At last the major fast-food corporations are at least being pressured to eliminate "artery-clogging trans fats and partially hydrogenated vegetable oils" in their cookies and crackers.[153] Sadly, it has to take the threat of legal action before manufacturers come around to providing a healthier way of life. We can only hope they follow through with this and that this "pressure" will extend to other foods they serve our children.

With all these concerns and cautions one wonders if there is any viable fat or oil in today's market. The answer to this question brings us to one of the most overlooked and misjudged oils available: pure, unrefined, organic coconut oil. One's first response to this might be to remind the authors that coconut oil is known to be saturated and unhealthy and, therefore, should be avoided at all costs. That, at least, is the message of many manufacturers and all too many doctors and health care advocates. The misconception here is in confusing the organic, unrefined coconut oil with the processed, refined variety in common use. They are not one and the same at all. Making that mistake is like confusing natural progesterone with synthetic progesterone or progestins such as Provera, DepoProvera, etc.

But once again nature herself has provided a solution. We need look no further than tropical oils. The molecular components of these plants have the advantage of growing in the hotter, equatorial regions, and over eons of time they have so adapted to the consistently warmer growing temperatures that they can sit unrefrigerated for up to two years and not go rancid. To avoid organic coconut oil because it is highly saturated is to disregard one of nature's safest and healthiest oils.

Barbara Joseph, M.D., in her book *My Healing from Breast Cancer*, counsels that "there is no greater way to impact the health of the planet than through our daily food choices. . . . Our pantries are filled with cancer-causing partially hydrogenated oils."[154] These have been altered to give them a more stable shelf life, in the process creating dangerous trans-fatty acids. These devitalized oils[155] impair the immune system response by interfering with the T-lymphocytes—the fighters against allergies, infection, cancer, and inflammatory joint disease.[156–159] It is also documented that the use of such refined hydrogenated and/or partially hydrogenated oils is shown to raise blood cholesterol levels.[160] In addition, the destructive processing of oils for consumer consumption includes carcinogenic preservatives such as BHT, BHA, and TBHQ.[161]

A Swedish trial published in 1998 verified a positive risk association of dietary polyunsaturated fat (omega-6) with breast cancer. In a 1986 study, unsaturated free fatty acids in plasma increased the biologically available estradiol, which the authors postulated as related to an increased risk for breast cancer.[162] Studies show that a high maternal consumption of corn oil consisting mainly of linoleic acid (omega-6 polyunsaturated fatty acid) increases circulating estradiol (E2) levels during pregnancy and the risk of developing carcinogen-induced mammary tumors.[163]

Dr. Peat has made a comprehensive study of, as he puts it, "the whole history of research on the biological effects of dietary fats."[164] He writes that when the LDL cholesterol (the supposedly bad kind) is *too* low, the body may be hindered from producing enough progesterone.[165]

Another connection between high dietary fat consumption and estrogen is known as the "enterohepatic reuptake of circulating estrogens."[166] This is the recycling of estrogenic molecules from the colon to the liver. This occurs in the absence of adequate amounts of fiber in the diet relative to dietary fat, which is most often the norm. It is now understood that estrogen binds to fiber and in this manner is removed from our colon. As stated elsewhere, one of progesterone's roles is to burn fat for energy thus releasing our stored estrogens into the bloodstream for possible elimination from the colon. Thus, a high fiber diet plays an essential role in allowing progesterone to assist the body in restoring hormonal balance.

Given that the standard American diet is definitely higher in fat than fiber, most adults, as well as children, are recirculating their estrogen overload rather than eliminating these toxins. Thus, and once again, dietary and lifestyle changes become imperative issues in our effort to balance our hormones and fight disease, especially breast cancer.[167]

On the basis of his extensive research, Dr. Peat challenges some of the modern-day assumptions about the so-called "essential fatty acids" that he says originated with faulty interpretation of certain tests performed on rats in the 1930s. In fact, he says, "it is now known that polyunsaturated fats interfere with thyroid hormone in just about every conceivable way"[168]—and they have a strong estrogen-promoting action.[169] In fact his research shows how polyunsaturated fats "synergize with estrogen" and their effects "can be seen in the offspring, as an increased tendency to develop breast cancer."[170] He emphasizes that excessive consumption of these types of fats leads directly to the development of such degenerative scourges as cancer, diabetes, heart disease, arthritis, osteoporosis, and connective tissue disease.

In fact, the evidence against an excess of polyunsaturated fats, used in most restaurants and processed foods found on the grocery shelves, is quite alarming as it shows how omega-6 oils in the diet, as well as an overweight condition in general, appear to increase the risk of breast, prostate and other hormonal cancers.[171] Dr. Peat states that "the best argument for a role of omega-3 fats in protecting against cancer is that they are the main fat in grass, and as a result, animals that graze have very little omega-6 fat in their tissues and milk"[172, 173] The diet of most farm-raised animals in the U.S. is now based on corn and soybeans rather than grass, which has unfavorably changed the balance of fatty acids in their meat to contain mainly the omega-6 unsaturated fats. Unfortunately, the establishment still thinks this is good, even though studies to the contrary date back at least to the 1990s.[174, 175]

Dr. Bruce Fife's research confirms, "Many vegetable oils promote cancer because they are easily oxidized to form carcinogenic free radicals."[176] With reference to osteoporosis, we are learning from researchers at Purdue University that the free radicals from unsaturated oils interfere with normal bone formation. On the other hand, healthy saturated fats protect bones[177] and also function as antioxidants. Therefore when dealing with osteoporosis, we should be avoiding all denatured, processed vegetable oils and use only the safe oils previously mentioned, such as coconut and palm.

When polyunsaturated oils predominant in our diet, or when we use commercially processed salad oil, mayonnaise, or common oil-based skin lotions (ingredients of which are absorbed into our body), the unhealthy fatty acid molecules contained in them will eventually interfere with the natural detoxification processes that are ongoing in the liver.[178] This causes the liver to become overloaded and congested and impairs its efficiency as the body's filtration system. Studies even show that the negative effects of the oil's harmful properties can be exacerbated by exposure to radiation.[179, 180]

But what is equally startling, and exciting because it offers a way to reverse these frightening effects, is that Dr. Peat has discovered much-maligned coconut oil to be part of the solution. This product, unfortunately, is currently out of favor, again because of unscientific studies and inaccurate "bad press." Today, studies are available that are independent of those done by a multitude of industries that are mainly interested in promoting processed foods. Fortunately, we now have access to research that shows how unrefined "coconut oil . . . inhibits the induction of carcinogenic agents that cause colon as well as mammary (breast) tumors in test animals"[181–185] by means of its antioxidant properties.

What more evidence do we need before embracing such a healthy food? The therapeutic nature of coconut oil reduces stress on the immune system by permitting white blood cells to function more efficiently.[186] Tropical oils (i.e., palm and coconut) contain tocotrionols, which inhibit the growth of cancer cells.[187, 188] Consumption of coconut oil has also been reported to reduce the risk of heart disease,[189] decrease body fat,[190] and improve "immune response to pathogenic bacteria."[191] It's unfortunate to learn about the increase in cancer and heart disease among the natives who had given up eating coconut oil in favor of polyunsaturated vegetable oils.[192, 193]

Incidentally, coconut oil also contains the same sterol found in pregnenolone,[194] the parent and major hormone from which all other hormones are made and are dependent upon.[195, 196] (See illustration on page 186.) Dr. Fife tells us that coconut oil is composed of the following medium chain fatty acids:

48 percent lauric acid (a 12-chain saturated fat)
7 percent capric acid (a 10-chain saturated fat)
8 percent caprylic acid (an 8-chain saturated fat)

All these triglyceride molecules have similar antimicrobial properties, which are normally "absent from all other vegetable and animal oils, with the exception of butter."[197] Consuming unrefined tropical oils provides improved immune response not only to pathogenic bacteria but it also provides us with immune protection by means of their antibacterial, antiviral, antifungal, and antiprotozoal properties.[198–207]

Coconut oil also contains the immune-boosting lauric acid (an essential component in breast milk), which is considered to be one of its vital nutrients and protectors. This MCFA, the primary fat in coconut oil, destroys lipid-coated bacteria and encourages friendly intestinal bacteria.[208] It also helps in the absorption and enhancement of other nutrients (i.e., calcium, magnesium, and amino acids). For these reasons, coconut oil, consisting of 48 percent lauric acid, is included in the healthier baby foods.[209] MCFAs are even beneficial in "reducing epileptic seizures in children" as seen from a study done at the University of Minnesota Medical School.[210]

I have found that it's hard to find skin-care lotions and products that are soy-free, thus I will often make my own therapeutic natural skin cream using unrefined coconut oil as the base. I found that it's not only a safe sunscreen, but it's healthy for the skin due to its multiple benefits. Melt two ounces of coconut oil and ten 30 mg capsules of CoQ10. It feels wonderful and is excellent for the skin, as is extra virgin olive oil.

One interesting illustration in the use of coconut comes to us from Hawaii where the native islanders give their weaning infants the jelly-like, easy-to-eat substance found inside the immature coconut as their first food because of its superior nutritional value. As the coconut matures, this jelly food separates into a clear sweet liquid (the milk in the middle of the shell) and a hardened white substance that adheres to the inside shell. It's interesting to note that this latter component is eventually used in commercial products such as shredded coconut—where preservatives, coloring, and other additives are often added. Needless to say, the more this product is processed, the less healthy it becomes for the consumer.

Coconut oil can also aid in defending against lung infections and ulcers.[211] The properties in this tropical oil have been found to kill candida and other fungal infections.[212] Dr. Fife explains how this oil is "the most potent non-drug or natural yeast-fighting substance," and is an invaluable food for fighting other infections,[213] such as kidney and bladder infections, due to its antimicrobial effects.[214] Further research shows coconut oil as one of the healthiest fats to use in combating chronic inflammatory problems.[215] It may also be a good source in fighting chronic fatigue syndrome, which is "affecting approximately 3 million Americans."[216]

In fact there's an incredible amount of documentation that shows how the easily oxidized short- and medium-chain saturated fatty acids (MCFAs) found in unrefined coconut oil can protect our tissues against the toxic effects of the unsaturated fats and can even reduce the harmful effects they have on the thyroid gland. For these reasons, its regular use offers protection against disease and premature aging. Dr. Peat recommends about an ounce a day.[217, 218]

One way to use coconut oil is as a salad dressing, mixed with extra virgin olive oil, apple cider vinegar, and sea salt.[219] (See more information about the healthiest form of sodium in chapter 6.) Coconut oil can be safely used in cooking without posing any health risks. Unknown to many of us is the fact that when the polyunsaturated, hydrogenated, or partially-hydrogenated vegetable/seed oils are stored at room temperatures or when they are heated to extremely high temperatures in cooking (or even warmed by our internal metabolic digestive processes), they are subject to rancidity and free-radical formation. What we need to realize is that as long as we purchase oils that are organic, unrefined, extra virgin, or tropical, we have turned from denaturized oils that only rob us of our health to those that have a multitude of hormonal and nutritional benefits.

Although many professional chefs sauté, grill, or fry with extra virgin olive oil, I personally would not put this therapeutic oil through such a denaturing process. I would rather choose to utilize all of its beneficial enzymatic qualities—most especially its antioxidant polyphenols that are responsible for the reduction of blood pressure in patients.[220] This beneficial effect could very well be reduced or even destroyed in the heating process. L. Aldo Ferrara, M.D., tells us about a study done on high blood pressure. He says "daily use of olive oil, about 40 grams* per day, markedly reduces the dosage [of blood pressure medication] by about 50 percent in hypertensive patients on a previously stable drug dosage."[221]

So why not continue to make the most of nutritional benefits found in olive oil's extra virgin natural state by not cooking with it at all?[222] Instead, I use unrefined coconut or palm oil and salt-free organic butter for all my cooking needs with no loss of nutrients and with no health risks whatsoever. Unfortunately, we have been so convinced that their "saturated" nature was a reason to avoid these oils that we have been programmed to overlook some of the healthiest foods available.

An added bonus via its naturalizing effect on the thyroid is that coconut oil, in spite of being a fat, has been known to bring about an amazing loss of excess weight. Farmers, in fact, who thought it would be an inexpensive way to fatten their animals, found it had just the opposite effect![223]

---

* Approximately ¹/₂ cup

How will such a diet affect humans? In his *Healing Miracles of Coconut Oil,* Dr. Bruce Fife researched more than one hundred studies that validate coconut oil's beneficial effect on elevated cholesterol levels[224] and how it can actually aid in weight loss.[225-227] Dr. Fife tells how the MCFAs found in coconut oil actually stimulate our metabolism and produce energy, whereas the commercial "vegetable" oils do just the opposite to our metabolism and thus trigger weight gain.[228] MCFAs are not stored as body fat as they "go to the liver where they are converted to energy"[229] to improve endurance as well as increase our metabolism.[230] In contrast, the polyunsaturated oils only function to further suppress the body's metabolic rate.[231, 232]

We all know that we get antioxidants from consuming fresh fruits and vegetables. However, many of us are not aware that coconut oil is also considered to be an antioxidant as it combats free radical formation and thus reduces the risk of many chronic disorders, including high blood pressure and heart disease. Other researchers such as Mary G. Enig, Ph.D., and Raymond Peat, Ph.D., have also confirmed the above and have enlightened us as to the difference between the healthy properties found in coconut oil as compared to the unhealthy ones found in unsaturated vegetable oils.[233-237] Indian folk remedies as well as Ayurvedic medicine use coconut oil to treat burns, ulcers, kidney stones, and even dysentery.[238]

Of great importance is the fact that consuming MCFAs, as found in coconut oil, can aid in many ways after gallbladder surgery because the "metabolism of MCFAs does not require bile or any pancreatic fat-digesting enzymes."[239] In other words, the fatty acid in coconut oil doesn't need the special enzymes that are required by long chain fatty acids (LCFAs) found in commercial vegetable (nut and seed oils). Considering how many women (and men) have had their gallbladders removed but are never told about the beneficial properties of organic coconut oil, is it any wonder these individuals tend to have so many digestive problems and so much difficulty losing weight?

In certain areas, grocery wholesalers may be able to get coconut oil for you quite inexpensively. Ask for "unrefined 76-degree melt," and you will be getting a natural product. Other sources are certain herb shops, health food stores, or ethnic markets and restaurants. High-quality organic products can also be obtained by contacting Virgin Oil de Coco-Crème at (877) 441-9479 or Omega Nutrition at (800) 661-3529.

As for the other oils—we have a right to feel confused! Some, of course, are better than others. In *Fats That Heal, Fats That Kill,* Udo Erasmus, who is an internationally known writer on the subject of fats and oils, stresses that some cold-water fish and northern marine animals contain the high-quality omega-3 oils EPA (eicosapentaenoic acid) and DHA (docosahexaenoic acid). These two fatty acids, constituents of our own cells,[240] help to keep our arteries open and prevent cholesterol disorders, strokes, and dangerous clot formation. From the fatty acid EPA the body can manufacture certain prostaglandins,[241] which are hormonelike materials that control all of our cells.

A deficiency of beneficial prostaglandins, according to Dr. John Lee, can "promote heart disease, immune system dysfunction, inflammation, pain, and PMS."[242] Although fish oils, like other oils, can easily become rancid, in studies using the very fresh oils of certain types of fish, it was observed that they "inhibited growth and metastasis of tumors."[243]

The omega-3 fatty acids (found in deep-water fish such as salmon, mackerel, tuna, cod, haddock, and sardines)[244, 245] and oils containing a high ratio of monounsaturates (such as extra-virgin olive, flaxseed, and high-oleic sunflower) have gotten a lot of publicity for their reputed ability to enhance immune function and reduce LDL cholesterol.[246] Adelle Davis writes that avocados, walnuts, and almonds are some of the foods that contain fatty acids that help burn excessive fat.[247]

You may also have read promising things about flaxseed oil and its use in cancer treatment. Additionally, some research confirms that the alpha-linoleic acid (ALA) in flax seed, an omega-3 fatty acid, actually decreases many inflammatory conditions[248] such as arthritis, pancreatitis, and tendonitis.[249] It will be wonderful if these things turn out to be true. But just how much of the information has been promulgated by manufacturers of flaxseed products? Dr. Paavo Airola warned about the strong tendency of this oil to rancidity.[250] The safest way to buy and consume flax without being concerned about its rancidity is to obtain a bag of whole organic flax seed and keep it in the freezer. When ready to use, pulverize just the amount you need in a coffee grinder. Sprinkle this fresh powder immediately on foods such as salads, cereals, drinks, and so forth. Use up what you grind so that you eliminate the chance of it becoming rancid. Also, store the remaining flax seeds in your freezer for future use. Consuming this concentrated omega-3 oil, along with its fiber, both of which are lacking in most diets, provides powerful medicinal health benefits. Other safer fats/oils include animal-based fats such as lamb and unsalted butter (if from organic sources).[251, 252, *]

---

* Keep in mind not to eat too much of any food or fat. It's always wise to check your pH level so that you continue to have your acid/alkaline ratio in proper balance.

THE FIGHT FOR NATURAL HEALING—
A BATTLE YOU CAN'T LOSE

The more we begin to understand what the body needs, the more we can support its innate design for utilizing natural foods to cleanse and regenerate tissue. By choosing from the many health care approaches those that meet our individual requirements, we can transform infirmity into vitality. So, before considering yet another drug for a condition that is still festering, why not take advantage of the unadulterated forms of healing that are gentle, yet powerful in addressing the cause of disease? Nature already offers us curative substances that will help us achieve optimum energy and make us less vulnerable to the effects of environmental stress. Making such an important personal effort will influence much more than just our physical health.

The simplified diagram below shows the conversion of cholesterol to pregnenolone. After conversion it follows two pathways branching out to either progesterone or DHEA, from which the remaining steroid hormones are manufactured.[253]

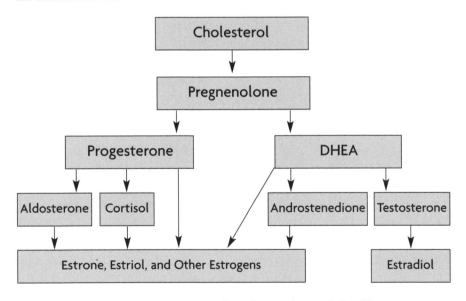

Figure 1. Cholesterol/Pregnenolone Conversion to Other Hormones

SEVEN

Planning a Personal Approach

*You need to be the instigators. . . . You cannot expect your
doctor to assume control and solve all your problems—
M.D. does not stand for Medical Deity.*
Christiane Northrup, M.D.[1]

The best way to avoid the "midlife crisis" experienced by many women may well be to take a saner approach to health. This involves learning about natural therapies, unknown to so many, that will restore the body's internal balance. Looking back over the years I wonder why I didn't take time to educate myself sooner about the many forms of alternative health care. In justifying my case, I reflect on how much easier it was just to let the medical doctor make all the decisions. How easy it is to become dependent on the advice of others, especially when we feel sick and tired! Unfortunately, that's not a wise attitude, as many of us can attest in hindsight.[2, 3]

Being unaware of our options, however, we accept, largely on faith alone, the standard medical treatment currently in vogue. Unfortunately, the relief it offers may be only temporary. Worse, its multiple side effects often force us to deal with future disorders that are routinely treated with biopsies, mastectomies, hysterectomies, and drugs. We go through years of confusion, wondering where to turn.

In retrospect, I realized the imprudence of being completely dependent on what my doctor prescribed, which was based on the "standard medical treatment" he was authorized to provide. Unhappy with the results, I went from one doctor to the next only to be given a different estrogen prescription or a different hormone-combo regime. There seemed to be as many points of view as there were doctors. I learned eventually that their information about drugs comes largely from the pharmaceutical companies and, in turn, the sales force that is promoting specific products. Down the road the patient's hope for a cure will hinge upon which drug, hormone, or combination of medications was being marketed when she received her prescription.

Some doctors are taught that estrogen is the only hormone that's necessary for the treatment of osteoporosis. And when the patient asks about the warnings listed on the estrogen (or progestin) packet, the advice she receives is this: "Not to worry—remember, there are more benefits than risks when using this hormone!" After my appointment with the particular gynecologist, internist, or endocrinologist of the day, I would always return home with the same kind of frustrations and fears, wondering why the subject of risks was never fully discussed.

BLIND ACCEPTANCE

My sole reliance on this system kept me at a low ebb during my early menopausal years. However, this was nothing compared with the ordeal of the women I knew who had been on synthetic hormones for several decades. Initially, some of these women had felt tremendous relief when estrogen was prescribed. However, as time went on, complications began to surface. Nevertheless, they decided to endure the fluid retention, weight gain, and other problems with the thought that it was better than trying to tolerate the menopausal symptoms. Too bad, because these signals in response to HRT are the body's way of crying out for us to STOP—and for very good reasons!

Nevertheless, many of us continue to consult orthodox medical practitioners. Although the process is expensive and time-consuming, we go along with it because we need help. One has to wonder how long this system of dependence, chaos, and sometimes intimidation will persist.

Expressing many women's discouragement with synthetic HRT, Gail Sheehy refers to Germaine Greer, who "properly faults the medical establishment for conspiring to make women dependent on pills and patches that have been woefully undertested."[4] And we ask, "Why is this, when medical research is supposed to be so infallible?" The answer may lie in an examination of where the profits are coming from. As we have already demonstrated, a synthesized commercial compound that requires a doctor's prescription for its sale commands a much higher market value—not to mention that it will not have an identical action to that of its natural counterpart and will often create toxic responses.[5, 6] Additionally, these responses will too often lead to more testing, more medication, and, very often, surgical intervention. The warnings in the *Physicians' Desk Reference* list the many unwanted and often serious side effects. But unaware of any of this, we may come home from a medical doctor's office exasperated once again, feeling more and more frustrated.

I see a real need for women to be more alert to the barriers and sometimes even incompetence that stand in the way of our health. As we seek that path less traveled, more and more of us will realize that the remedy we have been waiting for has already been found and is presently being utilized by many doctors and their patients. This information was discovered as far back as 1930, so it saddens me that all women today are not informed about NHRT. We should be given the chance to *first* try a natural product that has been shown, even proven,[7–12] to relieve persistent afflictions without side effects. Instead, synthetic compounds are prescribed and so often complicate our already stressful lives.

Hysterectomy . . . endometriosis . . . osteoporosis . . . breast, cervical, or uterine cancer—these no longer have to be specters overshadowing our lives. Dis-ease of the body, mind, and spirit can be a thing of the past as we begin to focus on prevention: proper diet, exercise, supplemental natural hormones. Once we experience for ourselves the impressive results, we'll be zealous to spread the good news about NHRT and to fight for our health and our well-being.

By listening to the wisdom of our own bodies and taking advantage of the evaluation tools that are available to us, we can learn whether there are deficiencies or excesses in our hormone levels and thus avoid the ordeals just mentioned. However, not everyone has the time, energy, or funds to have expensive tests done at a medical specialist's office. Just thinking about the difficulty of finding a doctor who understands the difference between the natural and the synthetic—not to mention trying to find time in an already busy and stressed-filled agenda to schedule an appointment—can be discouraging.

DIAGNOSTIC TESTING: WHAT? WHERE? WHY?

When you are making the transition to a more self-directed program, you'll be faced with some choices. The question often arises whether to have a blood or saliva test to measure hormone levels. Saliva tests are claimed by some to be a more reliable measure of hormones that are biologically active and available than the more commonly ordered serum blood tests,[13] which are, nevertheless, preferred by Dr. Peat.

Companies such as Aeron LifeCycles, (800) 631-7900, make saliva test boxes that can be sent to you for use in your own home. You can perform a convenient and noninvasive test (no needles) that will measure any or all of the following hormones: estradiol, progesterone, DHEA, and testosterone. Dr. Debbie Moskowitz says that this simple procedure "gives women the ability to monitor changes associated with various alternative approaches, such as diet, herbs, or creams [and] get information regarding baseline hormone levels, or to test hormone levels during a certain phase of the menstrual cycle."[14] For more information, call Transitions for Health at (800) 888-6814.

You can also ask your doctor about the comprehensive hormone balance evaluations that are performed by Diagnos-Techs, Inc. on the basis of saliva specimens collected at the patient's convenience. Kits are supplied to practitioners such as medical doctors, chiropractors, naturopaths, acupuncturists, and any other licensed doctors at no cost; your samples are sent to their lab. Diagnos-Techs will determine your baseline levels and evaluate the degree of deficiency in any of the hormones (estradiol, estriol, progesterone, testosterone, or DHEA). They will then report to your doctor the type and amount of hormonal support you may require. For this service, contact Diagnos-Techs, Inc., 6620 South 192nd Place, J-104, Kent, Washington 98032, or call (206) 251-0596.

You can also contact Dr. David Zava of ZRT Laboratory (12505 N.W. Cornell Road, Portland, OR 97229). He has developed a saliva hormone ratio assay for evaluation of your saliva test results to determine the presence of estrogen overload. He suggests that optimal protection against estrogenic overstimulation occurs at the midpoint of the luteal phase during a normal menstrual cycle (midway between ovulation and the onset of menses). This is when our ovarian progesterone levels should be at their highest concentration. Dr. Zava advises to check the ratio between estradiol and progesterone and advises that if estradiol "is greater than 1 pg/ml in a saliva test, progesterone should be at least 200 times higher (at least 0.2 ng/ml). . . . Maintaining this ratio should provide good protection against the harmful effects of estrogen."[15]

Even with this guideline for evaluating your saliva tests results, don't hesitate to call the lab, (503) 469-0741, or your doctor if you need assistance in determining your current ratio. If your estrogen is consistently lower than 1 pg/ml, is this indicative of a true estrogen deficiency? Not necessarily. We might not want to jump to this conclusion when we hear about

Dr. Nan Kathryn Fuchs' experience. She tells us "there's a difference between blood levels and breast levels of estrogen. Blood levels show the amount of estrogens circulating in the blood. But fatty breast tissues produce estrogen, and even if your blood levels are low, you may, like me, have too much estrogen in your breast tissues."[16] She found that thermography testing provided a more accurate measure of the estrogen stored in her breast tissue. Two years later Dr. Fuchs tells us in the *Women's Health Letter* (August 2004) that these pre-cancerous changes in the breasts "would not have shown up on a mammogram for years. But with thermography, I was able to pick up the problem at its earliest and most treatable stage. . . . My doctors and I went to work immediately. We developed a cancer-fighting program that included natural progesterone cream."[17]

Even if you are diagnosed with low levels of estrogen, remember you always want to keep progesterone the dominant hormone to ensure appropriate balance and protection.[18, 19] The decision as to whether to have a hormone saliva test or not often brings up many questions. A lot of guesswork still seems to be involved in the administration and interpretation of the assays. Some doctors tell you not to take hormones for a couple of weeks prior to taking the saliva test, whereas others say eight to forty-eight hours, and some tell you to take the test along with your normal hormone replacement program. Furthermore, you may be told to pick a day when your stress levels will not be high (I'd like to meet the woman who can orchestrate such a day). Also, one's hormones can fluctuate quite a bit, and what's normal for one woman is not necessarily so for another.[20] These levels can even change from one month to another, depending on many factors.

With all of these variables, I wonder if saliva tests can truly be a reliable reflection of our daily hormonal status. In fact, Dr. Susan Love questions why a woman would want to go that route. She encourages patients to be more aware of their symptoms, which she considers the best indicator of an individual's appropriate level.[21] As Dr. Marcus Laux states,

> Many internists and gynecologists put women on HRT drugs without testing their hormone levels. Some just test a woman's LH and FSH levels. Although we recommend getting a full testing of all hormone levels—a full steroid panel, as it's called—if your doctor is unable to interpret the results, it won't be that helpful, and *the best measure will be how you feel.*[22] (Emphasis added)

Such a steroid panel is available in the form of a urine test that can be ordered by your doctor. This test, called the twenty-four-hour urine sex hormone profile, measures the average output of various hormones throughout the day. The continuous collection of your urine during a twenty-four-hour period avoids the inaccuracies of test results based on only one reading. Doctors interested in more information may call Meridian Valley Clinical Lab at (253) 859-8700.

Along with these specific tests, a baseline gynecological exam is important in ruling out any underlying pathology as the cause of your premenstrual, menopausal, or postmenopausal symptoms. Once you receive a clean slate as far as more serious disease is concerned, you can turn to a preventive program of hormone replacement. The key here is to find a physician supportive of the natural, nonsynthetic, noninvasive approach that recognizes that *dis-ease* and many female problems stem from an absence of hormonal balance.

For fertility testing, there is a product called the CycleView microscope that relies on the crystalline pattern of dried saliva. On fertile days there is a fernlike, branching pattern to the dried saliva, whereas on nonfertile days the pattern is random. With this knowledge, women now have a nondrug, nonsurgical means by which to promote or prevent conception. The pocket-sized microscope is a convenient way to monitor daily hormonal changes and can be used over and over, not just one time. To inquire about this fertility awareness tool, call (415) 389-5400 (and see page 78).

As for testing for bone mineral density, the lowest radiation dose is produced by DEXA screening, which also allows for a high degree of precision and accuracy (within 1 to 2 percent on tests of the lateral lumbar spine). These tests are available in most major cities throughout the United States. For the location closest to you, contact the National Osteoporosis Foundation at (800) 464-6700.

Another resource is the OsteoGram Analysis Center, which uses radiographic absorptiometry technology and computerized analysis of standard hand X-rays for measurement of the bone mass of the middle fingers. The analysis will show a patient's bone density measured in terms of a *T*-score (number of standard deviations above or below the reference bone mass for normal young adults). The company provides a starter kit for converting any standard X-ray unit into a bone densitometer. Ask your doctor to phone (800) 806-5639, or write for an application: P.O. Box 47058, Gardena, California 90248.

The Great Smokies Diagnostic Lab, (800) 652-4762, offers a service for women wishing to monitor the effectiveness of their treatment relative to possible ongoing bone density loss. The lab uses a simple, noninvasive urine collection system to diagnose candidates for antiresorption therapy. MetaMetrix Medical Laboratory also has available a simple urine test that identifies accelerated demineralization. It measures the collagen fragment in the urine that is thought to be specific to the resorption process and an indicator of progressive bone breakdown. According to the laboratory, "Recent research has demonstrated the clinical utility and sensitivity of this procedure." You can contact them at (800) 221-4640. More recently a home urine test has been developed that measures the presence of an enzyme that is associated with elevated levels of bone breakdown. Using this test kit, a woman can monitor the efficacy of her bone-loss prevention program. This kit can be obtained from Women's Health America at (800) 558-7046 or www.womenshealth.com.

By using these resources, growing numbers of women are taking responsibility for their own health and finding a sense of confidence, worth, and freedom. They are weaning themselves away from their traditional dependence on and continual use of synthetic drugs and are no longer accepting these prescriptions unquestioningly. Perhaps some day, with the trend toward self-evaluation and monitoring and more personal initiative in the quest for natural therapies, the often inappropriate and unnecessary prescribing of synthetic hormones to women will be labeled malpractice, and the recommendation of any form of estrogen unopposed by natural progesterone will be considered a violation of insurance codes.

WISER CHOICES

Better times are just around the corner. But even as it becomes easier to find that special doctor who is familiar with the latest research on plant-based hormones, we need to understand that there are as many viewpoints and outlooks as there are physicians when it comes to drugs versus natural hormones.

Once you have personally delved into and understood the various roles played by natural progesterone in the metabolic and physiologic operations of the body, you can better discuss your health needs with your physician. You alone can feel the good or bad signals the body communicates, and you are the one who has to live with any side effects. How empowering to learn about this on your own!

So when faced with having to decide between prescribed medication and natural solutions, stand by your convictions and common sense. Be prepared to be calm when approaching doctors who have spent years learning about drug therapy. I have found that some do not appreciate being told of treatments they have not been schooled in.

A Case of Intimidation

One of my friends went to great lengths to research, read, and copy scientific literature from medical journals regarding natural substitutes for synthetic hormones, and then presented the information to her doctor. She even took him a book on the subject, written by a medical doctor who had been using a natural progesterone cream for over twenty years with great success. Her doctor responded to all her efforts with this emphatic statement: "I'm not convinced! I will continue treating you according to *conventional medical standards.*" Women face this very attitude every day, and it leaves very little, if any, room for further patient-doctor discussion.

This form of belittling, however subtle, is not helpful, nor is it respectful. The patient I have just described is a nurse. She is an intelligent, well-respected woman, known for her many useful endeavors in the community. She is also interested in obtaining the very best health care for herself and her loved ones. Her experience could have made her unsure of herself and unwilling to pursue natural HRT any further. However, in spite of her doctor's attitude, she prudently followed her own instincts, and now feels better for it.

If you have had a similar experience, you need to keep in mind that there are always other health care providers to turn to—doctors who do not allow their egos to influence their judgment about the best treatment for their patients, and who will at least look into natural therapies that have proved to be effective in the long run. These are the ones we need to seek out to be our family physicians, and the ones we need to tell our friends about. Wise counselors with this propensity, in fact, are quoted often in this book. We cannot afford anything less than to be treated by a doctor who is informed in the most important areas of natural health care.

Communicating Your Needs

A number of years ago, in order to make my gynecologist aware that nonprescription progesterone creams were readily available from various sources, I mailed her the information in appendix F of this book. After receiving it, she actually called me on the phone herself to thank me for collecting so much research and sharing all the literature with her.

She then told me she would not only use this information herself but make it available to her other patients. She then called in a prescription for me for natural progesterone. Needless to say, I was delighted at her response and relieved that I was finally going to receive the desperately needed natural hormones.

Likewise, a friend who has been supplying her open-minded physician with literature was told, "I'm glad you're my patient. It's really made me look at natural hormones!" So the more that we, as patients, continue to speak out, the more the medical profession will begin to acknowledge the importance of natural progesterone over artificial drugs. An article under the auspices of ten M.D.s and eight Ph.D.s illustrates this in roundabout fashion, conceding: *"Oral micronized progesterone, a natural form of the hormone, may provoke fewer side effects than its synthetic cousins."*[23]

Encourage your own doctor to read the information from the *Journal of the American Medical Association*[24] and *Medical Hypotheses*[25] regarding the body's need for nonsynthetic hormone replacement. When the doctor reflects on the data, he or she will then recognize that such treatment is not only desirable but also endorsed by medical authorities—endorsed years ago when facts were not compromised or influenced by profits.

So forge ahead! And in your search for "Dr. Good," remember to be positive, be assertive, and don't forget there are other good doctors out there waiting to serve you. They will be quite excited about what you have found and will respect you for going the extra mile. When you find one who really listens and is open to a higher level of doctor-patient communication, you will feel as if you have found not only a doctor but a friend. And as doctor and friend she would agree, "The more you know, the healthier you will be."

Most physicians are well aware that synthetic HRT can create uncomfortable and dangerous side effects, so if a natural product has been observed to have remarkable results with other patients, they may be quite interested in introducing it in their practices. Accordingly, appendix E provides a suggested form letter, to be changed as fits your needs. Feel free to copy the accompanying pages and give them to your doctor. This will allow her to examine a sampling of the extensive research already completed and available, should she wish to pursue the subject further.

Sending a letter or calling the office first is more efficient than going to the expense and frustration of spending time in a waiting room, only to find once you get into the doctor's office that he or she is not open to the concept of natural therapies.

In such a letter you can ask for a short interview to discuss natural hormones and your philosophy concerning PMS, menopause, and perhaps even cancer. Every doctor's attitude is different. Some do not take kindly to their patients' relating to them information of which they were unaware. Then again, others, especially those who are not afraid of what their peers will think, may be quite receptive to natural options.

This is just the beginning of a portfolio outlining steps you can take to obtain NHRT through your medical doctor, who can call in a prescription (under your insurance coverage) to specialized pharmacies throughout the country. Appendix G provides a list of pharmacies that specialize in compounding natural hormones. Or, you can obtain the natural progesterone cream on your own, directly from any of the distributors listed in appendix F. This is especially convenient for those who do not have a medical doctor or insurance plans that cover such prescriptions. And remember what Stuart M. Berger, M.D., said in *What Your Doctor Didn't Learn in Medical School:*

> All of us do better, physically, psychologically, and even physiologically, when we take an active, involved role in our own process of getting better—the exact opposite of "handing it over to the experts and hoping for the best."[26]

Ways and Means
of Hormone Application

All hormones can be dispensed as tablets, creams, implants, injectable solutions, suppositories, or skin patches. Some of these products can only be administered by your medical doctor (be sure to request only natural hormones), while others you can obtain and use on your own. Many of the progesterone and estrogen creams, for example, come with written instructions on when, how, and where to use them. If you need further information, this appendix includes resources that can answer most of your questions. For more information, call any of the manufacturers or pharmacies listed in appendix G.

USP Progesterone Versus Wild Yam Creams

It is important to clarify that the progesterone cream used in the studies of Dr. Ray Peat, Dr. John Lee, Dr. Norman Shealy, Dr. Alan Gaby, and others, as well as research cited herein, specifically contains USP progesterone, which is referred to as "natural" progesterone or simply "progesterone" on the labels. The major difference between this and the many wild yam creams available is in the laboratory processing, which converts the sapogenin molecule (most commonly from either the wild yam or the soybean) to a substance that duplicates the activity of the progesterone normally produced by the ovaries at the time of ovulation. It also acts as a precursor to other hormones as they are needed.[1]

Although there is some controversy about the effectiveness of products made with wild yam alone, many of these creams appear to be bioactive and able to provide some measure of hormonal balance especially in younger women or those whose symtoms are less severe. In fact, many women have reported relief of their debilitating and draining symptoms of PMS, peri-menopause, and menopause using products without this conversion. Indeed the wild yam supplementation is quite therapeutic for relieving many of the less severe female disorders, but it has not proven to be as potent as USP progesterone, nor has it been proven to aid in building bone density as has USP progesterone. Thus, Dr. Norman Shealy tells us that the laboratory con-version of diosgenin to natural progesterone must be made in order for this molecule to be able to provide the full spectrum of physiological benefits and for it to function in a bioidentical manner.[2]

Speaking of wild yam creams, many young girls who have not started their menses are complaining of symptoms relating to high estrogen levels. Their mothers are asking whether or not they should give their daughters proges-terone cream. This would not be a good idea because you would not want to alter the onset of normal menarche. But there are several things we can do as mothers to help our daughters avoid the estrogen overload that's causing them so much distress.

First of all, make every effort to purchase organic foods. If you are not a vegetarian, consume only organic vegetables and meats free of antibiotics and hormone additives. Synthetic estrogens are given to farm animals to fatten them up for market. Our young daughters in turn consume these animal prod-ucts and then they wonder why they gain weight or feel bloated, why their periods have become irregular, why they have headaches, and why they are plagued with acne problems. So, for our daughters' and family's protection, be sure to purchase organic meats free of antibiotics and free of estrogenic hor-mones. Additionally, when avoiding foods that promote high levels of estro-gen, stay away from soy products. (See chapter 6 for the rest of this story.) Be sure to read all the ingredients on food labels. We need to do everything we can to prevent unhealthy conditions, such as thyroid and other endocrine dis-orders, which are becoming rampant in today's world of food fads.

Even though dietary changes work very well, our daughters still may have high estrogen levels due to other environmental causes. Perhaps a wild yam cream supplement may help. Please remember, however, that USP proges-terone should only be used after the onset of puberty and menses. Also, she might want to include some phyto-progestogenic herbs in her diet (see list on page 166), which will aid in balancing the glandular system, especially adrenal activity. Also it may be helpful to use condiments such as nutmeg, turmeric, oregano, thyme, and yarrow to oppose high estrogen levels.

It's extremely disturbing to find the many so-called solutions or alterna-tives to HRT offered in TV ads, on the Internet, and in popular magazines, which are often so neglectful in their suggestions. As Todd Mangum tells us, "No one has mentioned using the real ones to combat hormone deficiencies. Instead, recommendations include Prozac for depression, Lipitor for cholesterol, high blood pressure drugs to treat hot flashes, and, of course, the recently patented (and profitable) designer estrogens and biophosphonates to treat osteoporosis."[3]

HEALTHY HORMONAL CHOICES: WHICH PROGESTERONE FORMS TO USE

Progesterone has been found to be most effective when administered transdermally, and this is the form recommended by many doctors practicing natural alternative therapies. When applied to the skin, the 15 to 30 mg per day (based on your height-to-weight ratio) are well absorbed in target tissues and thus can aid in achieving what Dr. John Lee calls "physiologic hormone balance"[4, 5]—in other words, the amount each woman's body needs. Dr. Lee says it's preferable to the pill form because the high doses that are given orally (100 to 400 mg) not only pass through the liver first, but also are converted there into metabolites that can have unwanted side effects.

Katharina Dalton, M.D., considered by some to be the foremost authority on PMS, also confirms that the pill form of progesterone is not as effective because it apparently "passes to the liver, the site of numerous progesterone receptors, where it is broken down and metabolized, instead of being transported in the blood in its bioactive form to the other target sites,"[6] such as the brain, nasopharyngeal passages, lungs, eyes, breasts, and lining of the womb. These are some of the areas where progesterone is needed, but, unfortunately, by the time oral progesterone reaches the systemic blood and brain, its concentration is quite low.[7]

Dr. Raymond Peat prefers progesterone to be taken sublingually because it is efficiently absorbed through the mucosa in the mouth (especially under the tongue). Sublingual progesterone, being fat-soluble, is more effective when dissolved in vitamin E. He says that it "will stimulate the ovaries . . . to produce progesterone" if the ovaries are still functioning and will even energize the adrenals and thyroid.[8]

FROM WILD YAM TO PREGNENOLONE

Many doctors are hesitant to recommend or prescribe pregnenolone or progesterone as hormone replacement therapy. Yet these two natural supplements are the ones synthesized from cholesterol and are converted into other hormones by the body on an as-needed basis.[9] The illustration on page 186 shows the role each hormone plays in this conversion and how the hormone pregnenolone is the first steroid produced from cholesterol. This information is documented in more detail in *Preventing & Reversing Arthritis Naturally* where we explain how low levels of pregnenolone exaggerate arthritic pain, memory loss, and endocrine imbalance.* Pregnenolone has been found to be a precursor to the hormone DHEA. Many inflammatory diseases have been found to be associated with low levels of DHEA.[10] Dr. David Lamson found that it may relieve arthritic symptoms, such as pain and morning stiffness, and may reduce the need for anti-inflammatory medication.[11-13]

Pregnenolone is well assimilated when taken orally or sublingually in powdered form. It dissolves well in water and in saliva. Dr. Peat says it is also absorbed efficiently by the intestines and recycled throughout the body. It lasts longer in the body than progesterone and "improves the body's ability to produce its own pregnenolone as well as progesterone. It tends to improve function of the thyroid and other glands, and this 'normalizing' effect on the other glands helps to account for its wide range of beneficial effects."[14] Interestingly, the sterol found in coconut oil is similar to the sterol found in pregnenolone.[15]

GUIDELINES FOR USE OF TRANSDERMAL PROGESTERONE CREAMS

In determining how much transdermal progesterone cream to use, we need to take into account the uniqueness of each individual and the fact that optimal ovarian production of progesterone is somewhere in the range of 15 to 30 mg per day from ovulation to menses. This varies from woman to woman based on her height-to-weight ratio as well as her health history. However, if a woman becomes pregnant, the placenta also begins a steadily increasing production of progesterone, reaching an upper limit of 300 to 400 mg per day during the third trimester. It is this wide margin, in contrast to the narrow thresholds of many of the body's other physiological ranges, that accounts for the inherent safety of natural progesterone.

As progesterone only lasts in the body for six to eight hours, it's important to apply $1/8$ teaspoon (stronger cream) to $1/2$ teaspoon (weaker cream) at least

---

* Years ago (in the 1940s) pregnenolone was used quite successfully instead of cortisone, with no side effects, in treating rheumatoid arthritis.

once in the morning and once in the evening. However, it is recommended that you use a smaller amount more often rather than an all-at-once approach. Progesterone cream can be massaged directly into the skin almost anywhere it's thin or soft—such as the wrists, inner arms, back of the hands, chest, breasts, lower abdomen, inner thighs, buttocks, back, soles of the feet, face, neck, and shoulders. It is preferable to alternate application among these various areas of the body to retain receptor sensitivity and to avoid wasteful oversaturation of any one area.

The progesterone travels through the skin into the subdermal fat and then into the bloodstream in approximately 20 to 30 minutes, where Dr. Peat says it is transported via the red blood cells, lipoproteins, and albumin.

Progesterone cream is available either by prescription or in nonprescription form. Potency will vary, depending on your doctor's prescription or the individual manufacturer. As the potency or strength of a cream depends on the amount of progesterone per ounce, we suggest calling the individual manufacturer as listed on the various products. Be sure to inquire how many milligrams are in the recommended $1/8$ to $1/2$ teaspoon used at each application. You want to be using from 15 to 30 mg each time in order to achieve a normal physiological dose.

Just remember you may need to vary this amount (more or less) because of individual variations in body size, nutritional status, stress levels, and customary amount of exercise. You also need to take into consideration the severity of your initial symptoms and/or any chronic condition you may have such as endometriosis, fibroids, and so forth. Then, over time, the dose can be adjusted according to your response, age, and changing health-related needs.

(See appendix G for telephone numbers to obtain specific creams or literature.)

Premenstrual Syndrome (PMS)

Some instructions say that the amount needed by a cycling female will vary according to the degree of symptoms. If a woman is still having periods and is in her childbearing years, progesterone works effectively when administered just prior to ovulation through just prior to menses. Normally, this pattern of use is from day 12 to day 26. To determine when you are ovulating, please refer to the specific details in chapter 3. In more severe cases of PMS, start using the cream on day 7 to 10, counting the first day of your last menstrual period as day 1, and continue its use until day 26. It is the sudden decrease in progesterone levels that triggers the menses a day or two later.

For minor symptoms, use the cream for fewer days, such as only ten days per month (count to day 16 from your last menstrual period and use $1/8$ to $1/2$ teaspoon once or twice daily until day 26). This would provide the minimal amount and length of time necessary to begin buildup of adequate progesterone levels.

Usually, cream is not used during menses. However, if you have severe cramping or heavy bleeding and/or clotting, apply to the abdomen as frequently as every half hour as needed for relief. If you suffer from menstrual migraines, you can apply the cream to your temples and to the back of your neck every half hour until the pain eases. This application is very effective but should only be used until the severity decreases. Usually this takes only three to four applications until relief is evident.

Perimenopause/Menopause/Postmenopause/Posthysterectomy

Many perimenopausal women are not experiencing optimal results in their use of the cream. This is due in great part to the fact that they are only using it for two weeks per month and thus not getting enough for their particular needs at that critical time of transition. Apply the cream daily for approximately three weeks out of every month. Abstaining for a week (or at least four days) each month helps maintain the body's ability to absorb it and reap maximum benefits. Normal use is approximately one jar or tube per month. If you do not notice a reduction of your symptoms within one to three monthly cycles of use, evaluate how often and how much cream you are using at each application. Many women, upon questioning, admit that they are inconsistent in their use of the cream, and many report dabbing it as if it were a rare perfume; sporadic or scant application can prevent the desired relief.

Calculating your approximate daily amount is easier to do when using a USP progesterone cream because the total active amount is listed in milligrams. Many jars or tubes contain 2 ounces, with 400 mg or more of progesterone per ounce. If you divide the total number of mg by the total number of days you use the cream each month (e.g., twenty to twenty-one days for menopausal women) and use one tube or jar each month, you will get approximately 20 mg or more per day. This daily amount can then be divided into two applications (three only if symptoms are severe), providing for a more continuous release of progesterone into the bloodstream.

Just remember that supplemental estrogen in any form (synthetic, bioidentical, or environmental) can keep us out-of-balance with respect to our levels of natural progesterone, which in fact need to be significantly higher than that of our total circulating and stored estrogens. This must be kept in mind now that we have learned that our endogenous estrogen continues to be manufactured in the fat cells as we enter the stage from peri- to postmenopause. This is also the case if we have had either a partial or complete hysterectomy or if we're on birth control.

TABLETS OR CAPSULES

With your doctor's guidance, follow the above instructions (as appropriate to your situation) for this delivery system also. Years ago, natural progesterone taken orally in pill form disintegrated in the stomach and never entered into the system. Now, certain pharmacies (see appendix G) have developed micronized progesterone in an oil base. The oil protects it from the acids in the stomach, and this process helps the progesterone make its way into the system for a better blood level.

You will notice when taking the capsule form of progesterone that the prescribed daily dosage is much higher (100 to 200 mg) than the cream form (20 to 30 mg). This higher amount compensates for the large percentage that's excreted by the liver. Its absorbability depends on many factors, such as the general health of a woman, how well her digestive system is functioning, and how well her liver is functioning. As Dr. Lee says, "Oral doses of progesterone (even in micronized version) must be greater than transdermal doses to create the equivalent biologic effects."[16] However, as previously discussed on page 199, Katharina Dalton, M.D., informs us that the pill form of progesterone is not as effective as the transdermal cream or the sublingual drops because it first "passes to the liver, the site of numerous progesterone receptors, where it is broken down and metabolized, instead of being transported in the blood in its bioactive form to the other target sites."[17]

IMPLANTS

This surgical procedure is done by your medical doctor. Once the hormone is implanted under the skin, women do not have to come back more than three times a year. However, if using the synthetic hormone, keep in mind what the authors of *Women on Menopause* say: "Once the implant is in place, you cannot get rid of it until the full six months is up, however badly you react to it."[18] Even after six months, some implants are reportedly difficult to remove.

A nineteen-year-old with a hormone implant came to my home in desperation because of the agonizing pain and pressure in her breasts. She claimed to no longer have any periods and was experiencing severe depression. The frightening physical symptoms and emotional instability that these toxic implants had brought on made her run for help in search of a natural alternative. But, unfortunately, the side effects from this drug will remain in her body for quite some time. The risks clearly do not seem to be worth any benefit she thought she was receiving.

It would take another book to tell of the horrendous consequences of having the synthetic drug implanted under the skin. Just a few obvious signs are excessive weight gain and extreme inflammation of the breast. My concern is for those women in similar situations who are not able to find supportive help. Hearing the horror stories of young girls on synthetic birth control implants would make anyone understand why we need to address this often overlooked issue.

PATCH

This is a transdermal agent (that is, applied to the skin). It usually comes in an estrogen form prescribed by your medical doctor. With this method the estrogen is released through the skin in a consistent manner. The alcohol in the patch drives the hormone through the skin and into the blood vessels.

INJECTIONS

Hormones are injected deep into the muscle. Some women are receiving progestins this way. One of the more commonly used sythetic forms comes under the name of DepoProvera. Also, in case you are considering the injections as a lifetime approach, they are just plain inconvenient. Naturally, this is marketed as the most convenient type of birth control because you only have to have the shots every three months. But buyers beware: Women are paying a huge price for this co-called "convenience." Some of the side effects are mild to severe weight gain, increased risk of strokes, hypothyroid symptoms, liver dysfunction, and difficulty getting pregnant once the chemical is out of your system.

SUPPOSITORIES

Progesterone suppositories made with spermaceti wax are not considered very efficient by many medical doctors. Dr. Raymond Peat warns that "the bulk of the progesterone goes out of the solution very quickly, forming crystals which are essentially insoluble in body fluids. . . . Consumers are paying a high price for a minimal effect."[19]

SUBLINGUAL OIL

Dr. Richard Kunin reports that his patients experience relief from their PMS symptoms in less than fifteen minutes with a sublingual dosage of oil-based progesterone. Dr. Martin Milner also recommends an oil-based suspension for his pre-, peri-, and postmenopausal patients. Dr. Betty Kamen suggests use of sublingual progesterone for hot flashes and migraines, as well as cramping (at fifteen-minute intervals until symptoms disappear). This therapy can be used in conjunction with $1/4$ to $1/2$ teaspoon of cream if symptoms are severe.[20]

CREAMS FOR VAGINAL ATROPHY

Vaginal dryness and the accompanying infections that can cause severe pain during intercourse can now be a condition of the past. As previously discussed in chapter 3 and elsewhere, you can apply your progesterone or wild yam cream intravaginally (please check first for purity of ingredients), along with vitamins A and E at bedtime or as needed. Such information can contribute to a happier and more relaxed life!

❧

The above application suggestions have been extracted from various educational materials and are based on the experiences of women in treating their premenstrual or menopausal problems. Of course, the dosage and method will vary according to individual needs, lifestyles, and preferences. The natural over-the-counter and prescription remedies can be obtained from any of the distributors or pharmacies listed in appendix G. Call their toll-free numbers for information on the ingredients in their creams, doctors, locations, or other questions you may have concerning any of the above topics. We encourage you to ask questions and seek out supportive health care providers who can guide you on your journey to optimal health and peace of mind.

Synthetic Compounds: A Sampling by Chemical or Brand Name

The pharmaceutical industry influences medical doctors to recommend the use of contraceptives as early as possible. Who hasn't seen the TV ad campaigns in which our teenagers are told it will help clear up their acne? Todd Magnum, M.D., tells us "the kiddy version of Prempro, otherwise known as birth control pills, nearly ensures these mis-informed women a lifetime of hormonal problems. These pills are artificial versions of both estrogen and progesterone, whose list of side effects parallel the problems found with conventional HRT."[1] Unbeknownst to most women, birth control pills have a stronger concentration of synthetic hormones than standard HRT. As the warning on the leaflets tell us, whether taking contraceptive pills or estrogen/progestins for PMS or menopausal disorders, you run the risk of cancer, liver tumors, gallbladder disease, or blood clots. And if that is not enough, many other adverse reactions are listed below. This critical information should be in large (not small) print and read aloud to each consumer.

Below is just a handful, selected from the huge number of synthetically produced hormones and related compounds that are on the market today. Names continue to be added to the list periodically as women prove unable to tolerate the ones formerly prescribed. With the aid of William Boyd's *Textbook of Pathology*,[2] the *Physicians' Desk Reference* (PDR),[3] *Goodman and Gilman's The Pharmacological Basis of Therapeutics*,[4] and *Facts and Comparisons* ("the pharmacist's Bible"—updated monthly),[5] we have isolated some specific names that might be indicated on prescription labels, along with associated warnings about their use. For updated information on new hormones or current prescriptions, contact the organization Wolters Kluwer at (800) 223-0554. Following are some of the popular terms:

ESTROGENS

Conjugated estrogens (Premarin, Cenestin)
Estrone (Estrone Aqueous, Estronol, Theelin Aqueous, Kestrone, Estroject-2, Gynogen, Kestrin Aqueous, Wehgen)
Estradiol (Estraderm, Estrace)
Estradiol valerate (Delestrogen, Valergen 10, Valergen 40 Dioval, Duragen-20, Estra-L 20, Estra-L 40, Deladiol-40)
Esterified estrogens (Estratab, Menest)
Estropipate (Ogen, Ortho-Est, Estropipate)
Quinestrol (Estrovis)
Ethinyl estradiol (Estinyl)
DES (diethylstilbestrol)
Chlorotrianisene (Trace)
Estradiol cypionate (depGynogen, Depo-Estradiol Cypionate, Depogen, Dura-Estrin, Estra-D, Estro-Cyp, Estroject-L.A.)
Ortho Dienestol, DV, and many more.

Warnings and Adverse Reactions: "There is now evidence that estrogens increase the risk of carcinoma of the endometrium."[6] Other risks include excessive reproduction of normal cells on the inside lining of the uterus (endometriosis), breast cancer, gallbladder disease, and fluid retention, influencing the conditions of asthma, epilepsy, and cardiac or kidney dysfunction. Excess estrogen could bring on nausea, bloating, cervical discharge, polyp formation, skin discoloration, hypertension, migraine headache, breast tenderness, or edema. If contemplating surgery, discontinue use of estrogen at least four weeks prior to surgery to avoid the risk of blood-clotting complications.[7]

PROGESTINS

Medroxyprogesterone acetate (Provera, DepoProvera, Amen, Curretab, Cycrin)
Hydroxyprogesterone caproate (Duralutin, Gesterol L.A., Hylutin, Hyprogest 250)
Norethindrone (Norlutin)

Norethindrone acetate (Norlutate, Norgestrel, Aygestin)
Megestrol acetate (Megace)
Micronor, Nor-Q.D., Ovrette, and many more.

Warnings and Adverse Reactions: (1) May cause insomnia, weakness, abdominal discomfort, flatulence, nausea, fever, vomiting, bleeding irregularities, erosion and abnormal secretions of the cervix, jaundice, severe itching, rash, acne, brown spots; also, risk of thrombophlebitis and thromboembolic disorders (blood clots in the lung, brain, or heart); cerebral hemorrhage and other cerebrovascular disorders; mental depression; impaired liver function; carcinoma of the breast. (2) Other risks include partial or complete loss of vision and retinal blood clots. Discontinue use if migraines, double vision, astigmatism, subluxated lens, apparent derangement of extraocular muscles, cataract, or edema should occur, or inflammation of the optic nerve at its point of entry into the eyeball. (3) Exposure to the progestins listed above that are prescribed during pregnancy can cause genital deformity in male and female fetuses (e.g., urethra abnormality). On the other hand, natural progesterone has been used successfully in premature labor to avoid spontaneous abortions and is of benefit to both mother and embryo (see chapter 3). (4) Careful observation should be paid to conditions brought on by fluid retention. Edema can affect epilepsy, migraine, asthma, and cardiac or renal dysfunction. Progestins in excess can cause weight gain, fatigue, abnormal menstrual flow, acne, hair growth or loss, depression, candida vaginitis.[8]

PROGESTIN/ESTROGEN COMBINATONS

Prempro, Premphase, Comblpatch, Femhrt, Ortho-Prefest, and many more.

Precautions: Two-drug combination hormone replacement therapy (estrogen and progestin) "can infrequently cause breast cancer, heart disease (CHF,[*] MI[†]), stroke, or blood clots in the lung (PE[‡]) or leg especially if used for a long period of time . . ." (A direct quote from drugstore printout, which should accompany the above-mentioned drugs.)

---

[*] congestive heart failure

[†] myocardial infarct

[‡] pulmonary embolism

For more names and details, call *Facts and Comparisons,* or look up the most recent *Physician's Desk Reference* in your local library.

Warnings and Adverse Reactions: According to *Facts and Comparisons,* these are much the same as for "Estrogens" and "Progestins," above.

CONTRACEPTIVES (PROGESTIN/ESTROGEN)

Monophasic oral contraceptives

Necon, Norinyl, Ortho-Novum, Ovcon, Demulen, Ovral, Nelova, Brevicon, Modicon, Ortho-Cyclen, Loestrin, Lo/Ovral, Desogen, Ortho-Cept, Levlen, Levora, Nordette, Zovia, Alesse, Levite, Loetrin

Biphasic oral contraceptives

Jenest, Ortho-Novum, Necon, Nelova, Mircette

Triphasic oral contraceptives

Tri-Norinyl, Tri-Levlen, Triphentasil, Ortho TriCyclen, Triphasil, Trivora, Ortho-Novum, Estrostep

Warnings: Clots in blood vessels to the heart and lungs may cause strokes or heart failure, retinal thrombosis, and optic neuritis. Other risks: gallbladder disease; insulin resistance; breast pressure or pain; cervical, endometrial, ovarian, and breast cancer; depression; abdominal pain and tenderness; elevated blood pressure; decreased glucose tolerance; excessive calcium in the blood. In chapter 4 we learned that natural micronized progesterone builds bone mineral density. On the other hand, "Medroxyprogesterone may be considered among the risk factors for development of osteoporosis."[9] Other side effects: photosensitization, abnormal or excessive uterine bleeding, fluid retention and related conditions of asthma, epilepsy, migraine, and heart, kidney, and liver disorders (benign or malignant tumors which may rupture or hemorrhage and cause severe abdominal pain, shock, or death).[10] Likewise, if one already suffers from hypertension, obesity, or diabetes, the prescription of contraceptives may cause sickness or even death.[11]

APPENDIX C
Natural Formulas for Infants

Adult allergies, as well as thyroid disorders, which are both so prevalent these days, may have been exacerbated for those who were given soy formula as infants.[1-3] Doctors should be aware of the increased risk of developing abnormal thyroid functioning with the use of soy infant formula.[4,5] Studies continue to confirm that adult onset autoimmune thyroid disease is often linked to those children who consumed soymilk formula on a regular basis.[6] Researchers have compared consumption of soy formula in diabetic vs. non-diabetic children and found those who drank it as infants are prone to diabetes.[7] Others who consumed soy formula in infancy developed a variety of allergies stemming from immune deficiency disorders.[8]

Perhaps I should tell my own story of when I became partially paralyzed two months after the birth of my son. I was no longer able to nurse my baby and was told to immediately put him on soy formula. My son, now in his thirties continues to have multiple food allergies, and I continue to live with guilt of doing exactly what my doctor told me.

We are not told that "the amount of phytoestrogens that are in a day's worth of soy infant formula equals that of 5 birth control pills," says Mary G. Enig, Ph.D., president of the Maryland Nutritionists Association. In fact, the Swiss health service estimated that approximately 300 grams of soy protein (about 2 cups) provided the estrogenic equivalent of the Pill.[9]

Nutritional experts believe that such a high amount of phytoestrogenic exposure can be linked with early puberty in girls and hinders physical maturation in boys.[10, 11] In 1998, the FDA received warnings from the British government about the harmful effects resulting from consuming such an overload of phytoestrogens.[12] These effects can be seen in a Johns Hopkins study where it was found that when pregnant rats were fed soy, their male offspring were born with enlarged prostates. The researchers from Johns Hopkins Bloomberg School of Public Health in Maryland also found that when rats were given moderate amounts of daily soy genistein (a phytoestrogen found in soy) testes were underdeveloped as they grew older.[13]

Soybeans have one of the highest phytate levels of any grain or legume that has been studied,[14] and even long periods of cooking at high temperatures will not completely eliminate the phytate levels.[15] The problem created is due to the fact that phytates (an organic acid found within the outer portion of all seeds) block the absorption of essential minerals (e.g., calcium, magnesium, iron, and especially zinc). Soy-induced zinc deficiencies occurring during pregnancy and lactation are thought to be responsible for congenital abnormalities in infants. In children, "insufficient levels of zinc have been associated with lowered learning ability, apathy, lethargy, and mental retardation."[16] The USDA references a study of 372 Chinese school children with very low levels of zinc in their bodies. The children who received zinc supplements had the most improved performance—especially in perception, memory, reasoning, and psychomotor skills such as eye-hand coordination.

As early as 1967, researchers found soy formulas to have a negative effect on zinc absorption and also a strong correlation between increased phytate content and poor growth. Author Sally Fallon warns "a reduced rate of growth is especially serious in the infant as it causes a delay in the accumulation of lipids in the myelin sheath, and hence jeopardizes the development of the brain and nervous system."[17] But for reasons beyond any kind of rationality, the FDA has engaged in a "rigorous approval process" for soy protein isolates (S.P.I.).[18] Perhaps it's now up to us to learn more about what's behind these bureaucratic and inconsistent reports and how we can protect ourselves from the political propaganda concerning healthy foods.

In chapter 6 we discussed soy allergies and particularly why people seem more sensitive to highly processed soy products. Sally Fallon, M.A., a member of the Price Pottenger Nutrition Foundation Advisory Board, and Mary Enig, Ph.D., nutritionist and expert in the field of lipid chemistry, provide some excellent recipes for baby formula. More information on their work can be found in their book *Nourishing Traditions: The Cookbook That Challenges Politically Correct Nutrition and the Diet Dictocrats*, as well as in their well-researched articles published in *Health Freedom News*.[19]

When making baby formula, the authors encourage the use of whole foods instead of isolated soy protein. And according to the Community Nutrition Institute, "Scientists assert that neonatal infants are particularly vulnerable to estrogens and that insufficient research on the long-term health effects of phytoestrogens warrants a ban on the nonprescription sale of soy formula."[20]

The following are some nourishing baby formulas. It's interesting to note that gelatin added to cow's milk not only emulsifies the fat, but it balances the casein (milk protein). This improves the absorption of the fat and also its digestibility. Studies show that "milk containing gelatin is more rapidly and completely digested in the infants" (N. R. Gotthoffer, *Gelatin in Nutrition and Medicine*).[21]

Joel Robbins, D.C., N.D., M.D., author of *Pregnancy, Childbirth & Children's Diet,* tells us that pasteurized milk "doesn't have enough nutrition, due to the pasteurization process, to sustain life. . . ."[22] Furthermore, cow's milk can upset an infant's mineral balance. It's too high in calcium and protein content and can cause digestive problems such as colic and diarrhea. Dr. Robbins advises that if you do use milk, "diluting it with carrot juice and [pure] water helps to offset this problem."[23] Make sure the juice is fresh and organic.

Many nutritionists are now using fresh, unpasteurized goat's milk (where available) instead of cow's milk, because it's closer to human milk than any other milk. Others add green barley or fresh celery juice, maintaining that such living foods provide the necessary enzymes and nutrition that the baby needs if not breast-feeding.

Soy-Free Infant Formula with Milk[24]

> 2 cups (16 oz) raw organic milk or cultured milk, not homogenized
> 1/4 cup whey
> 4 T. lactose
> 1 tsp. cod liver oil
> 1 tsp. unrefined sunflower oil
> 1 tsp. extra virgin olive oil
> 2 tsp. coconut oil
> 2 tsp. brewer's yeast
> 2 tsp. gelatin
> 1 3/4 cup filtered water
> 1 100 mg tablet vitamin C, crushed
> (Never heat formula in a microwave oven!)

Soy-Free, Milk-Free Infant Formula[25]

3^1/$_2$ cups homemade broth (beef, lamb, chicken—hormone- and
    antibiotic-free—or fish)

2 ounces organic liver (liquefy)

5 T. lactose

^{1}/$_4$ cup whey

3 T. coconut oil

1 tsp. cod liver oil

1 tsp. unrefined sunflower oil

2 tsp. extra virgin olive oil

1 100 mg tablet vitamin C, crushed

APPENDIX D
Resources for Cancer Patients

Myths of the Mammogram

Again and again we are asked to have yearly mammograms, but you might want to think twice the next time you see TV ads leading you to believe that regular screening may "add years to your life." Who would think that it might actually take years away from your life? The problem is that we can't observe any major side effects immediately after having a mammogram. However, these may begin to arise as time goes on. Thus, it is extremely important for women to educate themselves so that they can face the barrage of misleading information on the subject.

But this can be a confusing task. The leading cancer organizations have flip-flopped repeatedly over the years on their advice to women in various age groups. Despite what their most recent recommendation might be, note that back in 1976 the *New England Journal of Medicine* reported that the National Cancer Institute (NCI) and the American Cancer Society had "terminated the routine use of X-ray mammography for women under the age of fifty because of its detrimental effects."[1] And in 1994, the National Cancer Institute reported "no difference in the fatality rate [among women in their forties] between those whose breast cancer was detected by mammogram or those diagnosed by touch or palpation alone . . . therefore, in the NCI's judgment, there's no advantage in subjecting these women to regular screening."[2]

William C. Bryce, M.D., founding director of the Well Breast Foundation in California, also suggests the alternatives of thermography and diaphanoscopy, or transillumination of the breast, in his article "The Truth About Breast Cancer" *(Health Freedom News)*. Says Dr. Bryce, "Until the question of lifetime risk due to radiation can be resolved, mammography . . . should not be used in regular routine screening procedures. . . . A few years ago the National Cancer Institute stated that for every fifteen cancers diagnosed by mammography in women under thirty-five, another seventy-five were caused [by mammograms]."[3] Even biostatisticians at the National Cancer Institute and National Academy of Sciences "admit that mammography promotes cancer."[4]

The preventive measures proposed by medical doctors can be costly in more ways than one. Marcus Laux, N.D., reminds us that radiation damage to the cells of the body is cumulative over time. "There is increasing evidence," he says, "that the ionizing radiation used in mammograms is not only harmful, but can even cause the very cancer it's supposed to detect! William Douglas, M.D., further explains that "ionizing radiation mutates cells, and the mechanical pressure can spread cells that are already malignant."[5] *The New England Journal of Medicine* alerts physicians to educate women concerning the risk of "false positive results of a screening test for breast cancer."[6] Screening for breast cancer in this manner is "unjustified . . . and there is no reliable evidence that screening decreases breast-cancer mortality."[7] In fact "data suggest that increased detection [procedures] accounts for some [between 25 and 40 percent] but not all the rising incidence of breast cancer in the United States."[8]

Research from various sources shows that women who have had mammograms are more prone to cancer than those who have never had a mammogram. Look at the studies that show mammograms to be more harmful than beneficial.[9–14] Many pre-eminent cancer researchers, like Dr. John Bailar III, former editor of the *Journal of the National Cancer Institute*, predict that routine mammogram screening over a period of 10 to 15 years may induce breast cancer."[15] Dr. Laux reports that animal studies have shown that pressure on and manipulation of tumors (as might occur during mammography) causes an 80 percent increased chance that they will grow and metastasize![16]

Lorraine Day, M.D., a pathologist and respected orthopedic surgeon, speaks out in her talk "Cancer Doesn't Scare Me Anymore!"[17] She suggests several possible reasons why the regular use of mammography and radiation therapy are significant factors for an increased incidence of breast cancer. As a breast cancer survivor, thanks to holistic medicine, she draws attention to the fact that squeezing the breast repeatedly between the mammography plates may also exert pressure on any tumors that might be present and creates further risk of spreading cancer cells throughout the body.[18]

Through the periodical *Alternative Medicine* (1999) we learn that this information was discovered as far back as 1944 in an article published in *The Lancet* which reports that "mammography can rupture in-situ cysts in the breast and spread cancer cells into surrounding tissue."[19] The documentation for this comes from a study of 110 women in which it was observed that injury to the breast tissue during mammographic examination can lead to "overt invasive cancer" and metastases.[20]

Dr. Maureen Roberts wrote a powerful critique of mammographic screening prior to her own death from breast cancer. In the article "Breast Screening: Time for a Rethink?" published in the *British Medical Journal,* she stated her reservations—that mammography is an unfit screening test in that it's "technologically difficult to perform, the pictures are difficult to interpret, it has a high false positive rate, and we don't know how often to carry it out. We can no longer ignore the possibility that screening may not reduce mortality in women of any age. . . . If screening does little or no good, could it possibly be doing any harm?"[21]

The Lancet confirms that most of the "positive" readings are false positives, and "negative" reports don't guarantee the absence of breast cancer.[22] In fact, according to Charles B. Simone, M.D., founder of the Simone Protective Cancer Center, "about 80 percent to 90 percent are false positives that require excessive workups, such as unnecessary surgical biopsies, and even needless mastectomies."[23] Dr. Simone was a clinical associate in pharmacology and immunology at the National Cancer Institute. Women are not informed that these diagnostic methods can cause cancer "in a small but significant percentage of women."[24]

An earlier publication of *The Lancet* reported in 1985 that over 280,000 women were recruited in order to evaluate the potential risk of breast cancer by mammography. The conclusion was: "Even if you catch it early, with orthodox medicines and chemotherapy, you will not survive any better than if you catch it late,"[25] given the questionable outcome of conventional cancer therapy.

In this controlled trial for women below fifty, none was advised about the potential risks. Despite warnings by a committee of the United States' National Academy of Sciences, the women were exposed to doses that could possibly cause more cancer in the long run than could be prevented by the program.[26] In a ten-year follow-up of the mammography study, the women who refused screening (35 percent) had a lower incidence and mortality from breast cancer than either the mammography group or the control group.[27]

The article "How Mammography Causes Cancer" (*Alternative Medicine,* 1999) brings important data compiled by John W. Gofman, M.D., Ph.D., after forty years of investigation. As an authority on the effects of radiation, Dr. Gofman shows what even low-dose radiation can do to our bodies: 75

percent of breast cancer could be prevented by avoiding or minimizing exposure to the ionizing radiation from mammography, X-rays, and other medical sources.[28] Dr. Gofman strongly believes that there is no "safe threshold" for exposure to low-level ionizing radiation.[29] He additionally tells us that past exposure to ionizing radiation also increases our risk for breast cancer.[30] In fact, Dr. Peat states, "Estrogen and ionizing radiation are the most clearly documented causes of breast cancer."[31] And, for this reason, antiestrogenic hormones such as pregnenolone and progesterone can aid in compensating for the exposure to many estrogenic sources—helping to reduce our overall risk.[32]

There is so much information about the potential risks of routine mammograms that it is essential for all women to look into the matter for themselves and make informed decisions. For more about radiation levels in mammography, important questions to ask prior to scheduling a mammogram, and the funding and politics behind cancer treatments, I urge you to read Virginia M. Soffa's *The Journey Beyond Breast Cancer* as well as other related books in the suggested reading list at the end of this chapter. Also see appendix F for the list of studies reporting on the dangers of mammograms.

We can look to the discussion in *Healthy Healing* for an accurate answer to the question, "Should I or should I not have a mammogram?" Dr. Linda Rector-Page warns that "although mammograms have improved in the last twenty years both in clarity and amount of dosage, we still hear enough horror stories about swift fibroid onset to recommend that mammograms should not be done routinely or without suspected cause." She also notes that mammograms and low-dose X-rays may result in iodine depletion and thyroid problems.[33] She continues with the most prudent statement I have heard yet on the subject: "While early detection can mean less radical medical intervention, prevention through immune enhancement and a healthy lifestyle should be the primary goal—not early detection."[34]

One alternative to the mammogram is the sonogram (ultrasound imaging), which uses sound waves rather than electromagnetic waves and is, according to author Dee Ito, particularly accurate "in determining the presence of invasive cancers [and] cystic breasts."[35] Nonetheless, further studies are needed as there are preliminary indications that even sonography produces some cellular changes in the tissues. Another highly favored cancer detection test that we have already discussed in chapter 5 is called the AMAS (Anti-Malignin in Serum). This non-invasive test uses no x-rays and is quite accurate. For more information see page 147.

Thermography, another method of detection, was first used in the 1950s. Since then, the technology (also known as Thermal Imaging Processing) has been considerably improved. Philip Hoekstra, Ph.D., has performed thermography scanning on more than 50,000 women for a period of almost thirty years. He claims that in most cases this method is superior to mammography—especially for early detection of breast cancer.[36]

Although this screening technique has been proven to be noninvasive and nontoxic, you may question, "Why don't we hear more about thermography from our physicians?" The business of medicine views this type of technology as "competition" to the mainstream approach, which includes mammographic radiation, chemotherapy, and often multiple surgical procedures. We might consider here that profit often determines the choices made available to us—choices that do not always take into consideration our primary need of safely facilitating our recovery. The only way we will see significant changes in the methods made available for detecting abnormalities in the breasts will be for women themselves to insist on access to what they know is safer. This applies both to screening techniques and to hormone replacement therapy itself.

THERMOGRAPHIC BREAST IMAGING

As a Board Certified Clinical Thermographer, William C. Amalu, DC, DABCT, DIACT, FIACT, tells us that thermographic breast screening is brilliantly simple in its application, yet quite complex in its methodology. Thermography detects and measures the infrared heat emanating from the surface of the body and translates this information into anatomical images. With this type of breast cancer screening, the resulting images are analyzed for asymmetrical areas of increased heat and blood vessel activity (one breast compared to the other). These abnormal areas of heat, secondary to increased blood vessel activity are due to a process called neoangiogenesis (new blood vessel formation). Breast cancers create their own blood vessels to ensure a constant supply of nutrients to encourage more growth.

In order to enhance the detection of this process, an additional set of images is taken after the patient's hands are placed in ice-cold water for one minute. This causes an autonomic nervous system response. Our normal blood circulation is under the control of our autonomic nervous system, which governs our body functions without our conscious will. In response to the cold-water stress, our autonomic nervous system reduces the amount of blood going to the breast in order to maintain normal body core temperature. However, the blood vessels that cancerous and precancerous cells create are not under autonomic control, and are thus unaffected by the cold water stress. These blood vessels remain open and therefore stand out clearly on the thermographic image as a "hot spot." This in turn increases the suspicion that a cancerous process is present.

Another benefit of this technology is its role in primary breast cancer detection. Breast thermography indirectly gives us the ability to observe the influence of hormones on the breasts. Research has determined that the single greatest risk factor for the future development of breast cancer is lifetime exposure of the breasts to estrogen.[37] In fact, Dr. Raymond Peat's research shows that "estrogen is an important factor in aging and cancer . . ."[38] More than ever we now need to learn ways to evaluate and control the influence of estrogen on the breasts.

Thermography provides us with a safe method of primary breast cancer detection. When hormone activity in the breast is dominated by estrogen, a specific type of infrared image (as described above) is produced; thus, warning the patient of this condition.[39] Once this is identified, a woman can take a significant pro-active role in prevention. With this information in hand, many doctors start their patients on a regimen of progesterone cream applied directly to the breasts. The progesterone enters the breast tissue and counteracts the effects of excess estrogen. Using follow-up infrared imaging, the treatment can be monitored and changed if necessary to meet the needs of each woman's own unique response. Once the hormone balance has been restored to the breasts, a woman's overall breast cancer risk is greatly reduced. Dr. Amalu, Vice President of the International Academy of Clinical Thermology, and Member of the International Thermographic Society and member of the American Academy of Medical Infrared Imaging, and International Academy of Clinical Thermology, encourages us all to learn as much as we can about thermographic imaging, its safety, and the importance of every woman's ability to access this procedure.

You can find more information by calling (650) 361-8908, emailing Dr. Amalu at info@breastthermography.com, or writing 621 Middlefield Road, Redwood City, California 94063. Go to www.breastthermography.com for more information. In order to locate a qualified breast thermography center in your area go to www.iact-org.org/links.html. If you don't find a center near you, look back frequently as this list is updated often. For studies on the dangers of mammograms, see appendix F.

USEFUL READING

Betrayers of the Truth: Fraud and Deceit in the Halls of Science, by William Broad & Nicholas Wade (New York: Simon & Schuster, Inc., 1983).

Cancer Prevention and Nutritional Therapies, by Richard A. Passwater, Ph.D. (New Canaan, CT: Keats Publishing, Inc., 1994).

Cancer Therapy: The Independent Consumer's Guide to Non-toxic Treatment & Prevention, by Ralph W. Moss, Ph.D. (New York: Equinox Press, 1992).

Choices in Healing, by Michael Lerner (Cambridge, MA: The MIT Press, 1994).

The Healing of Cancer, by Barry Lynes (Ontario, Canada: Marcus Books, 1990).

How to Get Well, by Paavo Airola (Phoenix: Health Plus Publishing, 1985).

How to Prevent Breast Cancer, by Ross Pelton (New York: Simon & Schuster, 1995).

The Journey Beyond Breast Cancer, by Virginia M. Soffa (Rochester, VT: Healing Arts Press, 1994).

Love, Medicine & Miracles, by Bernie S. Siegel, M.D. (New York: Harper & Row, 1990).

My Healing from Breast Cancer, by Barbara Joseph, M.D. (New Canaan, CT: Keats Publishing, Inc., 1996).

Now That You Have Cancer, by Drs. Robert W. Bradford and Michael L. Culbert (Chula Vista, CA: Bradford Foundation, 1992).

The Persecution and Trial of Gaston Naessens, by Christopher Bird (Tiburon, CA: Krammer Inc., 1991).

The Scientific Validation of Herbal Medicine, by Daniel B. Mowrey, Ph.D. (New Canaan, CT: Keats Publishing, Inc., 1990).

Sex, Lies, and Menopause: The Shocking Truth about Hormone Replacement Therapy, by T. S. Wiley, Julie Taguchi, and Bent Formby (New York: William Morrow, 2003).

Sharks Don't Get Cancer, by William I. Lane and Linda Comac (New York: Avery Publishing Group, Inc., 1992).

Third Opinion, by John M. Fink (Garden City Park, New York: Avery Publishing Group, Inc., 1988).

The books listed above provide information on alternatives to conventional cancer treatment. I strongly recommend you also contact the organizations on page 221.

EDUCATIONAL WEB SITES

Hundred of articles, studies, and research papers regarding estrogen's role in the risk of cancer can be found on the following sites. These same links also provide valuable information about the harmful effects of soy on thyroid function and soy's estrogenic effect on breast tissue:

http://www.healthcentral.com/news/newsfulltext.cfm?ID=46067&src=n59
http://www.cumc.columbia.edu/news/in-vivo/Vol2_Iss10_may26_03/

http://www.westonaprice.org/index.html
http://www.soyonlineservice.co.nz/

ORGANIZATIONS

American Institute for Cancer Research
1759 R Street, N.W.
Washington, DC 20009
CANHELP, Inc.
Attn: Marketing Director
3111 Paradise Bay Road
Port Ludlow, WA 98365-9771

Foundation for Advancement in Cancer Therapy (F.A.C.T.)
Attn: Marketing Director
Box 1242 Old Chelsea Station
New York, NY 10113

The International Association of Cancer Victors and Friends, Inc.
Attn: Marketing Director
7740 West Manchester Avenue, Suite 110
Playa del Rey, CA 90293

Y-Me
Attn: Marketing Director
National Breast Cancer Organization
212 W. Van Buren
Chicago, IL 60607

BREAST CANCER AWARENESS

The multitudes of runs, hikes, walks, and other fund-raising events produce hundreds of millions of dollars to fight breast cancer, but unfortunately, breast cancer continues to be on the rise. When it comes to Breast Cancer Awareness Month, women must invest their time and money into other projects and treatments that will prevent cancer more effectively:

- Eat organic foods (free of harmful hormones and other toxic chemicals) as often as possible.

- Replace commercial household cleaners and garden pesticides with organic and biodegradable products.
- Drink pure (filtered or distilled) water.
- Eliminate synthetic hormone treatments such as HRT and the Pill (both known to promote breast cancer).
- Sustain hormonal and nutritional balance by opposing environmental xenoestrogens with botanical progesterone and phytonutrients.
- Detoxify the body and reduce stress.
- Investigate safe and more accurate screening techniques such as the AMAS or thermography exams.

A BRIEF INTRODUCTION TO NATURAL CANCER THERAPY

Progesterone demonstrates its beneficial physiological effects on the body much more productively when other areas are in balance. However, its effect is limited when long-term nutritional and dietary habits have created more highly concentrated levels of estrogen to progesterone, as is illustrated with the following example:

At this time there are an untold number of women (forty years and older) who have been on prescribed estrogen (any form—estradiol, estrone, estriol) for many years. One elderly lady (in her eighties) had been on oral estrogen and never had a problem until one day during a routine medical examination the doctors discovered she had breast cancer. The effects of our accumulation of estrogens can take a long time to appear. It can take six to eight years before breast, ovarian, or uterine cancer is detected. However, this diagnosis often comes at an earlier time in life because younger women are consuming large amounts of foods containing high levels of estrogens daily, for example, soy, dairy, or meats containing hormones and antibiotics.

Heavy meat consumption has been proven to stimulate high estrogen levels. "A nonsteroidal growth promoter with estrogenic activity that is used by the U.S. meat industry induces estrogenic responses in primary cultured breast cells and breast cancer cell lines."[40] Adding high dairy consumption to this type of dietary lifestyle causes a higher acidic internal environment pushing pH levels, as well as the hormonal levels, out of balance. Such eating habits make the small supplementation of competing progesterone not as effective at countering estrogen's abnormal stimulatory effect of cell growth.

Once nutritional, hormonal, and neurological approaches have been adopted, we can prevent or possibly reverse cancer through conscientiously combining some of the natural alternatives that are listed below. There are studies and untold numbers of documented cases that prove every one of these substances, found in their natural form, to be powerful in fighting cancer. According to Dr. E. T. Krebs Jr., co-discoverer and developer of laetrile-amygdalin, taking a drug or anything foreign to our cells has never been found to prevent or cure a disease. However, prevention and cures can result when using natural substances from our own environment—if the substances are bioidentical to the molecular forms in the body and therefore bioactive in addressing our deficiency.[41]

The following is a list of health remedies that have proven to work for so many in the fight against cancer and other diseases.

Plant-Based Dietary Elements—Organic, if Possible

Fresh, raw fruits and vegetables
Whole grains (including brown rice)
Vegetable protein; raw nuts and seeds
Raw (bitter) almonds (containing laetrile)
Olive and coconut oils
Soluble fiber
Fasting with fresh fruit juices in a.m. and vegetable juices in p.m. (lemon, apple, orange; carrot, beet, spinach, chard, cabbage, kale, parsley, asparagus, tomato, etc.)
Yams
Mushrooms (reishi, shiitake, etc.); Krestin (Japanese mushroom extract)
Onions

Aged garlic extract
Aloe vera
Sea vegetables, including kelp (laminaria)
Algae (chlorella, spirulina, dunaliella bardawil, sargassum, kjellmanianum)
Green barley
Wheatgrass
Chlorophyll
Lactobacilli (e.g., acidophilus, bifidis, and bulgaricus, in yogurt and other cultured milk products)
Amino acids (including l-carnitine, l-cysteine, l-glutathione, l-methionine, etc.)

Vitamins, Minerals, Antioxidants, Enzymes

Vitamins A, E, C, D, K, B-complex; natural carotenoid complex
Calcium
Magnesium
Zinc
Tellurium
Selenium

Pycnogenol
Germanium
Coenzyme Q 10
Superoxide dismutase (S.O.D.)
Proteolytic enzymes
l-Asparaginase
Bromelain

Herbs, Teas, Spices

Hoxsey herbs

Chinese medicine

Astragalus

Echinacea

Black radish

Chaparral

Dandelion

Silymarin (milk thistle)

Pau d'arco

Red clover

Rhubarb

Slippery elm

Suma

Iscador

Actinada

Kermesbeurro (as paste)

Jason Winters tea

Green tea

Essiac tea

Turmeric (circumin)

Basil leaves

Black pepper

Poppy seeds

Cinnamon

Asafoetida

Drumstick leaves

Kandathipili

Manathakkahli leaves

Neem flowers

Ponnakanni

Miscellaneous Natural Treatments

Antineoplastons (peptides that inhibit cancer growth)

Beta-1,3 glucan

Bovine cartilage

Camphor derivative (714-X)

Castor oil packs

Colon cleansing

Detoxification therapy

DMSO

EDTA chelation therapy

Electromagnetic treatment (Bjorn Nordenstrom)

Hydrazine sulfate

Intravenous amino acids/vitamins

Intravenous vitamin C

Hyperthermia

Homeopathic liver drainer

Laetrile-amygdalin*

Live cell therapy

Liver flushes

MGN-3 extract

Oxygen therapy

pH balancing

Phototherapy

Poly-MVA

Shark cartilage

STI571

Suramin

Thioproline

Tumostereone

---

* Vitamin B_{17} from apricot kernels; to read about why it is not legal to sell laetrile in the U.S. but it is elsewhere, see www.geocities.com/vialls/laetrile1.html/

This list is only a beginning. More importantly, it should be viewed in the context of the whole-body approach to creating *host resistance* to disease. There are many more counter-agents to cancer, as well as vaccines and drugs that contain synthetic components and therefore are not listed here. Please consult the references for more information and study all the pros and cons that may be involved.

Resources for Preventive Medicine

FINDING A DOCTOR

Hearing and seeing the multitude of influences that come into our lives by means of the Internet, radio, and TV—many of which are financed and approved by the pharmaceutical industry and the advertising monopolies—causes me to reflect on my past vulnerable state of needing help and obediently taking my prescribed medications. Back in those days I was completely oblivious to the politics behind high cost designer drugs, high tech medical equipment, or standard HRT, all of which generate enormous profits for those in the conventional medical field. Today, however, natural healthcare alternatives have provided me with a peace of mind never thought possible.

Having said this, here is a sample letter for those of you who want to take that first step toward finding an open-minded health care provider interested in alternative and preventive medicine.

DRAFT LETTER

(Your Name)
(Address)
(Phone number)

Dear Doctor_____,

I am interested in finding a physician who can guide me in the use of natural hormone supplementation. If you find that this approach to health care goes along with your program for treating women in your practice, and if you can relate to my need to find a doctor who does not wish to use synthetic hormones but to instead prescribe natural progesterone, please have your nurse or receptionist contact me for an appointment. Thank you for your attention to this important matter.

Sincere wishes,

_____

For the doctor who says, "Sorry, I just can't provide these natural hormones because we don't have enough information or studies in this area," you might want to hook up to the worldwide computer search network or provide him or her with some of the studies listed in appendix F. You or your doctor can order and receive abstracts and publications on any medical subject—which would include some of the natural alternatives referred to in this book. To support you in your freedom of choice, the following organizations can help you with your questions and your search for a doctor in your area who practices alternative medicine.

American Association of Naturopathic Physicians
601 Valley Street, Suite 105
Seattle, WA 98109
(866) 538-2267
www.naturopathic.org

American Chiropractic Association (ACA)
1701 Clarendon Boulevard
Arlington, VA 22209
(800) 986-4636
www.amerchiro.org

American Holistic Health Association
P.O. Box 17400
Anaheim, CA 92817-7400
(714)779-6152
www.ahha.org

American College for Advancement in Medicine
23121 Verdugo Drive
Laguna Hills, CA 92654
(800) 532-3688
www.acam.org/generalpub

American Institute for Cancer Research
1759 R Street, N.W.
P.O. Box 97167
Washington, DC 20090-7167
(800) 843-8114
www.aicr.org

American Osteopathic Association
142 E. Ontario Street
Chicago, IL 60611
(800) 621-1773
www.aoa-net.org

Center for Holistic Life Extension
482 W. San Ysidro Boulevard, Suite 1365
San Ysidro, CA 92713
(800) 664-8660
www.extendlife.com

International Chiropractors Association (ICA)
1110 N. Glebe Road, Suite 1000
Arlington, VA 22201
(800) 423-4690
www.chiropractic.org

National Center for Homeopathy
801 North Fairfax Street, Suite 306
Alexandria, VA 22314
(877) 624-0613
www.homeopathic.org

For more information on chiropractic science, education, techniques, and qualifications, as well as endorsements from the medical community, go to: www.healthcare-alternatives.com and click on the book: *Today's Health Alternative*.

SEEKING NATURAL ALTERNATIVES

Information about natural progesterone and related topics can be accessed on the Internet. Also, please see appendix G for sources of natural progesterone. And should you want to do an extensive search for progesterone and sources for preventive medicine, use your web browser to search for the term "natural progesterone." Be sure to include the word *natural* so you won't be inundated with information on the synthetic estrogen and progestin products.

Many women are finding this means of communication quite gratifying as they discover friends to talk to about health or nutritional problems similar to their own. Thanks to the electronic bulletin boards, women are hearing from other women who currently use progesterone. So today, in an instant, we can find out that we're not alone and that our situation is not unique. Often we can learn from the shared experiences of others. Be cautious, however, since online claims can so easily be made without any documentation or verification.

USEFUL READING*

Acid & Alkaline, by Herman Aihara (Ohsawa Macrobiotic Foundation, 1986).

Activate Your Immune System, by Leonid Ber, M.D. (Green Bay, WI: IMPAKT Communications, Inc., 1998).

Alternative Medicine, by The Burton Goldberg Group (Puyallup, WA: Future Medicine Publishing, Inc., 1993).

Aspartame (NutraSweet): Is It Safe?, by H. J. Roberts (Philadelphia: Charles Press, 1990).

The Bitter Truth About Artificial Sweeteners, by Dennis W. Remington and Barbara W. Higa (Provo, UT: Vitality House International, 1987).

The Chelation Way, by Dr. Walker Morton (New York: Avery Publishing Group, 1990).

Choices in Healing, by Michael Lerner (Cambridge, MA: MIT Press, 1994).

Coconut Oil for Health and Beauty, by Cynthia and Laura Hopfazel (Summertown, TN: Book Publishing Co., 2003).

Coenzyme Q-10 by William H. Lee, R.Ph., Ph.D. (New Canaan, CT: Keats Publishing, Inc., 1987).

Everybody's Guide to Homeopathic Medicines, by S. Cummings, M.D., and D. Ullman, M.P.H. (New York: J. P. Tarcher, Inc., 1980).

Everyday Miracles, by Linda Johnston, M.D. (Van Nuys, CA: Christine Kent Agency, 1991).

The Family Health Guide to Homeopathy, by Barry Rose, M.D. (Berkeley, CA: Celestial Arts, 1993).

Food Enzymes, by Humbart Santillo, B.S., M.H. (Prescott, AZ: Holm Press, 1991).

Forty Something Forever: A Consumer's Guide to Chelation Therapy, by Harold and Arline Brecher (Troup, TX: Health Savers Press, 1992).

Fresh Vegetable and Fruit Juices, by N.W. Walker, D.Sc. (Prescott, AZ: Norwalk Press, 1978).

---

* For books on NHRT, see appendix G.

Garlic: Nature's Original Remedy, by Stephen Fulder and John Blackwood (Rochester, VT: Healing Arts Press, 1991).

Garlic for Health, by Benjamin Lau, M.D., Ph.D. (Brushton, NY: Teach Services, 1988).

Green Barley Essence, The Ideal Fast Food, by Yoshihide Hagiwara, M.D. (New Canaan, CT: Keats Publishing, Inc., 1986).

The Healing Miracles of Coconut Oil, by Bruce Fife, N.D. (Colorado Springs, CO: HealthWise Publications, 2000).

Healthy Healing: A Guide to Self-Healing for Everyone, by Linda G. Rector-Page, N.D., Ph.D. (Soquel, CA: Healthy Healing Publications, 1997).

Healing Nutrients, by Patrick Quillin, Ph.D., R.D. (New York: Vintage Books, 1986).

Heart Frauds: Uncovering the Biggest Health Scam in History, by Charles T. McGee, M.D. (Colorado Springs, CO: HealthWise Publications, 2000).

Homeopathic Medicine for Pregnancy and Childbirth, by Richard Moskowitz, M.D. (Berkeley, CA: North Atlantic Books, 1992).

How to Get Well, by Paavo Airola, Ph.D. (Phoenix, AZ: Health Plus Publishers, 1980).

If It's Not Food, Don't Eat It, by Kelly Hayford (Lincoln, NE: iUniverse.com, Inc., 2004).

An Introduction to Young Living Essential Oils and Aromatherapy, by D. Gary Young, N.D. (Scottsdale, AZ: Essential Press, 1996).

Jane Brody's Nutrition Book, by Jane Brody (New York: Bantam Books, 1982).

Know Your Fats: The Complete Primer for Understanding the Nutrition of Fats, Oils and Cholesterol, by Mary G. Enig (Silver Spring, MD: Bethesda Press, 2000).

The Natural Pharmacy, by Skye Lininger, D.C.; Jonathan Wright, M.D.; Steve Austin, N.D.; Donald Brown, N.D.; Alan Gaby, M.D. (Rocklin, CA: Prima Health, 1998).

The Nutrition Desk Reference, by Robert H. Garrison, Jr., M.A.R., Ph.D., and Elizabeth Somer, M.A., R.D. (New Canaan, CT: Keats Publishing, Inc., 1990).

Prescription For Nutritional Healing, by James F. Balch and Phyllis A. Balch, C.N.C. (Garden City Park, NY: Avery Publishing Group Inc., 1990).

A Reference Guide for Essential Oils, compiled by Pat Leathan and Connie Higley (Topeka, KS: Abundant Health, 1996).

Saturated Fat May Save Your Life!, by Bruce Fife, N.D. (Colorado Spirings, CO: HealthWise Publications, 2001).

Seasalt's Hidden Powers, by Jacques de Langre, Ph.D. (Magalia, CA: Happiness Press, 1993).

Sunlight, by Zane R. Kime, M.D., M.S. (Penryn, CA: World Health Publications, 1980).

Take Control of Your Health and Escape The Sickness Industry, by Elaine
  Hollingsworth (Queensland, Australia: Empowerment Press International,
  2000).
Your Body's Many Cries for Water, by F. Batmanghelidj, M.D. (Falls Church, VA:
  Global Health Solutions, Inc., 1992).
What Your Doctor Didn't Learn in Medical School, by Stuart M. Berger, M.D.
  (New York: William Morrow and Company, Inc., 1988).
Women's Health Letter is a monthly, subscription-based newsletter for women
  over 40 written by health advocate and nutritionist Nan Kathryn Fuchs,
  Ph.D. It contains easy-to-understand, science-based articles of particular
  interest to pre- and postmenopausal women. For subscription information
  call (800) 728-2288.

FREE-RANGE AND ORGANIC MEAT PRODUCERS

For more information about organic meats, as well as the brands of meat
that are free of antibiotics, growth hormone stimulants, herbicides, and pesticides, contact the Organic Trade Association, (413) 774-7511,
www.ota.com. For further education on the subject, call (877) 773-1779 or
go to www.organic-center.org.

APPENDIX F

Clinical Studies and Research Reports

PROGESTERONE AND OSTEOPOROSIS

Medical Hypotheses states that "progesterone and not estrogen is the missing factor . . . effective in reversing osteoporosis. . . . The presence or absence of estrogen supplements [in subjects studied] had no discernible effect on osteoporosis benefits." The journal also claims that the use of natural progesterone is not only safer but less expensive than using Provera (medroxy-progesterone) and that "progesterone deficiency rather than estrogen deficiency is a major factor in the pathogenesis of menopausal osteoporosis."[1] We need to be aware of the frightening accounts and adverse effects of Provera and other synthetic progestins (nervousness, depression, insomnia, immune and circulatory disorders, and much more).

Progesterone works to stimulate bone production, even when estrogen activity is low or absent. Because progesterone appears to work on the osteoblasts (bone-building cells) to increase bone formation, it would complement estrogen's action of decreasing bone resorption, as stated by Dr. J. C. Prior, who explains further that progesterone fastens to receptors on the osteoblasts and "increases the rate of bone remodeling."[2] Estrogen helps to slow bone loss, but progesterone is proactive through its stimulatory effect on the osteoblasts and thus directly encourages bone buildup. Synthetic progestins diminish the supply of natural progesterone, which further accelerates the osteoporotic changes within the bone.

VITAMIN THERAPY TO COUNTER ESTROGEN DOMINANCE

Carlton Fredericks, Ph.D, suggests that the use of vitamin A and E cream for atrophic vaginitis is much safer than the synthetic estrogen creams so frequently prescribed by many medical doctors. He says that "both [Cynonal and Premarin] have side effects and may also irritate you."[3] Of much greater concern, however, is the fact that Premarin consists of estrone and estradiol, which have been shown to be carcinogenic.[4] Fortunately, there are companies who make the natural progesterone cream. Herbs such as maca root and Panax ginseng found in most health stores work wonders for vaginal dryness and many other conditions.

Dr. Fredericks, in his book *Guide to Women's Nutrition,* states that "vitamin B complex cuts down excess activity of estrogen, whether prescribed for menopause or birth control or produced by the woman's own ovaries." B complex, he emphasizes, "helps to counteract the effects of high levels of estrogen which has not been detoxified by the liver."[5]

THE ESTROGEN AFTERMATH

Evidence now shows estrogen to have harmful effects on the brain, causing stress, depression, and exhaustion due to overstimulation. While stimulating in the short term, over time it tends to be degenerative[6–8] We are currently being indoctrinated with the theory of estrogen's role in the prevention of Alzheimer's disease, but when examining the facts, we find the reverse to be largely the case—that it's an excess of estrogen coupled with a scarcity of progesterone that can bring on dementia.[9, 10] One study has shown that women on estrogen replacement have a higher rate of Alzheimer's than men,[11] and another that estrogen exposure in midlife elevates the risk for this disease in later years.[12]

And let's not overlook the positive correlation between "the pill" and breast cancer in younger women. In describing her personal experience with breast cancer, Barbara Joseph, M.D., emphasizes the need to avoid synthetic hormones. She especially encourages a diet of organically produced foods to reduce our exposure to the growth hormones that contribute to our estrogenic overload.[13] For brands of meats that are free of antibiotics, hormones, growth stimulants, herbicides, and pesticides, see appendix E.

The concerns of a great many other women who have been stricken with cancers are passionately echoed by authors such as Virginia Soffa *(The Journey Beyond Breast Cancer)* and Rose Kushner *(Alternatives: New Developments in the War on Breast Cancer).*[14] When Kushner calls pharmaceutical estrogens "fertilizers that stimulate and speed the growth of mammary carcinomas,"[15] we need to pay attention.

More and more women, in their search for safer choices, are standing their ground against the advertising campaigns. As role models they lead the way, directing light upon the dark barricade erected by big business and lending their peers the courage to help end this dangerous epidemic.

EVIDENCE-BASED CLINICAL STUDIES AND RESEARCH REPORTS (RECOMMENDED READING FOR YOUR DOCTOR)

Estrogen

"Effects of Estrone, Estradiol, and Estriol on Hormone-Responsive Human Breast Cancer in Long-Term Tissue," by Marc Lippman et al., *Cancer Research* 32, June 1977, 1901–07.

"The Cellular Effects of Estrogens on Neuroendocrine Tissues," by F. Naftolin et al., *J Steroid Biochem* 30, No. 1–6, 1988, 195–207.

"Androgens and Women's Health," by G. P. Redmond, *Int J Fertil Womens Med* 43, No. 2, 1998, 91–97.

"Drugged Waters: Does It Matter That Pharmaceuticals Are Turning Up in Water Supplies?," *Science News* 153, March 21, 1998.

"Microtubule and Plasmalemmal Reorganization: Acute Response to Estrogen," by C. M. Szego et al., *Am J Physiol* 254, No. 6, June 1988, E775–85.

"Estradiol Reduces Calcium Currents in Rat Neostriatal Neurons Via a Membrane Receptor," by P. G. Mermelstein et al., *J Neurosci* 16, No. 2, January 1996, 595–604.

"17 Beta Estradiol Potentiates Kainate–Induced Currents Via Activation of the cAMP Cascade," by Q. Gu and R. L. Moss, *J Neurosci* 16, No. 11, June 1996, 3620–29.

"Effect of Intrauterine Estriol on Reproductive Function in the Rabbit," by W. P. Dmowski et al., *Fertil Steril* 28, No. 3, 1977, 262–68.

"Estrogen Use and All-Cause Mortality: Preliminary Results From The Lipid Research Clinics Program Follow-up Study," by T. L. Bush et al., *Journal of the American Medical Association* 249, 1983, 903–06.

"Effects of Estrogen or Estrogen/Progestin Regimens on Heart Disease Risk Factors in Postmenopausal Women," by the Writing Group for the PEP Trial, *Journal of the American Medical Association* 273, No. 3, January 18, 1995.

"Estrogen in the Environment," by Rick Weiss, *Washington Post,* January 25, 1994, 10–13.

Progesterone

"Absorption of Oral Progesterone Is Influenced by Vehicle and Particle Size," by Joel T. Hargrove et al., *American Journal of Obstetrics and Gynecology* 161, No. 4, October 1989, 948–51.

"Observations on the Effect of Progesterone on Carcinoma of the Cervix," by R. Hertz et al., *Journal of the National Cancer Institute* 11, 1951, 867–73.

"Use of the Progestogen Challenge Test to Reduce the Risk of Endometrial Cancer," by R. D. Gambrell et al., *Obstetrics & Gynecology* 55, 1980, 732–38.

"The Use of Progesterone in the Treatment of PMS," by W. S. Maxson, *Clin. Obstet. Gynecol.* 30, 1987, 465–80.

"Long-Term Effect of Transdermal Hormonal Therapy on Aspects of Quality of Life in Postmenopausal Women," by I. Wiklund et al., *Muturitas* 3, March 14, 1992, 225–36.

"Diverse Modes of Action of Progesterone and Its Metabolites," by V. B. Mahesh et al., *J Steroid Biochem Molec Biol* 56, 1996, 209–19.

"Progesterone Inhibits Growth and Induces Apoptosis in Breast Cancer Cells: Inverse Effects on Bcl-2 and p53," by B. Formby and T. S. Wiley, *Annals of Clin and Lab Science* 28, 1998: 360–69.

"Progesterone Receptors and Human Breast Cells," by M. G. Clark, *Breast Cancer Research and Treatment* 3, 1983: 157–63.

"Prevention of Endometrial Hyperplasia by Progesterone During Long-Term Estradiol Replacement: Influence of Bleeding Pattern and Secretory Changes," by D. L. Moyer et al., *Fertility and Sterility* 59, 1993: 992–97.

"Progesterone: an Overview and Recent Advances," by M. B. Aufrere et al., *J Pharmaceut Sci* 65, 1976: 783.

"Natural Progesterone" (transcript), by John R. Lee, *Cancer Forum* 13, No. 5/6, Winter 1995–1995.

"Micronized Progesterone: Vaginal and Oral Uses," by J. A. Simon, *Clinical Obstetrics and Gynecology* 38, No. 4, 1995: 902–14.

"Breast Cancer Incidence in Women with a History of Progesterone Deficiency," by L. D. Cowan et al., *American Journal of Epidemiology* 114, 1981: 209–17.

"Serum Progesterone and Prognosis in Operable Breast Cancer," by P. E. Mohr et al., *British J Cancer* 73, 1996: 1552–55.

"The Efficacy of Progesterone in Achieving Successful Pregnancy: II. In Women with Pure Luteal Phase Defects," by Jerome H. Check and Harriet G. Adelson, *International Fertility* 32, No 21, 1987: 139–41.

"Antenatal Progesterone and Intelligence," by Katharina Dalton, *British Journal of Psychiatry* 114, 1968.

"The Premenstrual Syndrome," by Katharina Dalton, *British Medical Journal* 1, 1953.

"Prenatal Progesterone and Educational Attainments," by Katharina Dalton, *British Journal of Psychiatry* 129, 1976.

"Perimenopause: The Complex Endocrinology of the Menopausal Transition," by J. C. Prior, *Endocrine Reviews* 19, No. 4, August 1998, 397–428.

"Progesterone May Play a Major Role in the Prevention of Nerve Disease," by Warren E. Leary, *New York Times,* June 27,1995: C3.

Cancer

"Estrogen Replacement Therapy and Fatal Ovarian Cancer," by C. Rodriquez et al., *American Journal of Epidemiology* 141, 1995: 828-34.

"Medical Progress: Endometrial Carcinoma," by Peter G. Rose, *New England Journal of Medicine* 335, August 29, 1996: 640–49.

"Oral Contraceptives and Breast Cancer Risk Among Younger Women," by L. A., Brinton et al., *Journal of the National Cancer Institute* 98, No. 11, June 1995: 827–35.

"Molecular Origin of Cancer; Catechol Estrogen-3, 4-quinones as Endogenous Tumor Initiators," by E. L. Cavalieri et al., *Proc Natl Acad Sci* 94, 1994: 10937–42.

"Molecular Mechanisms of Estrogen Carcinogenesis," by J. D. Yager et al., *Ann Rev Pharmacol Toxicol* 36, 1996: 203–32.

"New Role for Estrogen in Cancer?," by Robert F. Service, *Science* 179, March 13, 1998: 1631–33.

"The Role of Estrogen in Mammary Carcinogenesis," by J. Fischman et al., *Annals of the New York Academy of Sciences* 768, No 91, 1995.

"New Drug Poses Risk of Ovarian Cancer," by Samuel S. Epstein and Pat Cody, *Chicago Tribune,* April 19, 1998.

"Reproductive Estrogens Linked to Reproductive Abnormalities, Cancer," by Beth Hileman, *Chemical and Engineering News,* January 31, 1994: 19–23.

"The Risk of Breast Cancer after Estrogen and Estrogen-Progestin Replacement," by L. Bergkvist et al., *New England Journal of Medicine* 321, 1989: 293–97.

Osteoporosis

"Endogenous Hormones and the Risk of Hip and Vertebral Fracture Among Older Women," by S. R. Cummings et al., *New England Journal of Medicine* 339, September 10, 1998: 733–38.

"Comparison of the Effects of Progesterone and Estrogen on Established Bone Loss in Ovariectomized Aged Rats," by E. L. Berengolts et al., *Cells and Materials* Supplement 1, 1991: 105–11.

"Effects of Progesterone on Post-Ovariectomy Bone Loss In Aged Rats," by E. L. Berengolts et al., *J Bone Min Res* 5, 1990: 1143–47.

"Spinal Bone Loss and Ovulatory Disturbances," by J. C. Prior et al., *International Journal Gynecol Obstet* 34, 1990: 253–56.

"Progesterone as a Bone-Trophic Hormone," by J. C. Prior, *Endocrine Reviews* 11, No. 2, 1990: 386–98.

"Significance of Molecular Configuration Specificity—The Case of Progesterone and Osteoporosis," by John R. Lee, *Townsend Letter for Doctors*, June 1993: 558.

"Influence of Estrogen and Progesterone on Matrix-Induced Endochondral Bone Formation," by C. C. Burnett et al., *Calcif. Tissure Int* 35, 1983: 609–14.

"Is Natural Progesterone the Missing Link in Osteoporosis Prevention and Treatment?," by John R. Lee, *Medical Hypotheses*, 1991: 35, 316, 318.

"Menopausal Hormone Replacement Therapy with Continuous Daily Oral Micronized Estradiol and Progesterone," by T. Joel Hargrove et al., *Obstetrics & Gynecology* 73, No. 4, April 1989: 606–12.

"Hormonal and Nutritional Aspects of Osteoporosis," by John R. Lee, *Health and Nutrition* 6, No. 7, 1991: 4.

"Effect of Fluoride Treatment on Fracture Rate in Postmenopausal Women," by B. L. Riggs et al., *New England Journal of Medicine* 322, 1990: 802–09.

"If Estrogens Retard Osteoporosis, Are They Worth the Cancer Risk?," by M. J. Halberstam, *Mod. Med.* 45, No. 9, 1977: 15.

"Progesterone and the Prevention of Osteoporosis," by J. C. Prior et al., *Canadian Journal of OB/Gyn & Women's Health Care* 3, No. 4, 1991: 181.

"Spinal Bone Loss and Ovulatory Disturbances," by J. C. Prior et al., *International Journal Gynecol. Obstet.* 34, 1990: 253–56.

"Progesterone Reported to Increase Bone Density 10 Percent in Six Months," by Joel Griffiths, *Med Tribune*, November 29, 1990.

"Osteoporosis Reversal: The Role of Progesterone," by John R. Lee, *International Clinical Nutrition Review* 10, No. 3, 1990: 384–91.

Progesterone in Orthomolecular Medicine, by Raymond F. Peat, Ph.D. (Portland, OR: Foundation for Hormonal and Nutrition Research, 1977).

"Osteoporosis!!," by M. T. Morter, Jr., D.C., *The Chiropractic Professional*, May/June 1987.

"Effects of Transdermal Versus Oral Hormone Replacement Therapy on Bone Density in Spine and Proximal Femur in Postmenopausal Women," by J. C. Stevenson et al., *The Lancet* 336, 1990: 265.

"Effect of Alendronate [Fosamax] on Risk of Fracture in Women with Low Bone Density but without Vertebral Fractures: Results from the Fracture Intervention Trial," by S. R. Cummings et al., *Journal of the American Medical Association*, Vol. 280, No. 24, December 1998: 1077–82.

"Throw Away Your Fosamax," by John R. Lee, *The John R. Lee, M.D. Medical Letter,* July 1998: 3.

"Cytoplasmic Glucocorticoid Binding Proteins in Bone Cells," by D. L. Feldman et al., *Endocrinology* 96, 1975: 29–36.

"Glucocorticoid Receptors and Inhibition of Bone Cell Growth in Primary Culture," by T. L. Chen et al., *Endocrinology* 100, 1977: 619–28.

"Detection of High Affinity Glucocorticoid Binding in the Rat Bone," by S. C. Manolagas et al., *Journal of Endocrinology* 76, 1978: 379–80.

Heart Disease

"Medroxyprogesterone Interferes with Ovarian Steroid Protection Against Coronary Vasospasm," by K. Miyagawa et al., *Nature Medicine* 3, 1997: 324–27.

"In Vitro Modulation of Primate Coronary Vascular Muscle Cell Reacivity by Ovarian Steroid Hormones," by R. D. Minshall et al., *FASEB J,* August 1998.

"Ovarian Steroid Protection Against Coronary Artery Hyperactivity in Rhesus Monkeys," by R. D. Minshall et al., *J Clin Endoc Metabol* 83, 1998: 649–59.

"Reactivity Based Coronary Vasospasm Independent of Atherosclerosis in Rhesus Monkeys," by K. Hermsmeyer et al., *J AM Col Cardiol* 29, 1997: 671–80.

"Myocardial Infarction and the Use of Estrogen and Estrogen-Progestogen in Postmenopausal Women," by S. Sidney et al., *Ann Int Med* 127, 1997:501–08.

"Magnesium and Cardiovascular Biology: An Important Link Between Cardiovascular Risk Factors and Atherogenesis," by B. M. Altura and B. T. Altura, *Cell Mol Biol Res* 41, No. 5, 1995: 347–59.

"Randomized Controlled Trial of Vitamin E in Patients with Coronary Disease: Cambridge Heart Antioxidant Study (CHAOS)," by N. Stephens et al., *The Lancet* 347, 1996: 781–86.

"Ascorbic Acid Induces a Favorable Lipoprotein Profile in Women," by L. Gatto et al., *J Am Coll Nutr* 15, No 2, 1996: 154–58.

"Homocysteine Metabolism and Risk of Myocardial Infarction: Relation with Vitamins B_6, B_{12} and Folate," by P. Verhoef et al., *Am J Epidemiol* 143, 1996: 845–59.

"What Dose of Viatmin E is Required to Reduce Susceptibility of LDL to Oxidation?," by L. A. Simons et al., *Australian New Zealand Journal of Medicine* 26, 1996: 496–503.

"Venous Thromboembolism," by D. Grady et al., Journal of the American Medical Associaton 13, August 1997.

"Risk of Idiopathic Cerebral Haemorrhage in Women on Oral Contraceptives with Differing Progestagen Components," by S. S. Jick et al., *The Lancet* 354, 1999: 302–03.

"Effect on Stroke of Different Progestogens in Low Oestrogen Dose Oral Contraceptive," by N. R. Poulter et al., *The Lancet* 254, 1999: 301.

"Randomized Trial of Estrogen Plus Progestin for Secondary Prevention of Coronary Heart Disease in Postmenopausal Women," by Stephen Hulley et al., *Journal of the American Medical Association* 280, 1998: 605–13.

"Heart and Estrogen/Progestin Replacement Study (HERS): design, methods and baseline characteristics," by D. Grady et al., *Control Clin Trials* 19, 1998: 314–35.

"Venous thromboembolic events associated with hormone replacement therapy," by D. Grady et al., *JAMA* 278, 1997: 477.

"Effects of hormone replacement therapy on reactivity of atherosclerotic coronary arteries in cynomolgus monkeys," by J. K. Williams et al., *J Am Coll Cardiol* 24, 1994: 1757–61.

"The Coronary Drug Project: initial findings leading to modifications of its research protocol," by Coronary Drug Project Research Group, *JAMA* 214, 1970: 1303–13.

"Findings leading to discontinuation of the 2.5-mg/day estrogen group," by Coronary Drug Project Research Group, *JAMA* 226, 1973: 652–57.

"Risk of Hospital Admission for Idiopathic Venous Thromboembolism Among Users of Postmenopausal Oestrogens," by H. Jick et al., *The Lancet* 348, 1996: 981–83.

"Risk of Venous Thromboembolism in Users of Hormone Replacement Therapy," by E. Daly et al., *The Lancet* 348, 1996: 977–80.

"Prospective Study of Exogenous Hormones and Risk of Pulmonary Embolism in Women," by F. Grodstein, et al., *The Lancet* 348, 1996: 983–87.

"Hormone Replacement Therapy and Risk of Venous Thromboembolism: Population Based Case-Control Study," by S. P. Gutthann et al., *BMJ* 314, 1997: 796–800.

"Mechanisms of Gallstone Formation in Women," by G. T. Everson et al., *J Clin Invest* 87, 1991: 237–46.

"Factors of Risk for Breast Cancer Influencing Post Menopausal Long-Term Hormone Replacement Therapy," by L. M. Chiechi et al., *Tumori* 86 (1), Jan-Feb 2000: 12–16.

Alzheimer's Disease

"Effect of Estrogen on Brain Activation Patterns in Postmenopausal Women During Working Memory Tasks," by S. E. Shaywitz et al., *Journal of the American Medical Association* 281, 1999: 1197–202.

"Breakdown of Membrane Phospholipids in Alzheimer Disease-Involvement of Excitatory Amino Acid Receptors," by A. A. Farooqui et al., *Mol Chem Neuropathol* 25, No. 2–3, 1995: 155–73.

"Failure of Nalmefene and Estrogen to Improve Memory in Alzheimer's Disease," by B. L. Weiss, *American Journal of Psychiatry* 144, 1987: 386–78.

Epilepsy

"Epileptic Seizure in Women Related to Plasma Oestrogen and Progesterone During the Menstrual cycle," by T. Backstrom, *Acta Neurol Scan* 54, 1976: 321–47.

"Intermittent Progesterone Therapy and Frequency of Complex Partial Seizures in Women with Menstrual Disorders," by A. G. Herzog, *Neurology* 36, 1986: 1607–10.

"Catamenial Epilepsy: Gynecological and Hormonal Implications: Five Case Reports," by K. A. Rodriguez Marcias, *Gynecology and Endocrinology* 10, 1996: 139–42.

Dietary Fats

"Influence of Unsaturated Fatty Acids on the Production of Tumor Necrosis Factor and Interleukin-6 by Rat Peritoneal Macrophages," by P. S. Tappia et al., *Mol Cell Biochem* 143, No. 2, 1995: 89–98.

"Dietary Polyunsaturated Fatty Acids and Composition of Human Aortic Plaques," by C. V. Felton et al., *The Lancet* 344, No. 8931, 1994: 1195–96.

"The Combined Effects of Dietary Fat and Estrogen on Survival, 7, 12-Dimethyl-benz(a)-Anthracene-Induced Breast Cancer and Prolactin Metabolism in Rats," by S. K. Clinton et al., *J Nutri* 125, No. 5, 1995: 1192–1204.

"Unsaturated Fats Directly Kill White Blood Cells," by E. A. Mascioli et al., *Lipids* 22, No. 6, 1987: 421.

"Nutritional-Physiological Effects of Dietary Fats in Rations for Growing Pigs, Effects of Sunflower Oil and Coconut Oil on Protein and Fat Retention: Fatty Acid Pattern of Back Fat and Blood Parameters in Piglets," by F. Berschauer et al., *Arch Tieremahr* 34, No. 2, East Germany 1984: 19–33.

"Experimental Diabetes and Diet," by B. A. Houssay and C. Martinez, *Science* 105, 1947: 548–49.

"Fish Oil Supplementation and Essential Fatty Acid Deficiency Reduce Nitric Oxide Synthesis by Rat Macrophages," by V. Boutard et al., *Kidney Int* 46, No. 5, 1994: 1280–86.

"Effect of Garlic and Fish Oil Supplementation on Serum Lipid and

Lipoprotein Concentrations in Hypercholesterolemic Men," by A. J. Adler et al., *Am J Clin Nutr* 65, 1997: 445–50.

"Effects of Interaction of RRR-a-tocopheryl Acetate and Fish Oil on Low-Density-Lipoprotein Oxidation in Post-Menopausal Women with and without Hormone-Replacement Therapy," by R. C. Wander et al., *Am J Clin Nutr* 63, 1996: 184–93.

"Inhibition by Polyunsaturated Fatty Acids of Cell Volume Regulation and Osmolyte Fluxes in Astrocytes," by Sanchez Olea et al., *American Journal of Physiology-Cell Physiology* 38, No. 1, 1995: C96-C102.

"Utilization of Polyunsaturated Fatty Acids by Human Diploid Cells Aging in Vitro," by R. D. Lynch, *Lipids* 15, No. 6, 1967: 412–20.

"Incidence of Cancer in Men on a Diet High in Polysaturated Fat," by M. L. Pearce and S. Dayton, *The Lancet* 1, 1971: 464–67.

"Binding of Unsaturated Fatty Acids to Na+, K+-ATPase Leading to Inhibition and Inactivation," by H. G. P. Swarts et al., *Biochem Biophys Acta* 1024, 1990: 32–40.

"A Reevaluation of Coconut Oil's Effect on Serum Cholesterol and Atherogenesis," by G. L. Blackburn et al., *The Journal of the Philippine Medical Association* 65, 1989: 144–52.

"Coconut oil and heart attack," by M. G. Eraly, from *Coconut and Coconut Oil in Human Nutrition*, Proceedings, Symposium on Coconut and Coconut Oil in Human Nutrition, March 27, 1994 (Kochi, India: Coconut Development Board, 1995), 63–64.

Coronary Heart Disease: The Dietary Sense and Nonsense, by G. V. Mann (London: Janus Publishing, 1993), 36–60.

For Additional Reading Material, see appendices D, E, and G.

Depression (Postpartum, PMS/Perimenopausal, and Menopausal)

"Should Premenstrual Syndrome be a Legal Defense," by Katharina Dalton, M.D., et al., Chapter in *Premenstrual Syndrome: Ethical Implications in a BioBehavioural Prospective,* 1986.

"Successful Prophylactic Progesterone for Idiopathic Postnatal Depression," by Katharina Dalton, M.D., *International Journal of Prenatal & Perinatal Studies,* September 1989.

"Postpartum Depression & Bonding," by Katharina Dalton, M.D., *International Journal of Prenatal & Perinatal Studies,* 1989: 225–26.

"Premenstural Syndrome and Postnatal Depression," by Katharina Dalton, M.D., *Health and Hygiene* 11, 1990: 199–201.

"Birth of the Blues: Postnatal Depression," by Katharina Dalton, M.D., *Chemist & Druggist*, March 1991: 34–36.

"Postnatal Depression and Prophylactic Progesterone," by Katharina Dalton, M.D., *British Journal of Family Planning* suppl. vol. 19, 1994: 10–12.

"Violence and the Premenstrual Syndrome," by Katharina Dalton, M.D., *Journal of Police Surgeons*, 1981.

"Legal Implications of Premenstrual Syndrome," by Katharina Dalton, M.D., *World Medicine*, April 17, 1982.

"Postnatal Depression," by Katharina Dalton, M.D., letter in *British Medical Journal*, November 1982.

"Premenstrual syndrome: A New Criminal Defense?," by Lawrence Taylor and Katharina Dalton, M.D., *California Western Law Review* 18 (2), 1983: 268–86.

"The Depression of PMS and Menstrual Distress," by Katharina Dalton, M.D., *Mimms*, March 1984: 32–33.

"Progesterone Prophylaxis Used Successfully in Postnatal Depression," by Katharina Dalton, M.D., *The Practitioner* 229, June 1985: 507.

"The Similarity of Symptomatology of Premenstrual Syndrome and Toxaemia of Pregnancy and Their Response to Progesterone," by Katharina Dalton, M.D., *British Medical Journal*, vol. II, November 6, 1954: 1071. (BMA Prize)

"Progesterone in Toxaemia of Pregnancy," by Katharina Dalton, M.D., *Medical World*, December 1955.

"Toxaemia of Pregnancy Treated with Progesterone During the Symptomatic Stage," by Katharina Dalton, M.D., *British Medical Journal*, vol. II, August 17, 1957: 378–81.

"Menstruation and Acute Psychiatric Illnesses," by Katharina Dalton, M.D., *British Medical Journal*, January 17, 1959.

"Menstruation and Crime," by Katharina Dalton, M.D., *British Medical Journal*, vol. II, December 30, 1961: 1752–53.

"Prospective Study into Puerperal Depression," by Katharina Dalton, M.D., *British Journal of Psychiatry* 118 (547), June 1971: 689-92.

"Puerperal and Premenstrual Depression," by Katharina Dalton, M.D., *Proceedings of the Royal Society of Medicine* 764 (12), December 1971: 1249–52.

"Migraine in General Practice," by Katharina Dalton, M.D., *Journal of the Royal College of General Practitioners* 23, 1973: 97–106.

"Menses and the Psyche," by Katharina Dalton, M.D., *General Practitioner*, May 1975: 20.

"Paramenstrual Baby Battering," by Katharina Dalton, M.D., *British Medical Journal*, May 1975.

"The Effect of Progesterone on Brain Function," by Katharina Dalton, M.D., Proceedings of the *Acta Endocrin* Congress, Amsterdam, August 1975.

"Prenatal Progesterone and Educational Attainments," by Katharina Dalton, M.D., *British Journal of Psychiatry* 129, 1976: 438–442. The Charles Olive Hawthorne, BMA Prize Essay, 1976.

"Premenstrual Syndrome with Psychiatric Symptoms," by Katharina Dalton, M.D., *Journal of the American Medical Association* 238 (25), December 19, 1977: 2729.

"Intelligence and Prenatal Progesterone: A reappraisal," by Katharina Dalton, M.D., *Journal of the Royal Society of Medicine* 71, 1979: 397–99.

"Cyclical Criminal Acts in Premenstrual Syndrome," by Katharina Dalton, M.D., *The Lancet,* November 15, 1980: 1070–71.

Soy Deception

"Meta-analysis of the Effects of Soy Protein Intake on Serum Lipids," by James W. Anderson et al., *New England Journal of Medicine* 333 (5), 1995: 276–82.

"Comparative Effects of Neonatal Exposure of Male Rats to Potent and Weak (Environmental) Estrogens on Spermatogenesis at Puberty and the Relationship to Adult Testis Size and Fertility: Evidence for Stimulatory Effects of Low Estrogen Levels," by N. Atanassova, *Endocrinology* 141 (10), 2000: 3898–907.

"An Extract of Soy Flour Influences Serum Cholesterol and Thyroid Hormones in Rats and Hamsters," by F. Balmir et al., *J Nutr* 126, 1996: 3046–53.

Excitotoxins: The Taste That Kills, by R. Blaylock, M.D. (Oxford: Health Press, 1997).

"Biological Effects of a Diet of Soy Protein Rich in Isoflavones on the Menstrual Cycle of Premenopausal Women," by A. Cassidy et al., *American Journal of Clinical Nutrition* 60, 1994: 333–40.

"The Effect of Phytoestrogens on the Female Genital Tract," by J. L. Burton et al., *J Clin Pathol* 55 (6), June 2002: 401–7.

"Dietary Genistein Inactivates Rat Thyroid Peroxidase in Vivo Without an Apparent Hypothyroid Effect," by H. C. Chang and D. R. Doerge, *Toxicol Appl Pharmacol* 168, 2000: 224–52.

"Persistent Hypothyroidism in an Infant Receiving Soy Formula," by P. A. Chorazy et al., Case Report Review and Review of the Literature. *Pediatrics* 96, 1995: 148–50.

"Vegetable Protein - A Delayed Birth?," by Richard J. Coleman, *Journal of the American Oil Chemists' Society* 52, April 1975: 238A.

"In Vitro and In Vivo: Mechanism for Anti-Thyroid Activity of Soy," presented at the November 1999 Soy Symposium in Washington, D.C., by the National Center for Toxicological Research.

"Dietary Estrogens Stimulate Human Breast Cells to Enter the Cell Cycle," by C. Dees et al., *Environmental Health Perspectives* 105 (suppl. 3), 1997: 633–36.

"Anti-thyroid Isoflavones from Soybean: Isolation, Characterization, and Mechanisms of Action," by R. L. Divi et al., *Biochem Pharmacol* 54 (10), Nov. 15, 1997: 1087–96.

"Inhibition of Thyroid Peroxidase by Dietary Flavonoids," by R. L. Divi et al., *Chem Res Toxicol* 9, 1996: 16–23.

"Goitrogenic and estrogenic activity of soy isoflavones," by D. R. Doerge and D. M. Sheehan, *Environ Health Perspect* 110 (suppl.3), June 2002: 349–53.

"Oestrogenic Activity of Soya-Bean Products," by H. M. Drane et al., *Food, Cosmetics and Technology* 18, 1980: 425–27.

"Tragedy and Hype: The Third International Soy Symposium," by M. G. Enig and S. A. Fallon, *Nexus Magazine* 7 (3), April-May 2000.

"Food Labeling: Health Claims: Soy Protein and Coronary Heart Disease," Food and Drug Administration 21 CFR, Part 101 (Docket No. 98P-0683).

"Breast and Soy-Formula Feedings in Early Infancy and the Prevalence of Autoimmune Thyroid Disease in Children," by P. Fort et al., *J Am Coll Nutr* 9 (2), April 1990: 164–67.

"Importance of Zinc in the Central Nervous System: The Zinc-containing Neuron," by C. J. Frederickson et al., *J Nutr* 130 (suppl. 5), May 2000: 1471S–83S.

"Quantification of Genistein and Genistin in Soybeans and Soybean Products," by M. Fukutake et al., *Food Chem Toxicol* 34, 1996: 457–61.

"Nutritional Status and Phytate: Zinc and Phytate X Calcium: Zinc Dietary Molar Ratios of Lacto-Ovovegetarian Trappist Monks: 10 Years Later," by B. F. Harland et al., *Journal of the American Dietetic Association* 88, December 1988:1562–66.

Cancer Rates and Risks, edited by Angela Harras, fourth edition, National Institutes of Health, National Cancer Institute, 1996.

"Secondary Sexual Characteristics and Menses in Young Girls Seen in Office Practice: A Study from the Pediatric Research in Office Settings Network," by Marcia E. Herman-Giddens et al., *Pediatrics* 99(4), April 1997: 505–12.

"Maternal Genistein Exposure Mimics the Effects of Estrogen on Mammary Gland Development in Female Mouse Offspring," by L. Hilakivi-Clarke et al., *Oncol Rep* 5(3), May-June1998: 609–16.

"Involvement of Intracellular Labile Zinc in Suppression of DEVD-Caspase Activity in Human Neuroblastoma Cells," by L. H. Ho et al., *Biochem Biophys Res Commun* 268(1), Feb 5, 2000: 148–54.

"Assessing Phytoestrogen Exposure in Epidemiologic Studies: Development of a Database (United States)," by P. L. Horn-Ross et al., *Cancer Causes Control* 11, 2000: 289–98.

"Phytoestrogens and Thyroid Cancer Risk: the San Fransisco Bay Area Thyroid Cancer Study," by P. L. Horn-Ross et al., *Cancer Epidemiol Biomarkers Prev* 11, 2002: 43–49.

"Prevalence and aetiology of hypothyroidism in the young," by I. Hunter et al., *Arch Dis Child* 83, 2000: 207–10.

"Occurence of Goiter in an Infant Soy Diet," by J. D. Hydovitz, *N Engl J Med* 262, 1960: 351–53.

"IEH Assessment on Phytoestrogens in the Human Diet," *Final Report to the Ministry of Agriculture,* Fisheries and Food, November 1997: 11.

"The Potential Adverse Effects of Soybean Phytoestrogens in Infant Feeding," by C. Irvine et al., *New Zealand Medical Journal,* May 24, 1995: 318.

"Phytoestrogens in soy-based infant foods: concentrations, daily intake, and possible biological effects," by C. H. G. Irvine, *Proc Soc Exp Biol Med* 217 (3), March 1998: 247–53.

"The Effects on the Thyroid Gland of Soybeans Administered Experimentally in Healthy Subjects," by Y. Ishizuki et al., *Nippon Naibunpi Gakkai Zasshi* 67 (5), May 20, 1991: 622–29.

"Dramatic Synergism Between Excess Soybean Intake and Iodine Deficiency on the Development of Rat Thyroid Hyperplasia," by T. Ikeda et al., *Carcinogenesis* 21, 2000: 707–13.

"Abnormal Thyroid Function Test in Infants with Congential Hypothyroidism: The Influence of Soy-Based Formula," by M. A. Jabbar et al., *J Am Coll Nutr* 16, 1997: 280–82.

"Serum estrogen levels, cognitive performance, and risk of cognitive decline in older community women," by K. Yaffe et al., *J Am Geriatr Soc* 46 (7), July 1998: 816–21.

"Food and Biocultural Evolution: A Model for the Investigation of Modern Nutritional Problems," by Solomon H. Katz, in *Nutritional Anthropology,* edited by F. E. Johnston (New York: Alan R. Liss Inc., 1987), 50.

"Studies of Marginal Zinc Deprivation in Rhesus Monkeys," by C. L. Keen, *Am J Clin Nutr* 47 (6), June 1988:1041–45.

"Dietary Oestrogenic Isoflavones are Potent Inhibitors of B-Hydroxysteroid Dehydrogenase of P. Testosteronii," by W. M. Keung, *Biochemical and Biophysical Research Committee* 215, 1995: 1137–44.

"Development of Malignant Goiter by Defatted Soybean with Iodine-free Diet in Rats," by S. Kimura et al., *Gann* 67, 1976: 763–65.

"Dietary Maladvice as a Cause of Hypothyroidism and Short Stature," by M. Labib et al., *Br Med J* 298, 1989: 232–33.

"Phytoestrogens: Adverse Effects on Reproduction in California Quail," by A. S. Leopold, *Science* 191, 1976: 98–100.

"Oestrogenic Activity of Soya-Bean Products," by H. M. Drane et al., *Food, Cosmetics and Technology* 18, 1980: 425–27.

"Phytoestrogens decrease brain calcium-binding proteins . . .," by E. D. Lephart et al., *Brain Res* 859 (1), March 17, 2000: 123–31.

Tofu, Tempeh, Miso, and Other Soyfoods: The "Food of the Future"—How to Enjoy Its Spectacular Health Benefits, by Richard Leviton (New Canann, CT: Keats Publishing, Inc., 1982), 14–15.

"Activation of skeletal muscle protein breakdown following consumption of soybean protein in pigs," by B. Lohrke, *Br J Nutr* 85 (4), April 2001: 447–57.

"The Oiling of America," by Mary G. Enig and Sally Fallon, *Nexus Magazine,* December 1998–January 1999 and February–March 1999; see www.WestonAPrice.org.

"Effect of Genistin on Growth and Development of the Male Mouse," by G. Matrone et al., *Journal of Nutrition,* 1956: 235–40.

"The Goitrogenic Action of Soybean and Ground-Nut," by R. McCarrison, *Indian J Med Res* 21, 1933: 179.

"Experimental rickets: The Effect of Cereals and Their Interaction with Other Factors of Diet and Environment in Producing Rickets," by Edward Mellanby, *Journal of the Medical Research Council* 93, March 1925: 265.

"Soy Intake and Cancer Risk: A Review of the In Vitro and In Vivo Data," by Mark J. Messina et al., *Nutrition and Cancer* 21 (2), 1994: 113–31.

"Plant Oestrogens in Soya-Based Infant Formula," by the UK Ministry of Agriculture, Fisheries, and Food, Food Surveillance Paper No. 167, 1998.

"Maternal-Fetal Thyroid Hormone Relationships and the Fetal Brain," by G. Morreale de Escobar et al., *Acta Med Austriaca* 15, 1988: 66–70.

"Copper, Iron, Zinc and Selenium Dietary Intake and Status of Nepalese Lactating Women and Their Breastfed Infants," by P. B. Moser et al., *American Journal of Clinical Nutrition* 47, April 1988: 729–74.

"Phytoestrogen Content of Processed Soybean Foods," by P. A. Murphy, *Food Technology,* January 1982: 60–64.

"Soy Based Infant Formula," by New Zealand Ministry of Health, 1998.

"Decreased Serum Total Cholesterol Concentration is Associated with High Intake of Soy Products in Japanese Men and Women," by C. Nagata et al., *Journal of Nutrition* 128, 1998: 209–13.

"Uterine Adenocarcinoma in Mice Treated Neonatally with Genistein," by R. R. Newbold, *Cancer Research* 61, 2001: 4325–28.

"Distribution of Phosphorus and Phytate in Some Nigerian Varieties of Legumes and Some Effects of Processing," by A. D. Ologhobo et al., *Journal of Food Science* 49(1), January/February 1984: 199–201.

"Oestrogenic Effect of Dietary Soybean Meal on Vitellogenesis in Cultured Siberian Sturgeon Acipenser baeri," by C. Pelissero et al., *General and Comparative Endocrinology* 83, 1991: 447–57.

"Effect of Soy Protein on Endogenous Hormones in Postmenopausal Women," by V. W. Persky et al., *Am J Clin Nutr* 75, 2002: 145–53.

"Stimulatory Influence of Soy Protein Isolate on Breast Secretion in Pre- and Post-Menopausal Women," by N. L. Petrakis et al., *Cancer Epid Bio Prev* 5, 1996: 785–94

"Zinc, The Brain, and Behavior," by C. C. Pfeiffer and E. R. Braverman, *Biol Psychiatry* 17 (4), April 1982: 513–32.

"Thyroid Refractoriness in an Athyreotic Cretin Fed Soybean Formula," by A. Pinchera et al., *N Engl J Med* 273, 1965: 83–87.

"Playing God in the Garden," by M. Pollan, *NY Times Sunday Magazine*, October 25, 1998.

"Low Maternal Free Throxine Concentrations During Early Pregnancy are Associated with Impaired Psychomotor Development in Infancy," by V. J. Pop et al., *Clin Endocrinol* 50, 1999: 149–55.

"Soy Protein Concentrate and Isolated Soy Protein Similarly Lower Blood Serum Cholesterol But Differently Affect Thyroid Hormones in Hamsters," by S. M. Potter et al., *J Nutr* 126, 1996: 2007–11.

"Evaluation of the Health Aspects of Soy Protein Isolates as Food Ingredients," by J. Rackis et al., prepared for FDA by Life Sciences Research Office, Federation of American Societies for Experimental Biology, Contract No. FDA 223-75-2004, 1979.

"The USDA Trypsin Inhibitor Study. I. Background, Objectives and Procedural Details," by Joseph J. Rackis et al., *Qualification of Plant Foods in Human Nutrition* 35, 1985: 232.

"Biological and Physiological Factors in Soybeans," by Joseph J. Rackis, *Journal of the American Oil Chemists' Society* 51, January 1974: 161A–170A.

"Endocrinology of Neoplastic Disease," by R. W. Rawson and J. E. Rall, *Recent Prog Horm Res* 11, 1955: 257–90.

"Effect of In-utero Exposure to Diethylstilbestrol on Age at Onset of Puberty and on Post-Pubertal Hormone Levels in Boys," by R. K. Ross et al., *Canadian Medical Association Journal* 128 (10), May 15, 1983: 1197–8.

"Effect of Protein Level and Protein Source on Zinc Absorption in Humans," by B. Sandstrom et al., *Journal of Nutrition* 119 (1), January 1989: 48–53.

"Chemical Carcinogens," edited by Charles E. Searle, *ACS Monograph* 173 (Washington, DC: American Chemical Society, 1976).

"Isoflavone Content of Infant formulas and the Metabolic Fate of These Early Phytoestrogens in Early life," by K. D. Setchell et al., *American Journal of Clinical Nutrition*, December 1998 Supplement: 1453S–1461S.

"Dietary Oestrogens—A Probable Cause of Infertility and Liver Disease in Captive Cheetahs," by K. D. R. Setchell et al., *Gastroenterology* 93, 1987: 225–33.

"Infant Feeding with Soy Formula Milk: Effects on the Testis and on Blood Testosterone Levels in Marmoset Monkeys During the Period of Neonatal Testicular Activity," by R. M. Sharpe et al., *Hum Reprod* 17 (7), July 2002: 1692–703.

"Soybean Goiter," by T. H. Shephard et al., *N Engl J Med* 262, 1960: 1099–1103.

"Lack of Modification by Environmental Estrogenic Compounds of Thyroid Carcinogenesis in Ovariectomized Rats Pretreated with N-bis (2-Hydroxypropyl) Nitrosamine (DHPN)," by H. Y. Son et al., *Japanese Journal of Cancer Research* 91, October 2000: 966–72.

"Lack of Modifying Effects of Environmental Estrogenic Compounds on the Development of Proliferative Lesions in Male Rats Pretreated with N-bis (2-Hydroxypropyl) Nitrosamine (DHPN)," by H. Y. Son et al., *Japanese Journal of Cancer Research* 91, September 2000: 899–905.

"Genistein Exerts Estrogen-Like Effects in Male Mouse Reproductive Tract," by L. Strauss, *Mol Cell Endocrinol* 144 (1–2), September 25, 1998: 83–93.

"Silicon to Soybeans," by M. Spicuzza, *Metro,* May 11, 2000: 21.

"The Availability of Minerals in Food, with Particular Reference to Iron," by Susan Tait et al., *Journal of Research in Society and Health* 103(2), April 1983: 74–77.

"Thyroid Stimulating Hormone (TSH)-Associated Follicular Hypertrophy and Hyperplasia as a Mechanism of Thyroid Carcinogenesis in Mice and Rats," by G. A. Thomas and E. D. Williams, *IARC Sci Publ* 147, 1999: 45–59.

"Comparison of Epidemiological Data on Congenital Hypothyroidism in Europe with Those of Other Parts in the World," by J. E. Toublanc, *Horm Res* 38, 1992: 230–35.

"Fetal thyroid function," by J. G. Thorpe-Beeston et al., *Thyroid* 2 (3), Fall 1992: 207–17.

"Nutritional Quality of Soybean Protein Isolates: Studies in Children of Preschool Age," by Benjamin Torum, in *Soy Protein and Human Nutrition,* edited by Harold L Wilcke et al. (New York: Academic Press, 1979).

"A Health Food Hits Big Time," by John Urquhart, *Wall Street Journal,* August 3, 1999: B1.

"The Effects of a Soybean Product on Thyroid Function in Humans," by J. J. Van Wyk et al., *Pediatrics,* 1959: 752–60.

"Nutritional Status of African Populations Predisposed to Esophageal Cancer," by C. E. Van Rensburg et al., *Nutrition and Cancer* 4, 1983: 206–16.

"Studies on the Processing and Properties of Soymilk," by G. M. Wallace, *Journal of Science and Food Agriculture* 22, October 1971: 526–35.

"Isoflavone Content in Commercial Soybean Foods," by H. J. Wang and P. A. Murphy, *J Agric Food Chem* 42, 1994: 1666–73.

"Association of High Midlife Tofu Consumption with Accelerated Brain Aging," by Lon White, The Third International Soy Symposium, November 1999: 26.

"Phytic Acid and Nutritional Rickets in Immigrants," by M. R. Wills et al., *The Lancet,* April 8,1972: 771–73.

"Biotech Food—What's on Our Shelves?," by R. Wolfson, Ph.D., *Alive: Canadian Journal of Health and Nutrition,* Nov 1996.

"Phytoestrogens and Parrots: The Anatomy of an Investigation," by D. J. Woodhams, *Proceedings of the Nutrition Society of New Zealand* 20, 1995: 22–30.

Dangers of Mammograms

"Case-Control Study of Factors Associated With Failure to Detect Breast Cancer by Mammography," by L. Ma et al., *J Nat Cancer Inst* 84, 1992: 781–85.

"High-Risk Mammographic Parenchymal Patterns, Hormone Replacement Therapy and Other Risk Factors: A Case-Control Study," by E. Sala et al., *Int J Epidemiol* 29, 2000: 629–36.

"A Tangled Web: Factors Likely to Affect the Efficacy of Screening Mammography," by C. J. Baines and R. Dayan, *J Natl Cancer Inst* 91, 1999: 833–38.

"Breast Tumor Characteristics as Predicators of Mammographic Detection: Comparison of Interval- and Sceeen Detected Cancers," by P. L. Porter et al., *J Natl Cancer Inst* 91, 1999: 2020–28.

"Ten-year Risk of False Positive Screening Mammograms and Clinical Breast Examinations," by Joann G. Elmore et al., *N Engl J Med* 338 (16), April 16, 1998: 1089–97.

"Is Screening for Breast Cancer with Mammography Justifiable?," by Peter C. Gotzsche et al., *The Lancet* 355 (9198), January 8, 2000: 129–34.

"Effect of Estrogen Replacement Therapy on the Specificity and Sensitivity of Screening Mammography," by M. B. Laya et al., *J Natl Cancer Inst* 88, 1996: 643–49.

"Does Increased Detection Account for the Rising Incidence of Breast Cancer?," by J. M. Liff et al., *Am J Public Health* 81 (4), April 1991: 462–65.

"Breast Cancer Induced By Radiation Relation to Mammography and Treatment of Acne," by N. Simon, *JAMA* 237 (8), February 21, 1977: 789–90.

APPENDIX G

Sources of Natural Progesterone

The natural progesterone in tablet or cream form, though approved by the FDA, is not available in most neighborhood drugstores. However, botanical hormones are accessible in various forms at dispensaries and health food stores around the country, some of which are listed on the following pages. As more and more physicians begin to understand their patients' needs for better assimilated hormones, additional pharmacies and stores will be encouraged to make these natural products available. The shift in consumer attitudes that is taking place has been noticed by these natural compounding pharmacies and their pharmacists, who report that women want natural products and "doctors are being forced to pay attention because women are bringing them the solution [to negative side effects]. They are demanding better treatment."[1]

Some of the larger firms listed here can also provide a variety of services that are usually not available in our neighborhood stores. For instance, regardless of which part of the country you live in, Women's International Pharmacy can (1) furnish you with at least a partial list of medical doctors located in your area who prescribe the natural hormones, (2) supply you with a list of local chiropractors or naturopaths who have ordered the nonprescription hormones (creams, gels, sublingual oils, etc.) for their patients' use, and (3) even file your insurance forms for you.

Not all of the druggists listed carry the nonprescriptive transdermal progesterone cream (labeled under a variety of different names). Nonetheless, these can be ordered through distributors and manufacturers, a number of which are listed here. Additionally, health food stores are carrying this natural progesterone cream, which they in turn obtain from the distributor or manufacturer. Be sure to encourage your local health store manager to stock these products.

A few of the pharmacies listed here also offer patient consultation and education. But they *all* supply progesterone, which comes in cream, tablet, and capsule form (dosage depending on what your doctor prescribes) and is compounded according to the physician's prescription by a licensed pharmacist using FDA-approved ingredients. All these pharmacies carry estriol as well. Some physicians prescribe simply the estriol along with progesterone, while others prescribe a "tri-estrogen" (80 percent estriol, 10 percent estradiol, 10 percent estrone) with progesterone. With many diverse philosophies and differing patient requirements, prescriptions can be customized in various ways.

If your doctor says he can't get natural progesterone, you might want to tell him that according to the *New York Times* (November 18, 1994), "The Upjohn Company in Kalamazoo, Michigan derives the finely particled progesterone from soybeans and sells it to pharmacies as a bulk powder. Pharmacies can then formulate it into capsules, tablets, suspensions or suppositories in various dosages according to a physician's prescription."[2] Your doctor can also obtain micronized progesterone from Schering-Plough Corporation in Madison, New Jersey, by requesting the soybean-derived hormone manufactured without the estrogen.

Today most USP progesterone is, in fact, extracted from soy. You will recall that neither USP nor human progesterone is present in either of the major plant sources (soybean or wild yam). Yams contain the sterol diosgenin, whereas soybeans contain the sterol stigmasterol—both of which have progesterone-like effects.[3] The substance sold as USP progesterone is produced in the lab by hydrolyzing extracts of soy or yam and converting saponins into sapogenins, from two of which, sarsasapogenin (soy) and diosgenin (yam), are derived the majority of natural progesterone produced for medical purposes. Actually, with the phytogenins from plants it is possible to manufacture not only progesterone but other hormones such as testosterone and estrogen.

It is also interesting to learn that diosgenin is quite concentrated in certain species of *Dioscorea*. While diosgenin (a plant steroid) may have some progestogenic or even phytoestrogenic action (a valid concern for some), the effect varies from one person to another.[5] Some doctors say that the human body cannot convert wild yam or diosgenin to hormones and that conversion to progesterone must take place in a laboratory. It is possible, however, that some women's bodies are better able to utilize plant-derived compounds than others. It is also important to remember that while the mechanism of phytogenic activity may not be clearly understood at this time, botanical supplementation continues to gain support among women, and their doctors, everywhere when it works for them.

Many nonprescriptive USP progesterone creams are available and often differ as to the concentration of bioavailable progesterone. Additionally, the other supportive ingredients (such as herbal extracts, essential oils, phytonutrients) vary from cream to cream.

For women wanting to compare specific ingredients, strengths, and bioactivity, we have listed many natural compounding pharmacies and manufacturers on the next several pages. These companies will answer your questions regarding their product(s) and may be able to assist you with any concerns you have regarding your individual requirements related to hormonal or nutritional rebalancing. Some will also provide a list of doctors in your area who focus on natural alternatives. And finally, the natural compounding pharmacies can customize prescription remedies for your specific needs.

In your search for natural hormone support be sure to ask any supplier (including compounding pharmacies) for an ingredient list so that you can confirm that there are no artificial ingredients or preservatives in the formulations you wish to use. Also be sure to ask them for the amount of active progesterone (in mg) per container (usually 2 oz) and per application.

You may hear charges that the use of wild yam to produce natural progesterone is threatening to make it an endangered species. I saw one such article just before going to press. Pharmacologist James Jamieson, however, assures me that this is definitely not the case. The wild yam is very common and grows all over the world in a wide variety of natural environments—Central America, Peru, China, Germany, and Afghanistan, to name a few. While it is possible that the plant may become scarce in particular locations, wildcrafting is very unlikely to have a serious impact on its worldwide distribution. In addition, these big, spongy tubers are easy to grow and are already cultivated commercially. Since we all need to be aware of the effect our personal decisions have on the environment, this information about the wild yam is reassuring.

My life has been greatly simplified now that I know where to call for my prescriptive or nonprescriptive hormone replacement. Furthermore, I waste no more time driving to and from the drugstore and waiting in line. You, too, will find life less stressful when your products arrive by UPS or the U.S. mail at your front door. What could be easier than having your natural hormone therapy delivered direct to your home? Give yourself a break—you deserve this service!

Natural Compounding Pharmacies, Manufacturers, and Distributors

In addition to helping you with prescription needs, compounding pharmacies and manufacturers on the following pages can often provide a doctor referral in your area.

Alabama

Florala Pharmacy, Inc., Florala, (800) 423-7847
Haisten Rexall Drugs, Trussville, (205) 655-3601
Medaus Compounding Pharmacy, Birmingham, (800) 526-9183
The Compounding Shoppe, Homewood, (800) 834-8666
Wellness Health & Pharmacy, Birmingham, (800) 227-2627

Alaska

Geneva Woods Pharmacy, Soldotna and Wasilla, (800) 478-0005
North Pole Prescription Laboratory, North Pole, (907) 488-8555

Arizona

Apothecary Shops of Arizona, Scottsdale, (877) 792-7684
Community Clinical Pharmacy, Mesa, (800) 729-8229
International Health, Scottsdale, (800) 481-9987
Life-Flo Health Care Products, Phoenix, (888) 999-7440
Living Healthier, Phoenix, (888) 796-4582
Prescription Lab Compounding Pharmacy, Tucson, (520) 886-1035
Professional Products, Phoenix, (888) 796-4582
Women's International Pharmacy, Sun City West, (800) 279-5708

Arkansas

Cantrell Drug & Wellness, Little Rock, (877) 666-5222
College Pharmacy, Conway, (800) 718-3588
Lee Pharmacy, Fort Smith, (800) 209-9940
Marshall Medic Pharmacy, Marshall, (888) 216-1117
Shinabery Pharmacy, Jonesboro, (866) 913-7238

California

Alternative Medicine Network, Temecula, (877) 753-5424
Broadmoore Labs, Inc., Ventura, (800) 822-3712
California Pharmacy & Compounding Center, Newport Beach, (800) 575-7776
Central Avenue Pharmacy, Pacific Grove, (800) 501-9715
Costa Mesa Pharmacy, Costa Mesa, (800) 564-1565
Homelink Natural Pharmacy, Torrance, (800) 272-4767

Kevala, a division of Karuna Corp., Novato, (800) 826-7225 or (888) 749-8643
Kokoro, LLC, Santa Ana, (800) 599-9412
Leiter's Park Pharmacy, San Jose, (800) 292-6773
Life Wellness Pharmacy, Carlsbad, (800) 210-9464
Med Specialties Compounding Pharmacy, Yorba Linda, (877) 373-2272
Myers Apothecary Shop, Ukiah, (888) 838-1444
Panorama Compounding Company, Lake Balboa, (800) 247-9767
Rancho Park Compounding Pharmacy, Los Angeles, (877) 2-COMPOUND
Roxsan Pharmacy, Beverly Hills, (888) 371-9919
Saint John's Medical Plaza Pharmacy, Santa Monica, (310) 453-6553
Santa Clara Drug The Compounding Shop, San Jose, (800) 646-2453
Springboard, Spring Valley, (619) 670-3860, or Huntington Beach, (800) 662-8045
Steven's Pharmacy, Costa Mesa, (800) 352-DRUG
The Compounding Pharmacy of Beverly Hills, (888) 799-0212
Triad Compounding Pharmacy, Cerrilos, (800) 851-7900
Valley Drugs, Encino, (818) 788-0635

Colorado

Belmar Pharmacy, Lakewood, (800) 525-9473
College Pharmacy, Colorado Springs, (800) 888-9358
Columbine Drugs, Loveland, (866) 560-3027
Monument Pharmacy, Monument, (800) 595-7565
Nature's Light, Bennett, (888) 281-8673
Spice of Life Compounding Pharmacy, Aurora, (303) 696-6301
Wise Pharmacy, Littleton, (303) 933-8181

Connecticut

Beacon Prescription Center, Willimantic, (860) 423-1125
Kaye's Pharmacy, Meriden, (203) 237-8997
Prescription Specialties, Inc., Cheshire, (800) 861-0933
Products of Nature International, Glastonbury, (800) 639-2449

Delaware

SaveWay Compounding Pharmacy, Newark, (302) 369-5520

Florida

Acology Prescription Compounding, Cape Coral, (800) 240-8958
Advanced Pharmacy Solutions, Inc., Largo, (888) 547-2654
Bokas Jordan Pharmacy, Gulf Breeze, (850) 932-2283
Family Pharmacy of Sarasota, Sarasota, (888) 245-5000

Health & Science Research Institute, Inc., Port Orange, (888) 222-1415
Naturally Eden, Inc., Ft. Walton Beach, (850) 243-5559
Nothin' But Herbs, Melbourne, (800) 242-1115
Pharmaceutical Specialties, Inc., Tampa, (800) 788-8123
Post Haste Pharmacy, Hollywood, (800) 230-5553
RxState, Clearwater, (888) 648-7250
Signature Pharmacy, Orlando and Casselberry, (877) 860-8171
Skip's Pharmacy, Boca Raton, (800) 553-7429
Specialty Pharmacy, Melbourne, (800) 499-7517
Sunshine Wellness Center, Brooksville, (352) 796-7200

Georgia

All Care Pharmacy, Lyons, (888) 833-3378
Angel Care, Atlanta, (800) 235-9732
Christian's Pharmacy, Forest Park, (404) 366-4321
Dixie PMS and Menopause Center, Marietta, (800) PMS-9232
Elation Therapy, Marietta, (888) 535-7632
HM Enterprises, Norcross, (800) 742-4773
Miller Compounding Pharmacy, Marietta, (800) 547-1399
Monfort Compounding Center Inc., Lawrenceville, (888) 540-2438
Pavilion Compounding Pharmacy, Atlanta, (800) 862-9812
Pure Health International, Atlanta, (800) 311-2186
Restored Balance, Inc., Cartersville, (800) 865-7499
Trumarx Drugs, Thomasville, (800) 552-9997

Idaho

AIM USA, Nampa, (800) 456-2462

Illinois

Lincoln Medical Apothecary, Aurora, (800) 391-9819
Marion Medical Pharmacy, Marion, (618) 997-6968
Martin Avenue Pharmacy, Inc., Naperville, (630) 355-6400
Schott's Pharmacy Care Center, Marseilles, (815) 795-2700
Snyder-Mark Roselle Drugs, Roselle, (800) PRO-GEST

Indiana

Cardinal HealthCare Pharmacy, New Castle, (800) 300-3159
Custom Dosing Pharmacy, Crown Point, (219) 662-5602
Easy Way International, Indianapolis, (800) 267-4522
Hook's Apothecary, Evansville, (812) 476-6194
Nora Apothecary & Alternative Therapies, Indianapolis, (800) 729-0276

Phillips Nutritional, Evansville, (800) 906-8874
The Medicine Shoppe, Munster, (800) 352-6337

Iowa

Carroll Apothecary, Carroll, (800) 786-4457
Sac City Drug and Custom Compounding, Sac City, (712) 662-7146

Kansas

Midwest Compounders Pharmacy, Overland Park, (888) 245-3012
Richardson's Custom Rx, Wichita, (800) 786-3431

Lousiana

Central Drugs, Hammond, (985) 345-5120
Kay's Hideaway Pharmacy, Monroe, (318) 343-4777
Line Avenue Pharmacy, Shreveport, (318) 221-5114
Muller Compounding Corner, Lacombe, (800) 479-0427

Maine

Beyond-A-Century, Greenville, (800) 777-1324
Kennebec Professional Pharmacy, Augusta, (888) 626-8163
Miller Drug, Bangor, (800) 427-8369
Portland Professional Pharmacy, Portland, (800) 850-9122

Maryland

Cape Drugs, Annapolis, (800) 248-5978
Family Pharmacy, Hampstead, (877) 726-7427
Professional Arts Pharmacy, Baltimore, (800) 832-9285

Massachusetts

Birds Hill Pharmacy, Needham, (888) 500-2660
Johnson Drug Co., Waltham, (888) 468-0481
NutrSupplies, Inc., Sudbury, (800) 906-8874

Michigan

Healthway Compounding Pharmacy, St. Charles, (800) 742-7527
Rx Solutions LLC, Monroe, (734) 240-0032
South Lyon Family Pharmacy, South Lyon, (877) 437-6225

Minnesota

Custom Rx Compounding and Natural Pharmacy, Richfield, (888) 303-9033

Missouri

Bellevue Pharmacy Solutions, St. Louis, (800) 728-0288

O'Brien Pharmacy, Kansas City, (800) 627-4360

Montana

Montana Compounding Pharmacy, Missoula, (800) 600-2009

Nebraska

Essential Pharmacy Compounding, Omaha, (888) 733-0300

Kubat Pharmacy, Omaha, (800) 782-9988

Nevada

Kronos Compounding Pharmacy, Las Vegas, (800) 723-7455

Medical Center Compounding Pharmacy, Las Vegas, (702) 873-8455

Pure Essence Laboratories, Inc., Las Vegas, (888) 254-8000

New Hampshire

Bedford Pharmacy, Bedford, (800) 662-6333

Emerson Ecologics, Inc., Bedford, (800) 654-4432

Sullivan Drug Store, Lancaster, (800) 442-4606

The Apothecary, Keene, (800) 626-4379

New Jersey

Atlas Drug and Nutrition Center, North Bergen, (888) 449-5990

Avenel Pharmacy, Avenel, (732) 634-1914

Far Hills Pharmacy, Bedminster, (908) 234-1101

Hopewell Pharmacy and Compounding Center, Hopewell, (800) 792-6670

Liberty Drug Compounding Center, Chatham, (800) 58-LIBERTY

Millers Pharmacy, Wyckoff, (888) 891-3334

Wedgewood Village Pharmacy, Sewell, (800) 331-8272

New York

At Last Naturals, Inc., Valhalla, (800) 527-8123

Barker's Pharmacy, Mattituck, (631) 298-8666

Bio-Nutritional Formulas, Mineola, (800) 950-8484

Dan Horn Pharmacy and Health Services, Olean, (716) 376-6337

Fallon Wellness Pharmacy, Clifton Park, (800) 890-1137

Master Compounding Pharmacy, LLC, Richmond Hill, (866) 630-5600

Medicine Shoppe, Canandaigua, (800) 396-9970

North Carolina

Sedna Specialty Health Products, Hendersonville, (800) 223-0858

Smith's Drugs Compounding, Forest City, (877) 441-4815

Triangle Compounding Pharmacy, Cary, (866) 858-0809

Ward Drug Company of Nashville, Nashville, (800) 721-5701

North Dakota

Heartland Products, Inc., Valley City, (888) 772-2345

Oklahoma

Claremore Compounding & Pharmacy, Claremore, (866) 370-3784
Innovative Pharmacy Solutions, Edmonds, (800) 441-8706
Lassiter Discount Drug, Del City, (888) 506-0636

Oregon

Broadway Apothecary, Eugene, (888) 644-9382
Emerita, Portland, (800) 648-8211
Kenogen, Eugene, (888) 818-5052
Pacific Compounds, Forest Grove, (877) 357-1771
Prescription Compounding Solutions, Medford, (866) 682-7979
Strohecker's Pharmacy, Portland, (503) 222-4822

Pennsylvania

Hazle Drugs Apothecary, Hazleton, (800) 439-2026
Burman's Pharmacy, Chester, (866) 872-5430
Suspenders Pharmacy Inc, Hershey, (800) 281-3146
THG Health Products, Inc., Oxford, (888) 623-4372

Tennessee

Cherokee Pharmacy, Cleveland, (423) 559-3000
Clark and Palin Pharmacy, Bristol, (800) 263-8890
Delk Pharmacy, Columbia, (615) 388-3952
Green Hills Health Wellness Pharmacy, Nashville, (800) 388-7994
Lakeside Pharmacy, Chattanooga, (800) 523-1486
People's Custom Rx, Memphis, (888) 900-6337

Texas

ApothéCure, Inc., Dallas, (800) 969-6601
Carie Boyd's Prescription Shop, Hurst, (800) 930-4360
International Academy of Compounding Pharmacies, Sugar Land, (800) 927-4227
Las Colinas Pharmacy, Irving, (972) 580-1814
National Association of Compounding Pharmacies, Amarillo, (800) 687-7850
Professional Compounding Centers of America, Houston, (800) 331-2498
Sarati International, Los Fresno, (800) 900-0701
Young Again Nutrients, Spring, (877) 205-0040

Utah

Jolley's Corner Pharmacy, Salt Lake City, (801) 582-1999
MedQuest Pharmacy, Salt Lake City, (888) 222-2956
Neways, Salem, (800) 998-7232

Vermont

Custom Prescription Shoppe, South Burlington, (800) 928-1488
PENRO Specialty Compounding, Colchester, (888) WE-MIX-4-U

Virginia

Leesburg Pharmacy, Leesburg, (800) 734-0502
The Medicine Shoppe, Boones Mill, (800) 852-5951
Vienna Drug Center, Vienna, (703) 938-7111
Hickman's Pharmacy, Princetown, (304) 425-1077

Washington

Beall's Pharmacy, Puyallup, (877) 845-0451
Bellgrove Pharmacy, Bellevue, (800) 446-2123
Clark's Pharmacy, Bellevue, (800) 480-DHEA
FirstPharma, Spokane, (888) 550-1566
Jim's Pharmacy, Port Angeles, (800) 421-0406
Kelley Ross Pharmacy, Seattle, (206) 622-3565
Key Pharmacy, Kent, (800) 878-1322
Professional Pharmaceutical Compounding, Poulsbo, (800) 882-2029
Union Avenue Pharmacy, Tacoma, (253) 752-1705

Wisconsin

Island Pharmacy Services, Woodruff, (800) 328-7060
Madison Pharmacy Associates, Madison, (800) 558-7046
Women's International Pharmacy, Madison, (800) 699-8144

Wyoming

Herbal Remedies, Casper, (866) 467-6444

Canada

Clinic Pharmacy, Oshawa, Ontario, (905) 576-9090
Courtesy Compounding Laboratories, Mississauga, Ontario, (905) 823-4664
Dauphin Clinic Pharmacy, Dauphin, Manitoba, (204) 638-4602
Falls Pharmacy, Niagara Falls, Ontario, (905) 354-3883
Habers Pharmacy, Toronto, Ontario, (877) 262-1084
Lemarchand Dispensary, New Edmonton, Alberta, (780) 482-3322
MacDonald's Prescriptions, Vancouver, British Columbia, (604) 872-2662

Marchese Pharmacy, Hamilton, Ontario, (905) 528-4201
Smith's Pharmacy, Toronto, Ontario, (800) 361-6624
Toronto Compounding Shoppe, Toronto, Ontario, (800) 201-8590
Victoria Compounding Pharmacy, Victoria, British Columbia, (877) 688-5181

Australia

Australian Pharmacy Compounding, Bankstown, New South Wales, (02)
    9793-1161
Redwood, Bondi Junction, New South Wales, (02) 9389-6400
Stenlake Compounding, Bondi Junction, New South Wales, (02) 9387-3205

New Zealand

Women's Balance Ltd., Howick, (64) 9-535-2020

If you are interested in using the Internet for more details about any of these companies' product lines, you can first go to: www.healthcare-alternatives.com (Web page for *The Estrogen Alternative: Natural Hormone Therapy with Botanical Progesterone*). Click on the book title, then onto "LINKS" and to any of the manufacturers' sites that are listed there. For a list of more compounding pharmacies nationwide or closer to you, call Professionals and Patients for Customized Care at (713) 933-8400.

As of this writing, I find that more manufacturers and distributors could be added daily to this list. Because of the popularity and diversity of the health benefits of phytohormones, it is virtually impossible to keep up with all the new companies marketing such products.

There has been a great deal of confusion pertaining to the progesterone content of various manufacturers' transdermal creams. The bioavailability of the progesterone in such products is of paramount importance. The quality of a formulation and its delivery system determines the absorption and effectiveness. It's essential that you know your product and your supplier and above all observe your body's response to the product of your choice.

It's important, when companies suddenly appear on the market, that we do our homework. Many would-be entrepreneurs are just now hearing about progesterone or wild yam extract and are jumping on what they consider a get-rich-quick bandwagon. Some of these organizations are not using the essential, natural ingredients that are necessary to achieve the results we speak about in this book. A company that will evaluate the ingredients in your product (milligrams per ounce) is Scientific Associates, Inc., (314) 487-6776.

Incidentally, James Jamieson, a pharmaceutical manufacturer and researcher, says that some companies' products may function more naturally than others as a result of enzymatic fermentation of the yam rather than actual pharmaceutical alteration. Thousands of years' experience, he says, has proven the effectiveness of the former process. Jamieson calls these yams modulators: they bring hormone levels to normal whether they are high or low. They do not build up in the body, and you cannot overdose on them. On the other hand, one manufacturer of so-called nutraceuticals for dietary use told me, in fact, that the more sophisticated the extraction processes for phytochemicals have become, the less effective these isolated plant fractions have proven to be.

Along these lines, the Reader's Digest's *Magic and Medicine of Plants* poses some very interesting questions that are relevant to our consideration of the use of any herbal products:

> Could the very purity of laboratory-isolated substances be a drawback?
> Do some natural plant medicines have ingredients that prevent danger-
> ous side effects in human use? . . . Is there sometimes a synergistic effect
> when the whole plant, as opposed to just the purified chemicals derived
> from it, is used? . . . Is the action of a whole plant sometimes more than
> the sum of its chemical parts?[6]

One might, therefore, want to work with manufacturers and pharmacies who are concerned with valid questions such as these. The substances that are often filtered out of the plant material do contain natural enzymes, alkaloids, peptides, phytosterols, etc. that interact with what is considered the "active" ingredient found in plants such as the wild yam. "They are part of the healing plant chemistry," says Dr. Richard Schulze. "To isolate the 'active ingredient' ignores all the OTHER ingredients that make an herb work."[7]

Plant compounds used in medicinal formulations are valuable, reliable, and easily assimilated sources of necessary building blocks, including proteins, carbohydrates, minerals, fatty acids, tannins, and many vitamins. These often function as precursors for our hormones and prostaglandins, and some even contain naturally occurring antibiotic elements. Barbara Griggs writes in *Green Pharmacy:* "Man and plant are close biological kin: the lifeblood of the plant, its green chlorophyll, has a chemical structure almost identical to the haemoglobin which is the central constituent of human blood; where chlorophyll has a molecule of magnesium in its structural pattern, haemoglobin carries a molecule of iron."[8] Marcia Jones, Director of the PMS and Menopause Center at Dixie Health, carries this analogy further, explaining that just as chlorophyll is nearly identical to hemoglobin, so diosgenin (from *Dioscorea*) is very similar to the molecular structure of progesterone and other hormones.

As a matter of course, we should seek out products whose manufacturers can assure us that the plants they use have been organically grown. Otherwise, residues of pesticides and other chemicals present in the end product could function as pseudo-estrogens and have the opposite from the desired effect, destroying hormonal balance.

Whatever the production method, it's worth mentioning that before purchasing any progesterone product, it pays to investigate whom you're buying from and what you are buying. The quality and potency of the ingredients can make a difference. And remember, each of us may have a unique way of responding to any particular progesterone formulation.

Some women feel the difference within a couple of weeks, others within several months. Again, what works for one person may not work as well for another—and it may be that all it takes is trying another brand, or using it long enough, or often enough, to give it a chance. And, as always is the case, if any unusual symptoms develop, consider consulting a health care practitioner knowledgeable in the use of natural hormone replacement therapy. Certain modifications in use are probably necessary to suit your own body's needs. (See appendix E for organizations that will help you find a physician who practices alternative medicine.)

USEFUL READING

Guide to Women's Nutrition, by Carlton Fredericks, Ph.D. (New York: The Putnam Publishing Group, 1989).

From PMS to Menopause: Female Hormones in Context, by Raymond F. Peat, Ph.D. (Eugene, OR: Kenogen, 1997).

Hormone Replacement Therapy: Yes or No?, by Betty Kamen, Ph.D. (Bel Marin Keys, CA: Nutrition Encounter, Inc., 1991).

The Journey Beyond Breast Cancer, by Virginia M. Soffa (Rochester, VT: Healing Arts Press, 1994).

Menopaws, by Martha Sacks (Berkeley, CA: Ten Speed Press, 1994).

The Menopause Industry: How the Medical Establishment Exploits Women, by Sandra Covey (Alameda, CA: Hunter House, 1994).

Natural Hormone Replacement (for Women Over 45), by Jonathan V. Wright, M.D., and John Morganthaler (Petaluma, California: Smart Publications, 1997).

Natural Progesterone: The Multiple Roles of a Remarkable Hormone, by John R. Lee, M.D. (Sebastopol, CA: BLL Publishing, 1993).

Natural Women, Natural Menopause, by Marcus Laux, N.D., and Christine Conrad (New York: HarperCollins, 1997).

Nutrition for Women, 5th ed., by Raymond F. Peat, Ph.D. (Eugene, OR: Kenogen, 1993).

Once a Month, by Katharina Dalton, M.D., F.R.C.G.P. (Pomona, CA: Hunter House, 1979).

Our Stolen Future, by Theo Colborn et al. (New York: Plume/Penguin, 1997).

PMS, Premenstrual Syndrome and You: Next Month Can Be Different, by Niels H. Lauersen, M.D. (New York: Simon & Schuster, 1983).

Pregnenolone, by Ray Sahelian, M.D. (Garden City, NY: Avery Publishing Group, 1997).

Preventing and Reversing Osteoporosis, by Alan R. Gaby, M.D. (Rocklin, CA: Prima Publishing, 1994).

Prostate Health in 90 Days Without Drugs or Surgery, by Larry Clapp, Ph.D., J.D. (Carlsbad, CA: Hay House, 1997).

The Silent Passage: Menopause, by Gail Sheehy (New York: Pocket Books, 1993).

The Super-Hormone Promise, by William Regelson, M.D., and Carol Colman (New York: Simon & Schuster, 1996).

What Your Doctor May Not Tell You about Menopause, by John R. Lee, M.D., with Virginia Hopkins (New York: Warner Books, 1996).

Without Estrogen: Natural Remedies for Menopause and Beyond, by Dee Ito (New York: Carol Southern Books, 1994).

Women's Bodies, Women's Wisdom, by Christiane Northrup, M.D. (New York: Bantam Books, 1994).

NOTES

Preface

1. Gina Kolata, "Many Taking Hormone Pills Now Face a Difficult Choice," *The New York Times*, July 15, 2002.
2. Sandra Coney, *The Menopause Industry, How the Medical Establishment Exploits Women* (Alameda, CA: Hunter House, 1994), 77, 108, 123, 195–99, 255, 258.
3. Book Review of *The Estrogen Alternative*, in *World Health News*, Vol. 1, No. 4, Fall 1997: 11.
4. Gina Kolata, "Many Taking Hormone Pills Now Face a Difficult Choice," *The New York Times*, July 15, 2002.
5. J. C. Prior et al., "Spinal Bone Loss and Ovulatory Disturbances," *International Journal Gynecol Obstet* 34, 1990: 253–56.
6. John R. Lee, "Osteoporosis Reversal: The Role of Progesterone," *International Clinical Nutrition Review* 10 (3), 1990: 384–91.
7. A. E. Roher et al., "Increased A beta peptides and reduced cholesterol and myelin proteins characterize white matter degeneration in Alzheimer's disease," *Biochemistry* 41 (37), September 17, 2002: 11080–90.
8. M. Michikawa et al., "Apolipoprotein E4 Induces Neuronal Cell Death Unnovo Cholesterol Synthesis," *J Neurosci Res* 54, 1998: 58–67.
9. J. Choi et al., "Lovostatin Induces Apoptosis of Spontaneously Immortalized Rat Brain Neuroblasts: Involvement of Nonsterol Isoprenoid Cells (3T3)," *Eur J Pharmacol* 301, 1996: 203–6.
10. M. Michikawa et al., "Inhibition of Cholesterol Production but Not of Nonsterol Isoprenoid Products Induces Neuronal Cell Death," *J Neurochem* 72 (6), June 1999: 2278–85.
11. Gina Kolata and Melody Petersen, "Hormone Replacement Study a Shock to the Medical System," *The New York Times*, July 10, 2002.

Introduction

1. Helen Keller, *Light in My Darkness*, revised and enlarged by Ray Silverman (West Chester, PA: Chrysalis Books, 2000), 124.

2. John R. Lee, *Natural Progesterone: The Multiple Roles of a Remarkable Hormone* (Sebastopol, CA: BLL Publishing, 1993).

3. John R. Lee, "Is Natural Progesterone the Missing Link in Osteoporosis Prevention and Treatment?" *Medical Hypotheses,* 1991.

4. Julian Whitaker, *Health & Healing: Tomorrow's Medicine Today*, Vol. 3, No. 6, June 1993.

5. P. A. Lehmann, "Russell E. Marker," *Journal of Chemical Education,* Vol. 50, March 1973, 195–99.

6. Katharina Dalton, "Ante-natal Progesterone and Intelligence," *British Journal of Psychiatry,* Vol. 114, 1968.

7. A. H. Follingstad, "Estriol, the Forgotten Estrogen?" *Journal of the American Medical Association,* Vol. 239, No. 1, January 2, 1978.

8. Joel T. Hargrove et al., "Menopausal Hormone Replacement Therapy with Continuous Daily Oral Micronized Estradiol and Progesterone," *Obstetrics & Gynecology,* Vol. 73, No. 4, April 1989, 606–12.

9. J. C. Prior, Y. Vigna, and N. Alojada, "Progesterone and the Prevention of Osteoporosis," *Canadian Journal of OB/Gyn & Women's Health Care,* Vol. 3, No. 4, 1991, 181.

10. John R. Lee, "Significance of Molecular Configuration Specificity—The Case of Progesterone and Osteoporosis," *Townsend Letter for Doctors,* June 1993, 558.

11. John R. Lee, *Natural Progesterone.*

12. John R. Lee, "Significance of Molecular Configuration Specificity," 558.

13. John R. Lee, "Natural Progesterone" (transcript), *Cancer Forum,* Vol. 13, No. 5/6, Winter 1994–1995.

14. Keller, *Light in My Darkness.*

Chapter 1: Sick and Tired of Being Tired and Sick

1. Macmillan Dictionary of Quotations (New York: Macmilllan, 1989), 358.

2. Richard A. Passwater, *Cancer and Its Nutritional Therapies* (New Canaan, CT: Keats Publishing, 1983).

3. Raquel Martin, *Today's Health Alternative* (Bozeman, MT: America West Publishers, 1992).

4. "Provera, Brand of Medroxyprogesterone Acetate Tablets, USP," Upjohn Company, Kalamazoo, MI, 1992.

5. Gail Sheehy, *The Silent Passage: Menopause* (New York: Pocket Books, 1993).

6. John R. Lee, "Is Natural Progesterone the Missing Link in Osteoporosis Prevention and Treatment?", *Medical Hypotheses,* 1991.

7. John R. Lee, *Natural Progesterone: The Multiple Roles of a Remarkable Hormone* (Sebastapol, CA: BLL Publishing, 1993).

8. John R. Lee, *What Your Doctor May Not Tell You About Menopause* (New York: Warner Books, 1996), 257.

9. John R. Lee, "Natural Progesterone," *Cancer Forum,* Vol. 13, No. 5/6, Winter 1994–1995, 9.

10. John R. Lee, *What Your Doctor May Not Tell You About Menopause*, 89, 197, 254.
11. C. Schairer et al., "Menopausal estrogen and estrogen-progestin replacement therapy and breast cancer risk," *Journal of the American Medical Association*, Vol. 283, 2000, 485–91.
12. R. D. Minshall et al., "In Vitro Modulation of Primate Coronary Vascular Muscle Cell Reactivity by Ovarian Steroid Hormones," *FASEB J*, August 1998.
13. K. Miyagawa et al., "Medroxyprogesterone Interferes with Ovarian Steroid protection Against Coronary Vasospasm," *Nature Medicine*, Vol. 3, 1997, 324–27.
14. Gina Kolata, "Many Taking Hormone Pills Now Face a Difficult Choice," *The New York Times*, July 15, 2002.
15. K. Miyagawa et al., "Medroxyprogesterone Interferes . . ."
16. S. Sidney et al., "Myocardial Infarction and the Use of Estrogen and Estrogen-Progestogen in Postmenopausal Women," *Annals of Internal Medincine*, Vol. 127, 1997, 501–8.
17. R. D Minshall et al., "Ovarian Steroid Protection Against Coronary Artery Hyperactivity in Rhesus Monkeys," *Journal of Clinical Endocrinology and Metabolism*, Vol. 83, 1998, 649–59.
18. K. Hermsmeyer et al., "Reactivity Based Coronary Vasospasm Independent of Atherosclerosis in Rhesus Monkeys," *Journal of the American College of Cardiology*, Vol. 29, 1997, 671–80.
19. B. Formby and T. S. Wiley, "Progesterone Inhibits Growth and Induces Apoptosis in Breast Cancer Cells: Inverse Effects on Bc1-2 and p53," *Annals of Clinical and Lab Science*, Vol. 28, 1998, 360–69.
20. L. D. Cowan et al., "Breast Cancer Incidence in Women with a History of Progesterone Deficiency," *American Journal of Epidemiology*, Vol. 114, 1981, 209–17.
21. B. Formby and T.S. Wiley, "Progesterone Inhibits Growth . . ."
22. R. Hertz et al., "Observations on the Effect of Progesterone on Carcinoma of the Cervix," *Journal of the National Cancer Institute*, Vol. 11, 1951, 867–73.
23. R. D. Gambrell Jr.et al., "Use of the Progestogen Challenge Test to Reduce the Risk of Endometrial Cancer," *Obstetrics & Gynecology*, Vol. 55, 1980, 732–38.
24. W. S. Maxson, "The Use of Progesterone in the Treatment of PMS," *Clinical Obstetrics and Gynecology*, Vol. 30, 1987, 465–80.
25. D. L. Moyer et al., "Prevention of Endometrial Hyperplasia by Progesterone During Long-Term Estradiol Replacement: Influence of Bleeding Pattern and Secretory Changes," *Fertility and Sterility*, Vol. 59, 1993, 992–97.
26. M. B. Aufrere et al., "Progesterone: an Overview and Recent Advances," *Journal of Pharmaceutical Science*, Vol. 65, 1976, 783.
27. John R. Lee, "Natural Progesterone," *Cancer Forum*.
28. I. Wiklund et al., "Long-Term Effect of Transdermal Hormonal Therapy on Aspects of Quality of Life in Postmenopausal Women," *Muturitas*, Vol. 3, March 14, 1992, 225–36.
29. Helen Keller, *Light in My Darkness*, revised and edited by Ray Silverman (Westchester, PA: Swedenborg Foundation, 1994).
30. Ibid.

31. Sandra Coney, *The Menopause Industry: How the Medical Establishment Exploits Women* (Alameda, CA: Hunter House, 1994), 270.

32. John R. Lee, *Natural Progesterone.*

33. John R. Lee, "Is Natural Progesterone the Missing Link in Osteoporosis Prevention and Treatment?" *Medical Hypotheses,* 1991.

34. John R. Lee, *Natural Progesterone,* iii, 33, 84–86.

35. Ibid., 46, 47.

36. Ibid., 26, 44, 45.

37. Ibid., iii, 4, 71–75, and John R. Lee, *What Your Doctor May Not Tell You About Menopause,* 207–14.

Chapter 2: The Myth of Estrogen Deficiency Versus the Reality of Progesterone Deficiency

1. John R. Lee, *Natural Progesterone: The Multiple Roles of a Remarkable Hormone* (Sebastopol, CA: BLL Publishing, 1993), 55.

2. Ibid., 5–6.

3. Norman Shealy, *Natural Progesterone Cream: Safe and Natural Hormone Replacement,* Keats Publishing, Los Angeles, 1999, 17.

4. J. C. Prior, "Perimenopause: The Complex Endocrinology of the Menopausal Transition," *Endocrine Reviews,* Vol. 19, No. 4, August 1998, 397–428.

5. S. R. Cummings et al., "Endogenous Hormones and the Risk of Hip and Vertebral Fracture Among Older Women," *New England Journal of Medicine,* Vol. 339, September 10, 1998, 733–38.

6. John R. Lee, *What Your Doctor May Not Tell You About Menopause* (New York: Warner Books, 1996).

7. Lita Lee, "Estrogen, Progesterone and Female Problems," *Earthletter,* Vol. 1, No. 2, June 1991.

8. Raymond F. Peat, "Progesterone: Essential to Your Well-Being," *Let's Live,* April 1982.

9. John R. Lee, "Is Natural Progesterone the Missing Link in Osteoporosis Prevention and Treatment?" *Medical Hypotheses,* 1991.

10. Peter S. Rhodes, *AIM* (Bryn Athyn, PA: New Will, 1991).

11. Gail Sheehy, *The Silent Passage: Menopause* (New York: Pocket Books, 1993), 29.

12. Shealy, *Natural Progesterone Cream,* 9.

13. Ibid., citing "Molecular Transformation of Plant sources to Progesterone," *Cancer Forum,* Vol. 13, No. 5/6, Winter 1994–95.

14. Lila Natchtigall and John Heilman, *Estrogen: The Facts Can Change Your Life* (Los Angeles: The Body Press, 1986).

15. Sandra Coney, *The Menopause Industry: How the Medical Establishment Exploits Women* (Alameda, CA: Hunter House, 1994), 77.

16. Ibid., 195.

17. Ibid., 199.

18. Ibid., 198.
19. Ibid., 21–22, 213.
20. John R. Lee, *Natural Progesterone*, 8, 54, 74.
21. Lita Lee, "Estrogen, Progesterone, and Female Problems."
22. Alvin Follingstad, "Estriol, the Forgotten Estrogen?" *Journal of the American Medical Association*, Vol. 239, No. 1, January 2, 1978.
23. Julian Whitaker, *Health & Healing*, Vol. 3, No. 3, March 1993.
24. Cummings et al., "Endogenous Hormones and the Risk of Hip and Vertebral Fracture."
25. Graham A. Colditz, "Type of Post-Menopausal Hormone Use and Risk of Breast Cancer: 12-Year Follow Up from the Nurses' Health Study," *Cancer Causes and Control*, Vol. 3, September 1992, 433–39.
26. M. A. J. McKenna, "Breast Cancer Risk Tied to Years of Menopausal Hormone Care," *Atlanta Journal/Constitution*, June 15, 1995.
27. John R. Lee, *Natural Progesterone*, 24, 33, 40, 43, 44, 84, 87.
28. Shealy, *Natural Progesterone Cream*, 20.
29. Lorrain Dusky, "Progesterone: Safe Antidote for PMS (Women's Health Report)," *McCall's*, October 1990.
30. Ibid.
31. Ibid.
32. I. Wiklund et al., "Long-Term Effect of Transdermal Hormonal Therapy on Aspects of Quality of Life in Postmenopausal Women," *Muturitas*, Vol. 3, March 14, 1992, 225–36.
33. Dusky, "Progesterone."
34. John R. Lee, *Natural Progesterone* and *What Your Doctor May Not Tell You About Menopause*.
35. Shealy, *Natural Progesterone Cream*.
36. Niels H. Lauersen, *PMS, Premenstrual Syndrome and You: Next Month Can Be Different* (New York: Simon & Schuster, 1983), 170.
37. John R. Lee, *Natural Progesterone*.
38. Ibid., 2.
39. Ibid., 35, 41, 54.
40. Lita Lee, "Estrogen, Progesterone, and Female Problems."
41. Katharina Dalton, "Premenstrual Syndrome and Postnatal Depression," *Health and Hygiene*, Vol. 11, 1990, 199–201.
42. Betty Kamen, *Hormone Replacement Therapy: Yes or No?* (Novato, CA: Nutrition Encounter, Inc., 1993), 4, 104, 210.
43. John R. Lee, *What Your Doctor May Not Tell You About Menopause*, 254.
44. Ibid., 197.
45. Ibid., 89.
46. Ibid., 24–33, 43–49.
47. John R. Lee, *Natural Progesterone*, 34, 35, 58, 65–70.
48. Alan R. Gaby, *Preventing and Reversing Osteoporosis* (Rocklin, CA: Prima Publishing, 1994), 9, 10, 21–22.

49. R. Martin and K. Romano, *Preventing and Reversing Arthritis Naturally: The Untold Story* (Rochester, VT: Healing Arts Press, 2000).

50. Raquel Martin, *Today's Health Alternative*.

51. John R. Lee, *Natural Progesterone*, 4–8.

52. Lita Lee, "Estrogen, Progesterone, and Female Problems."

53. Peat, "Progesterone."

54. Kamen, *Hormone Replacement Therapy*, 210.

55. Gaby, *Preventing and Reversing Osteoporosis*, 11.

56. Kamen, *Hormone Replacement Therapy*, 210.

57. John R. Lee, "Significance of Molecular Configuration Specificity."

58. John R. Lee, *Natural Progesterone*.

59. John R. Lee, *What Your Doctor May Not Tell You About Menopause*, 270.

60. Peat, *Nutrition for Women*, 5th ed. (Eugene, OR: Kenogen, 1993), 84–85.

61. "Natural Progesterone/Body Creams Vary in Potency," *Women's Health Advocate*, Vol. 3, No. 7, September 1996, 7.

62. John R. Lee, *Natural Progesterone*.

63. John R. Lee, *Natural Progesterone*, 79.

64. Christiane Northrup, *Women's Bodies, Women's Wisdom* (New York: Bantam Books, 1994), 76.

65. "Specific Estrogen Treatment for Atrophy Related Urogenital Complaints" (Ovestin estriol scientific information), The Netherlands, Organon International.

66. Ibid.

67. Gaby, *Preventing and Reversing Osteoporosis*, 135, 146, 261.

68. Raymond F. Peat, *Progesterone in Orthomolecular Medicine* (Eugene, OR, 1993).

69. Raymond F. Peat, Ph.D., *PMS to Menopause: Female Hormones in Context* (Eugene, OR: Kenogen, 1997), 80.

70. V. B. Mahesh et al., "Diverse Modes of Action of Progesterone and its Metabolites," *J. Steroid Biochem. Molec. Biol.*, Vol. 56, 1996, 209–19.

71. William Regelson, M.D. and Carol Colman, *The Super-Hormone Promise* (New York: Simon & Schuster, 1996), 41.

72. Koenigh, Schumacher M., Ferzaz B., Thi A., et al., "Progesterone Synthesis and Myelin Formation by Schwann Cells," *Science*, Vol. 268, No. 5216, 1995, 1500–03.

73. E. Henderson et al., "Pregnenolone," *J. Clin. Endocrinol.* Vol. 10, 1950, 455–74, in Ray Sahelian, M.D., *Pregnenolone* (Melatonin/DHEA Research Institute, Marina Del Rey), 1996.

74. Marcus Laux, *Naturally Well*, Vol. 2, No. 12, December 1995.

75. Sharon Gleason, "Menopause . . . It's Not a Disease," *The Rice Paper*, Summer 1994.

76. Coney, *The Menopause Industry*.

77. U. B. Ottosson, "Oral Progesterone and Estrogen/Progestogen Therapy: Effects of Natural and Synthetic Hormones on Subfractions of HDL Cholesterol and Liver Proteins," *Acta Obstet. Gynecol. Scand.* (supplement), Vol. 127, 1984, 1–37.

78. John R. Lee, *Natural Progesterone*, 8.

79. L. A. Brinton et al., "Oral Contraceptives and Breast Cancer Risk Among

Younger Women," *Journal of the National Cancer Institute,* Vol. 98, No. 11, June 1995, 827–35.

80. C. Shairer et al., "Menopausal estrogen and estrogen-progestin replacement therapy and breast cancer risk," *JAMA,* Vol. 283, 2000, 485–91.

81. E. L. Cavalieri et al., "Molecular Origin of Cancer: cathechol Estrogen-3, 4-quinones as Endogenous Tumor Initiators," *Proceedings of the National Academy of Science,* Vol. 94, 1994, 10937–942.

82. C. Rodriquez et al., "Estrogen Replacement Therapy and Fatal Ovarian Cancer," *American Journal of Epidemiology,* Vol. 141, 1995, 828–34.

83. John R. Lee, *Natural Progesterone,* 32–37, 71–75.

84. Ibid., 33.

85. Raymond F. Peat, *Nutrition for Women,* 5th ed., (Eugene, OR: Kenogen, 1993).

86. Ibid.

87. J. Fischman et al., "The Role of Estrogen in Mammary Carcinogenesis," *Annals of the New York Academy of Sciences,* Vol. 768, No. 91, 1995.

88. Brinton et al., "Oral Contraceptives and Breast Cancer Risk Among Younger Women."

89. B. Formby and T. S. Wiley, "Progesterone Inhibits Growth and Induces Apoptosis in Breast Cancer Cells: Inverse Effects on Bc1-2 and p53," *Annals of Clin and Lab Science,* Vol. 28, 1998, 360–69.

90. C. Rodriquez et al., "Estrogen Replacement Therapy and Fatal Ovarian Cancer."

91. John R. Lee, *Natural Progesterone,* 84.

92. Ibid., 70, 82, 85, 86.

93. The Burton Goldberg Group, *Alternative Medicine* (Puyallup, WA: Future Medicine Publishing, 1993), 675.

94. Nina Sessler, "Questions & Answers on Women's Health Issues: What Is Fibrocystic Breast Disease?" *Natural Solutions,* Vol. 1, Issue 1, Fall 1993.

95. Susan M. Love, *Dr. Susan Love's Breast Book* (New York: Addison-Wesley, 1990), 81–86.

96. John R. Lee, *Natural Progesterone,* 84.

97. Ibid., 87.

98. Resources to be found on: www.holyhormones.com/resources.htm

99. John R. Lee, *Natural Progesterone,* 87.

100. Northrup, *Women's Bodies, Women's Wisdom,* 220–24.

101. Ibid.

102. Gaby, *Preventing and Reversing Osteoporosis,* 154.

103. Majid Ali, "Chemical Conflict: The Age of Estrogen Overdrive," *Lifespanner,* December 1994.

104. Linda G. Rector-Page, *Healthy Healing: An Alternative Healing* (Soquel, CA: Healthy Healing Publications, 1992).

105. "The Estrogen Question," *The John R. Lee, M.D. Medical Letter,* November, 1998, 1.

106. Anne Dickson and Nikki Henriques, *Women on Menopause* (Rochester, VT: Healing Arts Press, 1988), 55.

107. Sari Harrar and Sara Altshul O'Donnell, *The Woman's Book of Healing Herbs*

(Emmaus, PA: Rodale Press, Inc., 1999), 226.

108. "News Update: Tampons and Dioxin," *Women's Health Advocate,* May 1998.

109. Harrar and Altshul O'Donnell, *The Woman's Book of Healing Herbs,* 227.

110. Ellen Brown and Lynne Walker, *Breezing Through the Change* (Berkeley, CA: Frog, Ltd. 1994), 77.

111. "Effects of Estrogen or Estrogen/Progestin Regimens on Heart Disease Risk Fractures in Postmenopausal Women; The Postmenopausal Estrogen/Progestin Intervention (PEPI) Trial," *Journal of the American Medical Association,* Vol. 273, January 18, 1995, 199–208.

112. Peter G. Rose, M.D., "Medical Progress: Endometrial Carcinoma," *New England Journal of Medicine,* Vol. 335, August 29, 1996, 640–49.

113. K. Boman et al., "The Influence of Progesterone and Androgens on the Growth of Endometrial Carcinoma," *Cancer,* Vol. 71, 1993, 3565–69.

114. Sheehy, *The Silent Passage.*

115. Ibid.

116. Ibid.

117. Ibid.

118. Tara Parker-Pope, "The Abortion Pill and Other Treatments that Could Help Avoid a Hysterectomy," *The Wall Street Journal,* February 25, 2003, D1.

119. T. S. Wiley, J. Taguchi, and B. Formby, *Sex, Lies, and Menopause: the Shocking Truth about Hormone Replacement Therapy* (New York: HarperCollins Publishers, Inc., 2003), 83.

120. Ibid., citing R. Fossati et al. "Cyotoxic and Hormonal Treatment for Metastatic Breast Cancer: A Synthetic Review of Published Randomized Trials Involving 31,510 Women," *J Clin Oncol,* Vol. 10, 1998, 3489–99.

121. Ibid., citing J. E. Rigby et al., "Can Physical Trauma Cause Breast Cancer?," *Eur J Cancer Prev,* Vol. 11, No. 3, June 2002, 307–11.

122. Ibid., citing J. P. Van Netten et al., "Physical Trauma and Breast Cancer," *The Lancet,* Vol. 343, No. 8903, April 16, 1994, 978–99.

123. Dickson and Henriques, *Women on Menopause,* 6.

124. Ibid.

125. John R. Lee, *Natural Progesterone,* 30.

126. Peat, "Progesterone."

127. John R. Lee, *What Your Doctor May Not Tell You About Menopause,* 89, 197, 198, 254.

128. C. Shairer et al., "Menopausal estrogen and estrogen-progestin replacement therapy and breast cancer risk."

129. Todd Mangum, M.D., "The Dangers of Hormone Replacement," Independent Media Institute, November 21, 2002.

130. Norman Shealy, *Natural Progesterone Cream.*

131. Evista 60Mg (Generic name: Raloxifene) prescription information (Medi Span, Inc. Database Edition 98.4, 1998).

132. Raymond F. Peat, "Progesterone and Ideas of Balance in Hormone Replacement Therapy: The Importance of Inhibition," *Ray Peat's Newsletter,* 2000, 2, 4.

133. Kamen, *Hormone Replacement Therapy*, 210.
134. Raymond F. Peat, "Estrogen: Simply Dangerous," *Ray Peat's Newsletter*, July 1995.

Chapter 3: The Seasons of a Woman's Life

1. José Ortega y Gasset, *The Revolt of the Masses* (1930).
2. Sterling Morgan, "Part II: PMS, Menopause, & Other Areas," *To Your Health*, September/October 1993, 19.
3. Katharina Dalton, *Once a Month* (Alameda, CA: Hunter House, 1994).
4. Stuart M. Berger, *What Your Doctor Didn't Learn in Medical School* (New York: William Morrow, 1988), 211–13.
5. Harriet Greveal, "Answers for PMS," *Total Health*, July 1985, 26.
6. Chakmakjian Zaren, "A Critical Assessment of Therapy for the Pre-Menstrual Tension Syndrome," *Journal of Reproductive Medicine*, Vol. 28, No. 8, August 1983, 532.
7. Dalton, "Premenstrual Syndrome and Postnatal Depression," *Health and Hygiene*, Vol. 11, 1990, 199–201.
8. Katharina Dalton, "Guide to Progesterone for Postnatal Depression" (pamphlet), 1990.
9. Ibid.
10. Katharina Dalton, "A Guide to Premenstrual Syndrome and Its Treatment" (pamphlet), 1990, 12.
11. Dalton, "Premenstrual Syndrome."
12. John R. Lee, *Natural Progesterone: The Multiple Roles of a Remarkable Hormone* (Sebastopol, CA: BLL Publishing, 1993), 33.
13. John R. Lee, "Natural Progesterone" (transcript), *Cancer Forum*, Vol. 13, No. 5/6, Winter 1994-1995, 61.
14. Betty Kamen, *Hormone Replacement Therapy: Yes or No?* (Novato, CA: Nutrition Encounter, Inc., 1993), 212.
15. Sterling Morgan, "Pregnancy & Natural Progesterone = Superior Baby," *To Your Health: The Magazine of Healing and Hope*, Vol. 5, No. 6, May/June/July 1993.
16. Raymond F. Peat, *Nutrition for Women*, 5th ed. (Eugene, OR: Kenogen, 1993).
17. Dalton, *Once a Month*, 53.
18. Ibid., 67.
19. Kamen, *Hormone Replacement Therapy*.
20. E. Tauboll, S. Linstrom, "The Effect of Progesterone and its Metabolite 5 Alpha-Pregnan-3 Alpha-ol-20-one on Focal Epileptic Seizures in the Cat's Visual Cortex in Vivo," *Epilepsy Research*, Vol. 14, No. 1, January 1993, 17–30. See also A.G. Herzog, "Reproductive Endocrine Considerations and Hormonal Therapy for Women with Epilepsy," *Epilepsia*, 32 Suppl. 6, 1991, S27–33.
21. Raymond Peat, *From PMS to Menopause: Female Hormones in Context* (International University, Eugene, Oregon, 1997), 74.
22. Norman Shealy, *Natural Progesterone Cream: Safe and Natural Hormone Replacement* (Los Angeles, CA: Keats Publishing, 1999).

23. John R. Lee, M.D., *Natural Progesterone: The Multiple Roles of a Remarkable Hormone* (Sebastopol, CA: BLL Publishing, 1993) citing R. D. Gambrell, "The Menopause: Benefits and Risks of Estrogen-Progestogen Replacement Therapy," *Fertil Steril*, Vol. 37, 1983, 457–474.

24. Niels H. Lauersen, *PMS: Premenstrual Syndrome and You—Next Month Can Be Different* (New York: Simon & Schuster, 1983).

25. Gail Sheehy, *The Silent Passage: Menopause* (New York: Pocket Books, 1993).

26. Peat, *Nutrition for Women*, 18.

27. Morgan, "Part II: Menopause."

28. Morgan, "Pregnancy and Natural Progesterone."

29. Ibid.

30. Raymond F. Peat, "Progesterone: Essential to your Well-Being," *Let's Live*, April 1982.

31. John R. Lee, *Natural Progesterone*, 29.

32. Ibid., 30.

33. J. C. Prior and Y. M. Vigna, "Spinal Bones Loss and Ovulatory Disturbances," *New England Journal of Medicine*, Vol. 223, 1990, 1221–27.

34. J. C. Prior, Y. M. Vigna, and N. Alojada, "Progesterone and the Prevention of Osteoporosis," *Canadian Journal of OB/GYN & Women's Health Care*, Vol. 3, 1991, 178–84.

35. Peat, "Progesterone."

36. C. Norman Shealy, *DHEA: The Health and Youth Hormone* (New Canaan, CT: Keats Publishing, 1996).

37. Alan R. Gaby, *Preventing and Reversing Osteoporosis* (Rocklin, CA: Prima Publishing, 1994), 165–68.

38. "Mother Knows Best! The Fascinating Healing Benefits of DHEA—The Body's "Mother Hormone!," *Bio/Tech News*, 1995, 5.

39. Shealy, *DHEA*.

40. John R. Lee, "Why Good Liver Function Makes for Better Hormone Balance," *The John R. Lee, M.D. Medical Letter*, September 1999, 6.

41. A. J. Morales et al., "Effects of Replacement Dose of Dehydroepiandrosterone in Men and Women of Advancing Age," *Journal of Clinical Endocrinology and Metabolism*, Vol. 78, No. 6, 1994, 1360–67.

42. Joe Glickman, Jr., "Hormone Holds Key to Aging Process," *Health Science Report*, Vol. 2, No. 1, 1996.

43. Elizabeth Barrett-Conner et al., "A Prospective Study of Dehydroepiandrosterone Sulfate, Mortality, and Cardiovascular Disease," *New England Journal of Medicine*, Vol. 315, No. 24, 1986, 1519–24.

44. D. M. Herrrington et al., "Plasma Dehydroepiandrosterone and Dehydroepiandrosterone Sulfate in Patients Undergoing Diagnostic Coronary Angiography," *Journal of the American College of Cardiology*, Vol. 16, No. 6, 1990, 862–70.

45. J. E. Nestler et al., "Dehydroepiandrosterone Reduces Serum Low Density Lipoprotein Levels and Body Fat but Does Not Alter Insulin Sensitivity in

Normal Men," *Journal of Clinical Endocrinology and Metabolism,* Vol. 66, No. 1, 1988, 57–61.

46. G. B. Gordon et al., "Reduction of Atherosclerosis by Administration of Dehydroepiandrosterone. A Study in the Hypercholesteroemic New Zealand White Rabbit With Aortic Intimal Injury," *Journal of Clinical Investigations,* Vol. 82, No. 2, 1988, 712–20.

47. Glickman, "Hormone Holds Key to Aging Process."

48. G. B. Gordon, "Reduction of Atherosclerosis."

49. A. G. Schwartz and L. L. Pashko, "Cancer Chemoprevention with the Adrenocortical Steroid Dehydroepiandrosterone and Structural Analogs," *Journal of Cellular Biochemistry* (Supplement), Vol. 17G, 1993, 73–79.

50. G. B. Gordon et al., "Serum Levels of Dehydroepiandrosterone Sulfate and the Risk of Developing Gastric Cancer," *Cancer Epidemiology,* Vol. 2, No. 1, 1993, 33–35.

51. G. B. Gordon, L. M. Shantz, and P. Talalay, "Modulation of Growth, Differentiation and Carcinogenesis by Dehydroepiandrosterone," *Advances in Enzyme Regulation,* Vol. 26, 1987, 355–82.

52. C. W. Boone, V. E. Steele, and G. J. Kelloff, "Screening for Chemopreventive (Anticarcinogenic) Compounds in Rodents," *Mutation Research,* Vol. 267, No. 2, 1992, 251–55.

53. L. Bologa, J. Sharma, and E. Roberts, "Dehydroepiandrosterone and its Sulfated Derivative Reduce Neuronal Death and Enhance Astrocytic Differentiation in Brain Cell Cultures," *Journal of Neuroscience Research,* Vol. 17, No. 3, 1987, 225–34.

54. Glickman, "Hormone Holds Key to Aging Process."

55. Ibid., 3.

56. Peat, "Progesterone."

57. Alfred Gilman, Louis Goodman, *Goodman & Gilman's Pharmacological Basis of Therapeutics,* 6th ed. (New York: Macmillan, 1980), 1420–38.

58. K. Miyagawa et al., "Medroxyprogesterone Interferes with Ovarian Steroid protection Against Coronary Vasospasm, *Nature Medicine,* Vol. 3, 1997, 324–27.

59. R. D. Minshall et al., "In Vitro Modulation of Primate Coronary Vascular Muscle Cell Reactivity by Ovarian Steroid Hormones," *FASEB J,* August 1998.

60. R. D. Minshall et al., "Ovarian Steroid Protection Against Coronary Artery Hyperactivity in Rhesus Monkeys," *J Clin Endoc Metabol,* Vol. 83, 1998, 649–59.

61. K. Hermsmeyer et al., "Reactivity Based Coronary Vasospasm Independent of Atherosclerosis in Rhesus Monkeys," *J Am Col Cardiol,* Vol. 29, 1997, 671–80.

62. S. Sidney et al., "Myocardial Infarction and the Use of Estrogen and Estrogen-Progestogen in Postmenopausal Women," *Ann Int Med,* Vol. 127, 1997, 501–8.

63. C. Schairer et al., "Menopausal estrogen and estrogen-progestin replacement therapy and breast cancer risk," *JAMA,* Vol. 283, 2000, 485–91.

64. Todd Mangum, M.D., "The Dangers of Hormone Replacement," Independent Media Institute, November 21, 2002.

65. Amanda Spake, "The Menopausal Marketplace," *U.S. News & World Report,* November 18, 2002, 48

66. www.mercola.com/2002/jul/13/estrogen.htm.
67. Spake, "The Menopausal Marketplace."
68. Ibid.
69. L. Cavalieri et al., "Molecular Origin of Cancer; Catechol Estrogen-3, 4-quinones as Endogenous Tumor Initiators," *Proc Natl Acad Sci,* Vol. 94, 1994, 10937–42.
70. L. Bergkvist, et al., "The Risk of Breast Cancer After Estrogen and Estrogen-Progestin Replacement," *New England Journal of Medicine,* Vol. 321, 1989, 293–97.
71. J. Fischman et al., "The Role of Estrogen in Mammary Carcinogenesis," *Annals of the New York Academy of Sciences,* Vol. 768, No. 91, 1995.
72. L. A. Brinton et al., "Oral Contraceptives and Breast Cancer Risk Among Younger Women," *J Natl Cancer Inst,* Vol. 98, No. 11, June 1995, 827–35.
73. C. Rodriquez et al., "Estrogen Replacement Therapy and Fatal Ovarian Cancer," *American Journal of Epidemiology,* Vol. 141, 1995, 828–34.
74. Writing Group for the PEP Trial, "Effects of Estrogen or Estrogen/Progestin Regimens on Heart Disease Risk Factors in Postmenopausal Women," *JAMA,* Vol. 273, No. 3, January 18, 1995.
75. Peter G. Rose, "Medical Progress: Endometrial Carcinoma," *New England Journal of Medicine,* Vol. 335, August 29, 1996, 640–49.
76. J. Raloff, "Hormone Therapy: Issues of the Heart," *Science News,* Vol. 151, March 8, 1997, 140.
77. Ibid.
78. Ibid.
79. Ibid.
80. Ibid.
81. D. Rodriquez et al., "Estrogen Replacement Therapy and Fatal Ovarian Cancer," *American Journal of Epidemiology,* Vol. 141, 1995, 828–35.
82. Raloff, "Hormone Therapy: Issues of the Heart," 140.
83. Spake, "The Menopausal Marketplace."
84. Stephen Hulley et al., "Randomized Trial of Estrogen Plus Progestin for Secondary Prevention of Coronary Heart Disease in Postmenopausal Women," *Journal of the American Medical Association,* Vol. 280, 1998, 605–13.
85. D. Grady et al., "Heart and Estrogen/progestin Replacement Study (HERS): Design, Methods, and Baseline Characteristics," *Control Clin Trials,* Vol. 29, 1998, 324–35.
86. Lauran Neergaard, "Study on risks of estrogen-progestin combination raises questions," AP Health Article, July 9, 2002.
87. Melody Petersen, "Heartfelt Advice, Hefty Fees," *New York Times,* August 11, 2002; Jenny Thompson, "The Color Purple," Health Sciences Institute e-Alert, September 23, 2003.
88. Sheehy, *The Silent Passage.*
89. Ibid.
90. Ibid.
91. Ibid.

92. Bert Stern et al., *The Pill Book* (New York: Bantam Books, 1986), 542.
93. D. T. Baird and A. F. Glasier, "Drug Therapy: Hormonal Contraception," *New England Journal of Medicine*, Vol. 328, No. 1543, 1993.
94. Kamen, *Hormone Repacement Therapy*, 35.
95. Anne Dickson and Nikki Henriques, *Women on Menopause* (Rochester, VT: Healing Arts Press, 1988), 67.
96. Lita Lee, "Estrogen, Progesterone and Female Problems," *Earthletter*, Vol. 1, No. 2, June 1991.
97. Elaine Hollingsworth, *Take Control of Your Health and Escape the Sickness Industry*, 6th edition (Australia: Empowerment Press International, 2000), 90, 92, 108, 109.
98. Carlton Fredericks, *Guide to Women's Nutrition* (New York: Putnam Publishing Group, 1989).
99. Amanda Ross, "Evening the Score," *Health eTips, Jonathan V. Wright's Nutrition & Healing*, April 1, 2003, www.wrightnewsletter.com.
100. John R. Lee, "Clinician of the Month," *The John R. Lee, M.D. Medical Letter*, May 1999, 5.
101. John R. Lee, "Why Good Liver Function Makes for Better Hormone Balance," 5.
102. Ibid.
103. James F. Balch, M.D., and Phyllis A. Balch, C.N.C., *Prescription for Nutritional Healing* (Garden City Park, NY: Avery Publishing Group Inc., 1997, 22.
104. John R. Lee, "Why Good Liver Function Makes for Better Hormone Balance," 6.
105. Patricia Andersen-Parrado, "Homeopathic Remedies to Ease Acute and Chronic Arthritis Pain," *Better Nutrition*, February, 1997, 26.
106. Marilyn Glenville, Ph.D., *Natural Choices for Menopause* (New York: St. Martins Press, 1999), 97, 98, 103.
107. John R. Lee, *Natural Progesterone*, 44.
108. Julian Whitaker, *Health & Healing Tomorrow's Medicine Today*, Vol. 4, No. 5, May 1994.
109. Ibid.
110. The Burton Goldberg Group, *Alternative Medicine* (Puyallup, WA: Future Medicine Publishing, 1993), 1014–15.
111. Ibid.
112. Joe Graedon, *The People's Pharmacy* (New York: Avon Books, 1977), 188–93.
113. "Dangers of Estrogen," Form P8263-01, Mead Johnson Laboratories, Princeton, NJ, December 1992.
114. John R. Lee, *What Your Doctor May Not Tell You About Menopause* (New York: Warner Books, 1996), 307.
115. Raquel Martin, *Today's Health Alternative* (Bozeman, MT: America West Publishers, 1992).
116. Sheehy, *The Silent Passage*, 124.
117. Skye Lininger, D.C., Jonathan Wright, M.D., Steve Austin, N.D., Donald Brown, N.D., Alan Gaby, M.D., *The Natural Pharmacy* (Rocklin, CA: Prima Health, 1998), 320. See also M. Araghiniknam et al., "Antioxidant Activity of

Dioscorea and Dehydroepiandrosterone (DHEA) in Older Humans," *Life Sci,* Vol. 11, 1996, 147–57.

118. Verina E. Palmer, "Women at Risk," *The Phoenix Tribune,* February 5, 1998, D1.

119. Donald J. Brown, *Herbal Prescriptions for Better Health* (Rocklin, CA: Prima, 1996), 181, 182, and D. Propping et al., "Diagnosis and Therapy of Corpus Luteum Insufficiency in General Practice," *Therapiewoche,* Vol. 38, 1988, 2992–3001.

120. Barbara Joseph, M.D., *My Healing from Breast Cancer* (New Canaan, CT: Keats Publishing Inc., 1996), 222.

121. Anthony J. Chichoke, "The Uniqueness of Women," *The Energy Times,* May/June 1994, 2.

122. Alfred Gilman and Louis Goodman, *Goodman and Gilman's Pharmacological Basis of Therapeutics,* 6th ed. (New York: Macmillan, 1980).

123. Ibid.

124. John R. Lee, *Natural Progesterone,* 40–41.

125. Shealy, *DHEA.*

126. Christine Ammer, *The New A-Z of Womens' Health: A Concise Encyclopedia* (New York: Facts on File, Inc., 1989), 357.

127. Coney, *The Menopause Industry.*

128. Dalton, "Guide to Progesterone."

129. Peat, "Progesterone."

130. Peat, *From PMS to Menopause: Female Hormones in Context,* 8.

131. S. N. Chatterjee, et al., "Effect of Intrauterine Contraceptive Suture on Corpora Lutea of Guinea-Pigs," *Indian Journal of Exp. Biol.,* Vol. 9, 1997, 105

132. Linda G. Rector-Page, *Healthy Healing: An Alternative Healing Reference* (Soquel, CA: Healthy Healing Publications, 1992), 166.

133. Raymond F. Peat, "Diabetes, Scleroderma, Oils and Hormones," *Ray Peat's Newsletter,* Issue 131, July 1995.

134. Joseph, *My Healing from Breast Cancer,* 12. See also K. Malone et al., "Oral Contraceptives in Relation to Breast Cancer," *Epidemiologic Reviews,* Vol. 15, No. 1, 1993, 80–97.

135. Virginia Soffa, *The Journey Beyond Breast Cancer* (Rochester, Vermont: Healing Arts Press, 1994), 33.

136. Joseph, *My Healing from Breast Cancer,* 248. See also L. A. Brinton et al., "Oral Contraceptives and Breast Cancer Risk Among Younger Women," *Journal of the National Cancer Institute,* Vol. 87, No. 11, June 7, 1995, 827–35.

137. John R. Lee, *Natural Progesterone,* 43.

138. "Prometrium (progesterone USP)," Solvay Pharmaceuticals, Inc., Marietta, GA, 1998.

139. Carol Landau, Michele G. Cyr, and Anne W. Moutlon, *The Complete Book of Menopause* (New York: Putnam Books, 1994), 153.

140. Gaby, *Preventing and Reversing Osteoporosis,* 149–150.

141. John R. Lee, *Natural Progesterone,* 46.

142. Lita Lee, "Estrogen."

143. Dalton, *A Guide to Premenstrual Syndrome.*
144. Dalton, *Once a Month,* 110.
145. Linda G. Rector-Page, N.D., Ph.D., *Healthy Healing: An Alternative Healing,* 310, 302.
146. Dalton, "Guide to Progesterone."
147. Luise Light, "How to Get Pregnant When All Else Fails," *Vegetarian Times,* July 1997.
148. Ibid.
149. John R. Lee, *What Your Doctor May Not Tell You About Menopause.*
150. Lindacarol Graham, "Do You Have a Hormone Shortage?" *Redbook,* February 1989, 16.
151. Jerome H. Check and Harriet G. Adelson, "The Efficacy of Progesterone in Achieving Successful Pregnancy: II. In Women with Pure Luteal Phase Defects," *International Fertility,* Vol. 32, No. 21, 1987, 139–41.
152. Ibid.
153. "Getting Pregnant and Staying Pregnant," *The John R. Lee M.D. Medical Letter,* September 1998, 3.
154. Dalton, *Once a Month,* 231.
155. Check and Adelson, "The Efficacy of Progesterone in Achieving Successful Pregnancy: II. In Women with Pure Luteal Phase Defects."
156. V. A. Tzingounis, S. Michalas, and D. Kaskerelis, "Effect of Oestriol on Cervical Mucus," *Clinical Trials Journal,* Vol. 19, 1982, 3844; "Specific Estrogen Treatment for Atrophy Related Urogenital Complaints," (Ovestin Estriol Scientific Information. Product Surveillance Department, Organon International, The Netherlands.
157. Jesse Hanley, M.D., "Using Herbs to Balance Hormones," (Interview) *The John R. Lee M.D. Medical Letter,* June 1998, 5.
158. Ibid.
159. Skye Lininger, D.C., Jonathan Wright, M.D., Steve Austin, N.D., Donald Brown, N.D., Alan Gaby, M.D., *The Natural Pharmacy* (Rocklin, CA: Prima Health, 1998), 317.
160. Ibid., 318.
161. Christiane Northrup, *Health Wisdom for Women,* Vol. 2, No. 11, November 1995, 6; October 1995.
162. Dalton, *Once a Month,* 163–64.
163. John R. Lee, *The John R. Lee M.D. Medical Letter,* September 1998, 3.
164. Dalton, "Ante-natal Progesterone and Intelligence," *British Journal of Psychiatry,* Vol. 114, 1968, 1377–82.
165. Ibid.
166. Dalton, *Once a Month,* 163–64, 246–47. See also BMA Prize, "The Similarity of Symptomatology of Premenstrual Syndrome and Toxaemia of Pregnancy and Their Response to Progesterone," *British Medical Journal,* 1954, Vol. II, 1071; "Progesterone in Toxaemia of Pregnancy," *Medical World,* December 1955; "Toxaemia of Pregnancy Treated with Progesterone During the Symptomatic

Stage," August 1957, *British Medical Journal*, Vol. II, 378–81; "Early Symptoms of Pre-eclamptic Toxaemia," *The Lancet*, January 23, 1960, 198–99.

167. Dalton, *Once a Month*, 163–64.
168. Ibid., 169, 232; "Premenstrual Syndrome"; and "Prenatal Progesterone and Educational Attainments," *British Journal of Psychiatry*, Vol. 129, 1976, 438–42.
169. John R. Lee, *Natural Progesterone*, 81, 87.
170. John R. Lee, *What Your Doctor May Not Tell You About Menopause*, 80.
171. Gaby, *Preventing and Reversing Osteoporosis*, 148.
172. Dalton, *Once a Month*, 163.
173. Gaby, *Preventing and Reversing Osteoporosis*, 261.
174. McKenna, "Darwin with a Twist," *The Atlanta Journal/Constitution*, April 25, 1995.
175. Raymond F. Peat, "Estrogen: Simply Dangerous," *Ray Peat's Newsletter*, July 1995, 3.
176. Associated Press, "Hormone Treatment Reduces Chance of Premature Births," *Washington Post*, Friday, February 7, 2003, A11.
177. John R. Lee, "Getting Pregnant and Staying Pregnant," *The John R. Lee M.D. Medical Letter*, September 1998, 1.
178. Lita Lee, "Estrogen."
179. Peat, *Nutrition for Women*.
180. Peat, "Progesterone."
181. Raymond F. Peat, "The Progesterone Deception," *Townsend Letter for Doctors*, November 1987.
182. Peat, *Progesterone in Orthomolecular Medicine*.
183. Lita Lee, "Estrogen."
184. Morgan, "Pregnancy and Natural Progesterone."
185. John R. Lee, *Natural Progesterone*, 25.
186. Ibid., 17, 41.
187. Dalton, "Guide to Progesterone."
188. Ibid.
189. Ibid.
190. Stern et al., *The Pill Book*, 351.
191. Dalton, "Ante-natal Progesterone."
192. George H. Malkmus, *God's Way to Ultimate Health* (Eidson, TN: Hallelujah Acres Publishing, 1997), 156–59.
193. Ibid.
194. Udo Erasmus, *Fats That Heal, Fats That Kill* (Burnaby, B.C., Canada: Alive Books, 1997).
195. Ibid.
196. Peat, *Nutrition for Women*, 16, 18.
197. Ibid., 16.
198. Mark Perloe and Linda Gail, *Miracle Babies and Other Happy Endings for Couples with Fertility Problems* (New York: Rawson, 1986). See www.ivf.com/tocmb.html.
199. Raymond F. Peat, *Progesterone in Orthomolecular Medicine* (Eugene, OR: Kenogen 1995).

200. Dr. William Campbell Douglass, *Second Opinion*, Vol. VIII, No. 4, April 1998, 1.
201. Ibid., 2. See also *Health Journal*, Price-Pottenger Nutrition Foundation (PPNF), Summer 1997. Email: ppnf@aol.com
202. Peat, *Nutrition for Women*, ii–iv, 17, 116.
203. Raymond F. Peat, Ph.D., *From PMS to Menopause: Female Hormones in Context* (Eugene, OR: Kenogen, 1997), 175–87.
204. B. A. Houssay and C. Martinez, "Experimental Diabetes and Diet," *Science*, Vol. 105, 1947, 548–49.
205. Raymond F. Peat, "Stress and Water," *Ray Peat's Newsletter*, February 1995.
206. Mohammed Kalimi and William Regelson, eds., *The Biologic Role of Dehydroepiandrosterone (DHEA)* (Hawthorne, NY: Walter de Gruyter, 1990).
207. Raymond, F. Peat, "Estrogen: Simply Dangerous," *Ray Peat's Newsletter*, July 1995.
208. John R. Lee, *What Your Doctor May Not Tell You About Menopause*, 307.
209. William Regelson, M.D., and Carol Colman, *The Super-Hormone Promise* (New York: Simon & Schuster, 1996), 188.
210. H. L. Koenig et al., "Progesterone Synthesis and Myelin Formation by Schwann Cells: A Newly Demonstrated Role of Progesterone," *Science*, Vol. 268, June 1995, 1500–03.
211. E. E. Baulieu and M. Schumacher, "Progesterone as a Neuroactive Neurosteroid, with Special Reference to the Effect of Progesterone on Myelination," *Hum Reprod*, Vol. 15, Suppl. 1, June 2000, 1–13.
212. E. E. Baulieu and M. Schumacher, "Neurosteroids, with Special Reference to the Effect of Progesterone on Myelination in Peripheral Nerves," *Hum Reprod*, Vol. 16, No. 8, August 2001, 1542.
213. Ibid.
214. Regelson and Colman, *The Super-Hormone Promise*, 188.
215. Koenig et al., "Progesterone Synthesis and Myelin Formation,1500–03.
216. Regelson and Colman, *The Super-Hormone Promise*, 188.
217. John R. Lee, *What Your Doctor May Not Tell You About Menopause*, 95.
218. Koenig et al., "Progesterone Synthesis and Myelin Formation, 1500–03.
219. John R. Lee, *What Your Doctor May Not Tell You About Menopause*, 95.
220. Regelson and Colman, *The Super-Hormone Promise*, 188.
221. "American Home Video Natural Medicine Update" (1995 TV program on the subject of Hormone Replacement Therapy with guest Betty Kamen, Ph.D. Hosts: Jeffrey and Valerie Donigan).
222. John R. Lee, *What Your Doctor May Not Tell You About Menopause*, 95.
223. Regelson and Colman, *The Super-Hormone Promise*, 188.
224. Peat, *Nutrition for Women*, 43.
225. John R. Lee, *What Your Doctor May Not Tell You About Menopause*, 252–54.
226. Claudia Kalb, "Hormones and the Mind," *Newsweek*, April 19, 1999.
227. John R. Lee et al., *What Your Doctor May Not Tell You About Premenopause* (New York: Warner Books, Inc., 1999), 53.
228. Peat, *From PMS to Menopause: Female Hormones in Context*, 70.

229. John R. Lee, "The Truth About Estrogen and the Brain," *The John R. Lee M.D. Medical Letter,* June 1999, 2.

230. Peat, *From PMS to Menopause: Female Hormones in Context,* 70.

231. Ibid.

232. "News Update," *Women's Health Advocate Newsletter,* Vol. 4, No. 11, January 1998, 1.

233. Ray Sahelian, M.D., *Pregnenolone* (Garden City, NY: Avery Publishing Group and Longevity Research Center Inc., 1997).

234. Peat, *From PMS to Menopause: Female Hormones in Context,* 122, 123.

235. T. I. Belova, "Structural Damage to the Mesencephalic Reticular Formation Induced by Immobilization Stress," *Bull. Ep. Biol. & Med.,* Vol. 1108, No. 7, 1989, 126030.

236. T. L. Bush et al., "Estrogen Use and All-Cause Mortality: Preliminary Results From The Lipid Research Clinics Program Follow-Up Study," *Journal of the American Medical Association,* Vol. 249, 1983, 903–06.

237. K. Savolainen et al., "Phosphoinositide Second Messengers in Cholinergic Activity," *Neurotoxicology,* Vol. 15, No. 3, 1994, 493–502.

238. Peat, "Estrogen: Simply Dangerous," July 1995.

239. Raymond F. Peat, Ph.D., "The Problem of Alzheimer's Disease as a Clue to Immortality," *Ray Peat's Newsletter,* 1996.

240. D. E. Brenner et al., "Postmenopausal Estrogen Replacment Therapy and the Risk of Alzheimer's Disease: A Population-Based Case-Control Study," *American Journal of Epidemiology* Vol. 140, 1994, 262–67.

241. Peat, *From PMS to Menopause: Female Hormones in Context,* 123. See also B. L. Weiss, "Failure of Nalmefene and Estrogen to Improve Memory in Alzheimer's Disease," *American Journal of Psychiatry,* Vol. 144, 1987, 386–87.

242. Peat, "The Problem of Alzheimer's Disease as a Clue to Immortality."

243. Peat, *From PMS to Menopause: Female Hormones in Context,* 123.

244. H. C. Liu et al., "Performance on a Dementia Screening Test in Relation to Demographic Variables Study of 5,297 Community Residents in Taiwan," *Arch Nerol,* Vol. 51, No. 9, 910–15.

245. Raymond F. Peat, "Food-Junk and Some Mystery Ailments: Fatigue, Alzheimer's, Colitis, Immunodeficiency," *Ray Peat's Newsletter,* 1988. See also B. J. Freedman, "Persorption of Raw Starch: A Cause of Senile Dementia?" *Med Hypotheses,* Vol. 35, No. 2, June 1991, 85–87.

246. Raymond F. Peat, "Estrogen Receptors: What Do They Explain?, *Ray Peat's Newsletter,* March 1999.

247. Richard P. Huemer, "Fibromyalgia: The Pain That Never Stops," *Let's Live,* November 1996, 34–35.

248. Betty Kamen, "Fibromyalgia: An Age-Old Malady Begging for Respect," *Let's Live,* November 1994, 31.

249. Ibid., 32, and I. Lorenzen, "Fibromyalgia: A Clinical Challenge," *Journal of Internal Medicine,* Vol. 235, no. 3, March 1994, 199–203.

250. Sandra Coney, *The Menopause Industry* (Alameda, CA: Hunter House, 1994), 61.

251. Colditz, K. M. Egan, and M. J. Stampfer, "Hormone Replacement Therapy and

Risk of Breast Cancer: Results from Epidemiologic Studies," *American Journal of Obstetrics and Gynecology*, Vol. 168, 1993, 1476–80.

252. Quoted in Ann Louise Gittleman, "Menopause and Nutrition," *The Energy Times*, September/October 1994.

Chapter 4: Can We Circumvent Osteoporosis?

1. Joseph E. Maynard, *Healing Hands* (Woodstock, GA: Jonorm Publishing, 1991).
2. John R. Lee, *Natural Progesterone: The Multiple Roles of a Remarkable Hormone* (Sebastopol, CA: BLL Publishing, 1993), 56.
3. John R. Lee, M.D., et al., *What Your Doctor May Not Tell You About Premenopause* (New York: Warner Books, Inc., 1999), 197.
4. Ibid.
5. Sandra Cabot, *Smart Medicine for Menopause* (Garden City Park, NY: Avery Publishing, 1995), 30.
6. John R. Lee, *Natural Progesterone*, 56.
7. J. C. Prior, "Progesterone as a Bone-Trophic Hormone," *Endocrine Reviews*, Vol. 11, No. 2, 1990, 386–98.
8. E. L. Berengolts et al., "Comparison of the Effects of Progesterone and Estrogen on Established Bone Loss in Ovariectomized Aged Rats," *Cells and Materials*, Supplement 1, 1991, 105–11; and E. L. Berengolts et al., "Effects of Progesterone on Post-Ovariectomy Bone Loss in Aged Rats," *Journal of Bone Mineral Research*, Vol. 5, 1990, 1143–47.
9. John R. Lee, *Natural Progesterone*, 32.
10. Ibid., 30, 59–69, and Lita Lee, "Estrogen, Progesterone and Female Problems," *Earthletter*, Vol. 1, No. 2, June 1991.
11. Leslie Lawrence, "Education Can Ward off Osteoporosis," *The Atlanta Journal/The Atlanta Constitution*, September 14, 1993.
12. *The Holistic Dental Digest*, No. 76, June 1992.
13. M. J. Halberstam, "If Estrogens Retard Osteoporosis, Are They Worth the Cancer Risk?" *Modern Medicine*, Vol. 45, No. 9, 1977, 15.
14. Gail Sheehy, *The Silent Passage: Menopause* (New York: Pocket Books, 1993), 180–81.
15. Ibid., 125–26.
16. J. C. Prior, Y. Vigna, and N. Alojada, "Spinal Bone Loss and Ovulatory Disturbances," *International Journal of Gynecology and Obstetrics*, Vol. 34, 1990, 253–56.
17. John R. Lee, "Is Natural Progesterone the Missing Link in Osteoporosis Prevention and Treatment?" *Medical Hypotheses*, 1991.
18. Majid Ali, "Chemical Conflict: The Age of Estrogen Overdrive," *Lifespanner*, December 1994.
19. Sheehy, *The Silent Passage*, 181–82.
20. Alan R. Gaby, *Preventing and Reversing Osteoporosis* (Rocklin, CA: Prima Publishing, 1994), 234.

21. Joel Griffiths, "Progesterone Reported to Increase Bone Density 10% in Six Months," *Medical Tribune,* November 29, 1990.
22. D. T. Felson et al., "The Effect of Postmenopausal Estrogen Therapy on Bone Density in Elderly Women," *New England Journal of Medicine,* Vol. 88, No. 8, Oct. 14, 1993.
23. Berengolts et al., "Comparison of the Effects of Progesterone and Estrogen,"105–11.
24. Berengolts et al., "Effects of Progesterone on Post-Ovariectomy Bone Loss in Aged Rats," 1143–47.
25. John R. Lee, *Natural Progesterone,* 54–55.
26. D.L. Feldman et al., "Cytoplasmic Glucocorticoid Binding Proteins in Bone Cells," *Endocrinology,* Vol. 96, 1975, 29–36.
27. T. L. Chen et al., "Glucocorticoid Receptors and Inhibition of Bone Cell Growth in Primary Culture," *Endocrinology,* Vol. 100, 1977, 619–28.
28. S. C. Manolagas et al., "Detection of High Affinity Glucocorticoid Binding in the Rat Bone," *Journal of Endocrinology,* Vol. 76, 1978, 379–80.
29. D. R. Rudy, "Hormone Replacement Therapy," *Postgraduate Medicine,* December 1990, 157–64.
30. "Osteoporosis," *Merck Manual of Medical Information* (New York, NY: Pocket Books, 1997), 220.
31. Gaby, *Preventing and Reversing Osteoporosis,* ix–x.
32. John R. Lee, *Natural Progesterone,* 54.
33. Ibid.
34. John R. Lee, "Osteoporosis Reversal: The Role of Progesterone," *International Clinical Nutrition Review,* Vol. 10, No. 3, 1990.
35. John R. Lee, "Fighting Osteoporosis with Natural Progesterone," *Natural Solutions,* Professional & Technical Services Inc., Vol. 1, Issue 1 Fall 1993).
36. John R. Lee, "Osteoporosis Reversal: The Role of Progesterone," 384–91.
37. Ibid.
38. Ibid.
39. Ibid.
40. John R. Lee, *Natural Progesterone,* 42, 54–55, and Prior, "Progesterone as a Bone-Trophic Hormone," 386–98.
41. Sheehy, *The Silent Passage,* 183.
42. Alan Cook, "Osteoporosis: Review and Commentary," *Journal of the Neuro-musculoskeletal System,* Vol. 2, No. 1, 1994.
43. John R. Lee, *Natural Progesterone,* 85.
44. Gaby, *Preventing and Reversing Osteoporosis,* 143–52.
45. John R. Lee, "Is Natural Progesterone the Missing Link in Osteoporosis Prevention and Treatment?"
46. Ibid.
47. Ibid., and John R. Lee, "Osteoporosis Reversal: The Role of Progesterone."
48. John R. Lee, "Is Natural Progesterone the Missing Link in Osteoporosis Prevention and Treatment?"

49. John R. Lee, "Osteoporosis Reversal: The Role of Progesterone."

50. John R. Lee, *Natural Progesterone*, 41, and "Is Natural Progesterone the Missing Link in Osteoporosis Prevention and Treatment?"

51. John R. Lee, *Natural Progesterone*, 59.

52. John R. Lee, "Is Natural Progesterone the Missing Link in Osteoporosis Prevention and Treatment?" and Sheehy, *The Silent Passage*, 98, 245.

53. Gaby, *Preventing and Reversing Osteoporosis*, 1–7.

54. Ibid.

55. Dee Ito, *Without Estrogen: Natural Remedies for Menopause and Beyond* (New York: Carol Southern Books, 1994), 6.

56. Joel Fuhrman, "Osteoporosis: How to Get It and How to Avoid It," *Health Science*, January/February 1992.

57. Ibid.

58. Ibid.

59. Prior, "Progesterone as a Bone-Trophic Hormone."

60. Fuhrman, "Osteoporosis: How to Get It and How to Avoid It."

61. M. T. Morter Jr., "Osteoporosis!!" *The Chiropractic Professional*, May/June 1987, and *Your Health, Your Choice: Guide to Nutrition and Disease Prevention* (Rogers, AK: B.E.S.T. Research, 1990), 3, 83, 167.

62. Nancy Appleton, Ph.D., *Healthy Bones: What You Should Know About Osteoporosis* (Garden City Park, NY: Avery Publishing Group Inc., 1991), 58–59.

63. James F. Balch, M.D., and Phyllis A. Balch, C.N.C., *Prescription for Nutritional Healing* (Garden City Park, NY: Avery Publishing Group Inc., 1997), 27.

64. Anne Dickson and Nikki Henriques, *Women on Menopause* (Rochester, VT: Healing Arts Press, 1988), 78.

65. Rosemary Gladstar, "A New Cycle of Life: Celebrating Menopause Herbally," *The Herb Quarterly*, Winter 1993, 42.

66. Joel Robbins, D.C., N.D., M.D., "Nutrition and Its Relation to Health," (Tulsa, OK: Health Dynamics Corporation, 1999), cassette.

67. Ibid.

68. Ibid.

69. Dr. Mary Ruth Swope, *Green Leaves of Barley* (Melbourne, FL: National Preventive Health Services, Inc., 1987), 148.

70. Balch and Balch, *Prescription for Nutritional Healing*, 109.

71. Betty Kamen, *Hormone Replacement Therapy: Yes or No?* (Bel Marin Keys, CA: Nutrition Encounter, 1991).

72. Cathy Perlmutter and Toby Hanlon, "Triumph over Menopause," *Prevention*, August 1994.

73. Ibid.

74. E. A. Mascioli et al., "Unsaturated Fats Directly Kill White Blood Cells," *Lipids*, Vol. 22, No. 6, 1987, 421.

75. R. D. Lynch, "Utilization of Polyunsaturated Fatty Acids by Human Diploid Cells Aging in Vvitro," *Lipids*, Vol. 15, No. 6, 1967, 412–20.

76. John R. Lee, *Natural Progesterone*, 60.

77. Anthony J. Cochoke, "What Your Customer Should Know," *Health Food Business Magazine,* September 1996.
78. John R. Lee, *What Your Doctor May Not Tell You About Menopause* (New York: Warner Books, 1996), 296.
79. Ibid.
80. John A. McDougall and Mary A. McDougall, *The McDougall Plan* (Piscataway, NJ: New Century Publishers, Inc., 1983).
81. Gaby, *Preventing and Reversing Osteoporosis,* 6.
82. David Williams, M.D., *Alternatives* (Potomac, MD: Mountain Home Publishing, April 2002), 75.
83. John R. Lee, *Natural Progesterone,* 60.
84. L. Cohen and R. Kitzes, "Infrared Spectroscopy and Magnesium Content of Bone Mineral in Osteoporotic Women." *Isr. Journal of Med. Sci.* No. 27, 1981, 1132–25.
85. Gaby, *Preventing and Reversing Osteoporosis,* 107.
86. Nancy Appleton, Ph.D., *Lick the Sugar Habit* (Garden City Park, NY: Avery Publishing Group Inc., 1996), 85.
87. G. E. Abraham and H. Grewel, "A Total Dietary Program Emphasizing Magnesium Instead of Calcium: Effect on the Mineral Density of Calcaneus Bone in Postmenopausal Women on Hormonal Therapy," *Journal of Reproductive Medicine,* 1990, 503–07.
88. Gaby, *Preventing and Reversing Osteoporosis,* 44.
89. Joseph Z. Schneider, "The Calcium to Phosphorus Ratio as Related to Mineral Metabolism." *International Journal of Orthodontists,* Vol. 16, No. 3, March 1930, 277–85.
90. Melvin E. Page et al., *Your Body Is Your Best Doctor* (New Canaan, CT: Keats Publishing, 1972).
91. Gaby, *Preventing and Reversing Osteoporosis,* 15.
92. B. O'Dell and E. Morris, "Relationship of Excess Calcium and Phosphorus to Magnesium Requirement and Toxicity in Guinea Pigs," *Journal of Nutrition,* 82, 1963, 175–81.
93. Robert Garrison Jr., *The Nutrition Desk Reference* (New Canaan, CT: Keats Publishing, 1997), 243.
94. Jason Elias and Katherine Ketcham, *In the House of the Moon* (New York: Warner Books, 1995), 292–93.
95. Gaby, *Preventing and Reversing Osteoporosis,* 108.
96. Ibid., 108, 109.
97. G. E. Abraham and H. Grewal, "A Total Dietary Program Emphasizing Magnesium Instead of Calcium: Effect on the Mineral Density of Calcaneous Bone in Postmenopausal Women on Hormonal Therapy," *Journal of Reproductive Medicine,* Vol. 35, 1990, 503–7.
98. *The John R. Lee M.D. Medical Letter,* (Interview), May 1999, 3.
99. Bernard Jensen, Ph.D., *Arthritis, Rheumatism and Osteoporosis: An Effective Program for Correction through Nutrition* (Escondido, CA: Bernard Jensen Enterprises, 1986), 10–15.

100. Appleton, *Lick the Sugar Habit.*

101. Balch and Balch, *Prescription for Nutritional Healing,* 27

102. Ibid., 7.

103. Morton Walker, *The Chelation Way* (New York: Avery Publishing Group, 1990), 26.

104. Carlton Fredericks, Ph.D., *Guide To Women's Nutrition* (New York: The Putnam Publishing Group, 1989), 42.

105. Raymond Peat, Ph.D., "Menopause and Its Causes," *Ray Peat's Newsletter,* Summer 1995; Raymond Peat, Ph.D., "Estrogen: Simply Dangerous," *Ray Peat's Newsletter,* Fall 1995; Raymond Peat, Ph.D., *Progesterone in Orthomolecular Medicine* (Eugene, OR, 1993).

106. Elaine Hollingsworth, *Take Control of Your Health and Escape the Sickness Industry,* 6th edition (Australia: Empowerment Press International, 2000).

107. Gaby, *Preventing and Reversing Osteoporosis,* 83.

108. John R. Lee, *Natural Progesterone,* 40.

109. Balch and Balch, *Prescription for Nutritional Healing,* 22, and Cedric Garland and Frank Garland, *The Calcium Connection* (New York: G. P. Putnam's Sons, 1988).

110. Garland and Garland, 65–66, 84.

111. Sheehy, *The Silent Passage,* 182.

112. Ibid., 183.

113. The Burton Goldberg Group, *Alternative Medicine* (Puyallup, WA: Future Medicine Publishing, 1993), 776.

114. Ruth Sackman, "Common Sense About Calcium," *Cancer Forum,* Vol. 13, No. 3/4, Fall 1994, 6.

115. John R. Lee, *Natural Progesterone,* 60.

116. Appleton, *Healthy Bones: What You Should Know About Osteoporosis,* 82–83.

117. Gaby, *Preventing and Reversing Osteoporosis,* 39, 109.

118. Appleton, *Healthy Bones: What You Should Know About Osteoporosis,* 58–59.

119. Suzanne M. Snedeker et al., "Effect of Dietary Calcium and Phosphorus Levels on the Utilization of Iron, Copper, and Zinc by Adult Males," *Journal of Nutrition,* 112, 1982, 136–43.

120. Balch and Balch, *Prescription for Nutritional Healing,* 7.

121. Ibid.

122. Appleton, *Lick the Sugar Habit,* 27.

123. Appleton, *Healthy Bones: What You Should Know About Osteoporosis,* 58, 59.

124. Ibid.

125. Garrison, *The Nutrition Desk Reference,* 242.

126. Appleton, *Healthy Bones: What You Should Know About Osteoporosis,* 58, 59.

127. Mona A. Calvo and Youngmee K. Park, "Changing Phosphorus Content of the U.S. Diet: Potential for Adverse Effects on Bone," *Journal of Nutrition,* 126, 1996, 1168S–80S.

128. Appleton, *Lick the Sugar Habit,* 26–27.

129. Kamen, *Hormone Replacement Therapy.*

130. J. C. Prior, Y. Vigna, and N. Alojada, "Progesterone and the Prevention of Osteoporosis," *Canadian Journal of OB/Gyn & Women's Health Care,* Vol. 3, No. 4, 1991, 181.

131. Ibid.
132. John R. Lee, *Natural Progesterone*, 57–58.
133. Kamen, *Hormone Replacement Therapy*.
134. Trien Susan Falmholtz, *Change of Life* (New York: Fawcett Columbine Books, 1986).
135. Balch and Balch, *Prescription for Nutritional Healing*, 214.
136. Raymond F. Peat, *Nutrition for Women*, 5th ed. (Eugene, OR: Kenogen, 1993).
137. Gaby, *Preventing and Reversing Osteoporosis*, 194.
138. John R. Lee, "Throw Away Your Fosamax," *The John R. Lee M.D. Medical Letter*, July 1998, 3.
139. Ibid.
140. D. M. Black et al., "Randomized Trial of Effect of Alendronate [Fosamax] on Risk of Fracture in Women with Existing Vertebral Fractures," Fracture Intervention Trial Research Group, *The Lancet*, Vol. 348, No. 9041, December 1996, 1535–41.
141. S. R. Cummings et al., "Effect of Alendronate [Fosamax] on Risk of Fracture in Women with Low Bone Density but without Vertebral Fractures: Results from the Fracture Intervention Trial," *Journal of the American Medical Association*, Vol. 280, No. 24, December 1998, 1077–82.
142. Sidney Wolfe, ed., "New Research: Who Benefits and How Much with Alendronate (Fosamax)?" *Worst Pills, Best Pills*, Vol. 5, No. 2, February 1999.
143. John R. Lee, "Throw Away Your Fosamax," 3.
144. Ibid.
145. www.uop.edu/pharmacy/asp/osteoprosis/pages/fosamax.htm (10/30/97).
146. Samuel S. Epstein, M.D., and Pat Cody, "New Drug Poses Risk of Ovarian Cancer," *Chicago Tribune*, April 19, 1998.
147. Raymond F. Peat, Ph.D., "Estrogen Receptors—What Do They Explain?," *Ray Peat's Newsletter*, March 1999.
148. Ibid. See also F. Naftolin et al., "The Cellular Effects of Estrogens on Neuroendocrine Tissues," *Journal of Steroid Biochem.*, Vol. 30, Nos. 1–6, 1988, 195–207; A. Maggi et al., "Role of Female Gonadal Hormones in the CNS: Clinical and Experimental Aspects," *Life Sci.*, Vol. 37, No. 10, September 1985, 893–906; P. G. Mermelstein et al., "Estradiol Reduces Calcium Currents in Rat Neostriatal Neurons Via a Membrane Receptor," *Journal of Neuroscience*, Vol. 16, No. 2, January 1996, 595–604; Q. Gu and R. L. Moss, "17 Beta Estradiol Potentiates Kainate-Induced Currents Via Activation of the cAMP Cascade," *Journal of Neuroscience*, Vol. 16, No. 11, June 1996, 3620–29; J. P. Wiebe, "Nongenomic Actions of Steroids on Gonadotropin Release," *Recent Prog. Horm. Res.*, Vol. 52, 1997, 71–99.
149. Eli Lilly and Company, Indianapolis, IN, PV 3141, December 10, 1997.
150. Evista 60Mg (Generic name: Raloxifene) prescription information (Medi Span, Inc. Database Edition 98.4, 1998).
151. Ibid.
152. Epstein and Cody, "New Drug Poses Risk of Ovarian Cancer."
153. Ibid.

154. Erasmus, *Fats That Heal, Fats That Kill,* 267.

155. Sydney Lou Bonnick, "Intensive Healing for Brittle Bones," *Prevention,* June 1994, 92–94.

156. Ibid.

157. Gaby, *Preventing and Reversing Osteoporosis,* 234.

158. Bonnick, "Intensive Healing."

159. Gaby, *Preventing and Reversing Osteoporosis,* 234.

160. *The Holistic Dental Digest,* No. 76, June 1992.

161. Danielson et al., "Hip Fracture and Fluoridation in Utah's Elderly Population," *Journal of the American Medical Association,* August 12, 1992.

162. Ibid., and Robert C. Olney, "Stop Fluoride Diseases: Remove Fluorides from Food, Water, Air and Drugs," *Cancer News Journal,* Vol. 9, No. 4, Fall 1955.

163. Nicholas Daflos, "A Tale of Two Federal Agencies," *Cancer Forum,* Vol. 13, No. 3/4, Fall 1994, 9–11.

164. Frederick B. Exner, *The American Fluoridation Experiment: The Case Against Fluoridation* (Sarasota, FL: Devlin-Adair Co., 1957).

165. L. Waldbott, "The Physiologic and Hygienic Aspects of the Absorption of Inorganic Fluorides," *Archives of Environmental Health,* Vol. 2, Issue 2, February 1961, 155–67.

166. Daflos, "A Tale of Two Federal Agencies."

167. Furhman, "Osteoporosis: How to Get It and How to Avoid It."

168. Garland and Garland, *The Calcium Connection,* and Nancy Appleton, *Lick the Sugar Habit,* 14–16.

169. Morter, "Osteoporosis!!" and "The Sodium Connection," *The Chiropractic Professional,* November/December 1987.

170. N. W. Walker, *Fresh Vegetable and Fruit Juices* (Prescott, AZ: Norwalk Press, 1978), 63.

171. Ibid., 63.

172. Ibid., 64.

173. Jean Carper, "As Greens Go, Kale's Best of Bunch," *The Atlanta Journal/The Atlanta Constitution,* August 4, 1994.

174. Gaby, *Preventing and Reversing Osteoporosis,* 116–119.

175. Sally W. Fallon and Mary G. Enig, "Why Butter is Better," *Health Freedom News,* Vol. 14, No. 6, November/December 1995; Earlyne Chaney, *The EYES Have It: A Self-Help Manual for Better Vision* (New York: Instant Improvement, 1993), 38–40; and Nathaniel Mead, "Don't Drink Your Milk," *Health Freedom News,* March 1995, 36–37.

176. Fallon and Enig, "Soy Products for Dairy Products? Not So Fast . . . ," *Health Freedom News,* Vol. 14, No. 5, September 1995; Mead, "Don't Drink Your Milk!"; and Chaney, *The EYES Have It,* 38–40.

177. Paavo Airola, *How to Get Well* (Phoenix, AZ: Health Plus, 1985), 190.

178. Ibid., 190.

179. Chaney, *The EYES Have It.*

180. Linda G. Rector-Page, *Healthy Healing: An Alternative Healing Reference* (Sonora, CA: Healthy Healing Publications, 1992).

181. Larry Doss, M.D., "Bone Health," *Journal of Longevity Research*, 12; and A. C. Goyton and J. E. Hall, *Textbook of Medical Physiology* (Philadelphia, PA: Saunders, 1996,) 989.

182. K. H. Nilsen et al., "Microcrystalline Calcium Hydroxyapatite Compound in Corticosteroid-Treated Rheumatoid Patients: A Controlled Study," *British Medical Journal* Vol. 2, No. 1124, 1978.

183. Julian Whitaker, M.D., *147 Medically-Proven Miracle Cures* (Phillips Publishing, Inc. 1996), 7.

184. Beth M. Ley, *How to Fight Osteoporosis and Win! The Miracle of Microcrystalline Hydroxyapatite (MCHC)*, (Aliso Viejo, CA: BL Publications, 1996), 51–55.

185. Gaby, *Preventing and Reversing Osteoporosis*, 73.

186. P. J. Benke et al., "Osteoporotic Bone Disease in the Pyridoxine Deficient Rat." *Biochem. Med.*, 6, 1972, 526–35.

187. T. M. Reynolds, "Hip Fractures in Patients May be Vitamin B_6 Deficient. Controlled Study of Serum Pyridoxal-5-phosphate," *Acta. Orthop. Scand.*, 63, 1992, 635–38.

188. Beth M. Ley, *How to Fight Osteoporosis and Win! The Miracle of Microcrystalline Hydroxyapatite (MCHC)* (Aiso Viejo, CA: BL Publications, 1996), 22.

189. Cathy Perlmutter and Toby Hanlon, "Triumph over Menopause," *Prevention*, August 1994.

190. Gaby, *Preventing and Reversing Osteoporosis*, 221–22.

191. Ibid., 220–22.

192. Raymond F. Peat, *Nutrition for Women*, 9, 28.

193. Peat, "Steroids," *Blake College Newsletter*, Vol. 1, No. 4, 3.

Chapter 5: The Risk of Cancer

1. C. Norman Shealy, M.D., Ph.D., *Natural Progesterone Cream: Safe and Natural Hormone Replacement* (Los Angeles, CA: Keats Publishing, 1999), 22.

2. John R. Lee, "Natural Progesterone" (transcript), *Cancer Forum*, Vol. 13, No. 5/6, Winter 1994-1995.

3. Allen B. Astrow, "Rethinking Cancer," *The Lancet*, February 26, 1994.

4. Richard A. Passwater, *Cancer and Its Nutritional Therapies* (New Canaan, CT: Keats Publishing, 1983), 39.

5. M. A. J. McKenna, "Chemicals that Mimic Estrogen May Be Causing Reproductive Ills," *The Atlanta Journal/The Atlanta Constitution*, March 8, 1995.

6. Chicago (AP) "American Girls Maturing Earlier Than Ever . . ." *Desert News*, April 5, 1997.

7. Ibid.

8. Theo Colburn et al., *Our Stolen Future* (New York: Plume/Penguin, 1997).

9. "Drugged Waters: Does it Matter that Pharmaceuticals Are Turning Up in Water Supplies?," *Science News*, Vol. 153, March 21, 1998.

10. J. Raloff, "Additional Source of Dietary Estrogens," *Science News*, June, 3, 1995.

11. Ibid.

12. Raf Casert, "Scandal Food Scare Spreading in Belgium: Cancer-Causing Agent Triggers Meat, Egg Alert," *International Sun Sentinel,* Florida, June 5, 1999.

13. "News Update: Tampons and Dioxin," *Women's Health Adavocate,* May 1998, 7.

14. Sari Harrar et al., *The Woman's Book of Healing Herbs* (Emmaus, PA: Rodale Press, Inc., 1999), 230.

15. John R. Lee, *Natural Progesterone.*

16. Ibid.

17. B. Formby and T. S. Wiley, "Progesterone Inhibits Growth and Induces Apoptosis in Breast Cancer Cells: Inverse Effects on Bcl-2 and p53," *Annals of Clinical and Laboratory Science,* Vol. 28, 1998, 360–69.

18. E. L. Cavalieri et al., "Molecular Origin of Cancer; Catechol Estrogen-3, 4-quinones as Endogenous Tumore Initiators, *Proc. National Academy of Science,* Vol. 94, 1994, 10937–42.

19. "Estrogens as Endogenous Carcingogens in the Breast and Prostate," National Cancer Institute Symposium, March 1998.

20. Lita Lee, "Estrogen, Progesterone and Female Problems," *Earthletter,* Vol. 1, No. 2, June 1991.

21. Ibid.

22. Epstein, "The Chemical Jungle: Today's Beef Industry," *International Journal of Health Services,* Vol. 20, No. 2, 1990, 277–80.

23. Lita Lee, "Estrogen, Progesterone and Female Problems."

24. Steve Sternberg, "Tracking Biological Sabotage" (Science, 4D), *USA Today,* September 16, 1997.

25. Robert F. Service, "New Role for Estrogen in Cancer?" *Science,* Vol. 179, March 13, 1998, 1631–33. See also J. Fischman et al., "The Role of Estrogen in Mammary Carcinogenesis," *Annals of the New York Academy of Sciences,* Vol. 768, No. 91, 1995.

26. Formby and Wiley, "Progesterone Inhibits Growth and Induces Apoptosis in Breast Cancer Cells," 360–69.

27. C. Rodriquez et al., "Estrogen Replacement Therapy and Fatal Ovarian Cancer," *American Journal of Epidemiology,* Vol. 141, 1995, 828–35.

28. "Estrogens as Endogenous Carcinogens in the Breast and Prostate."

29. Service, "New Role for Estrogen in Cancer?" 1631–33.

30. Ibid.

31. Rodriquez et al., "Estrogen Replacement Therapy and Fatal Ovarian Cancer."

32. J. D. Yager et al., "Molecular Mechanisms of Estrogen Carcinogenesis," *Ann. Rev. Pharmacol. Toxicol.,* Vol. 36, 1996, 203–32.

33. Neal D. Barnard, M.D., *Eat Right, Live Longer* (New York: Harmony Books, 1995). See also G. M. Heimer, "Estriol in the Postmenopause," *Acta. Obstet. Gynecol. Scand.* (Suppl.) Vol. 139, 1987, 3–23; U. Molander et al., "Effect of Oral Oestriol on Vaginal Flora and Cytology and Urogenital Symptoms in the Post-Menopause," *Maturitas,* Vol. 12, 1990, 113–20; D. K. Gerbaldo, et al., "Endometrial Morphology After 12 Months of Vaginal Oestriol Therapy in Post-Menopausal Women," *Maturitas,* Vol. 13, 1991, 269–74.

34. Julian Whitaker, *Health & Healing: Tomorrow's Medicine Today,* Vol. 3, No. 3, March 1993.

35. Stephanie Clements, "Prevention and Recovery Tied to Weight," *Denver Post,* Section #3F, September 27, 2004.
36. "Studies Document Pesticide Harm," *Science,* June 7, 1996 and *The Lancet,* July 1996.
37. John R. Lee, *Natural Progesterone,* 73, 75.
38. Alvin Follingstad, "Estriol, the Forgotten Estrogen?" *Journal of the American Medical Association,* Vol. 239, No. 1, January 2, 1978.
39. John R. Lee, *Natural Progesterone,* 73–75.
40. John R. Lee, "Natural Progesterone," 16.
41. Peat, *Ray Peat's Newsletter,* Sept. 1996, and R. C. Merrill, "Estriol: A Review," *Physiology Reviews,* Vol. 38, No. 3, 1958, 463–80.
42. M. van Haaften et al., "Intensification of 16 Alpha-Hydroxy-Estrone as a Metabolite of Estriol," *Gynecol. Endocrinol.,* Vol. 2, No. 3, September 1988, 215–21.
43. Raymond F. Peat, Ph.D., *From PMS to Menopause: Female Hormones in Context* (Eugene, OR: Kenogen, 1997), 137. See also W. P. Dmowski et al., "Effect of Intrauterine Estriol on Reproductive Function in the Rabbit," *Fertil. Steril.,* Vol. 28, No. 3, 1977, 262–68.
44. Marc Lippman et al., "Effects of Estrone, Estradiol, and Estriol on Hormone-Responsive Human Breast Cancer in Long-Term Tissue, *Cancer Research,* Vol. 32, 1901–07.
45. "Federal Panel: Add Estrogen to Cancer List," *USA Today,* Dec. 15, 2000.
46. Dawn M. Grabrick et al., "Risk of Breast Cancer with Oral Contraceptive Use in Women With a Family History of Breast Cancer," *JAMA,* Vol. 284, No. 14, October 11, 2000.
47. Bent Formby, Ph.D., et al., "Progesterone Inhibits Growth and Induces Apoptosis in Breast Cancer Cells: Inverse Effects on Bcl-2 and p53," *Annals of Clinical and Laboratory Science,* November 1998, Vol. 28, No. 6, 360–69.
48. Rodriquez et al., "Estrogen Replacement Therapy and Fatal Ovarian Cancer."
49. Follingstad, "Estriol."
50. John R. Lee, *Natural Progesterone,* 55.
51. Raymond F. Peat, "Progesterone: Essential to Your Well-Being," *Let's Live,* April 1982.
52. John R. Lee, "Natural Progesterone."
53. Ibid.
54. Raymond Peat, "Estrogen's Mechanisms in Aging and Cancer," *Ray Peat's Newsletter,* March 2003, 1, 6; M. E. Mendelsohn, "Nongenomic, ER-Mediated Activation of Endothelial Nitric Oxide Synthase," *Circulation Research,* Vol. 87, No. 11, November 2000, 956–60; L. L. Engel et al., "Some Kinetic Properties of Human Placental Estradiol-7 Beta Dehydrogenase: Patterns of Inhibition of Adenine Nucleotides," *Adv Enzyme Regul,* Vol. 17, 1978, 3463–71; S. Boljevic et al., "Carbon dioxide inhibits the generation of active forms of oxygen in human and animal cells and the significance of the phenomenon in biology and medicine," *Vojnosanit Pregl,* Vol. 53, No. 4, 1996, 261–74.
55. John R. Lee, *Natural Progesterone,* 36.

56. Peat, "Estrogen, Simply Dangerous," *Ray Peat's Newlsetter,* July 1995.
57. Passwater, *Cancer,* 24.
58. John R. Lee, "Natural Progesterone."
59. John R. Lee, *Natural Progesterone,* 33, 36, 74.
60. Lita Lee, "Estrogen."
61. Alan R. Gaby, *Preventing and Reversing Osteoporosis* (Rocklin, CA: Prima Publishing, 1994).
62. Lorraine Day, *Cancer Doesn't Scare Me Anymore!* (videotape) (Rancho Mirage, CA: Rockford Press, 1994).
63. Follingstad, "Estriol."
64. John R. Lee, "Natural Progesterone."
65. Barbara Joseph, M.D., *My Healing from Breast Cancer* (New Canaan, CT: Keats Publishing, 1996), 6.
66. "47 Epidemiological Studies in 30 Countries, Including 50,302 Women with Breast Cancer and 96,973 Women Without the Disease," *The Lancet,* Vol. 360, 2002, 187–95.
67. J. Brind et al., "Induced Abortion as an Independent Risk Factor for Breast Cancer: A Comprehensive Review and Meta-Analysis," *J Epidemiol Community Health,* Vol. 50,1996, 41–96.
68. J. Daling et al., "Risk of Breast Cancer in Young Women: Relationship to Induced Abortion," *J Natl Cancer Inst,* Vol. 86, 1994, 1584–92.
69. O. C. Hadjimichael et al., "Abortion Before First Livebirth and Risk of Breast Cancer," *Br J Cancer,* Vol. 53, 1986, 281–84.
70. J. Russo et al., "Susceptibility of Mammary gland to Carcinogenesis. Pregnancy Interruption as a Risk Factor in Tumor Incidence," *Am J Pathol,* Vol. 100, 1980, 497–512.
71. L. Vatten et al., "Pregnancy Related Protection Against Breast Cancer Depends on Length of Gestation," *Br J Cancer,* Vol. 87, 2002, 289–90.
72. Joseph, *My Healing from Breast Cancer,* 91.
73. Ibid., 45, 48.
74. Ibid.
75. Raymond F. Peat, Ph.D., *PMS to Menopause: Female Hormones in Context.*
76. Clark et al., "Progesterone Receptors as a Prognostic Factor in Stage II Breast Cancer," *New England Journal of Medicine,* Vol. 309, 1983, 1343–47.
77. W. L. McGuire, "Steroid Hormone Receptors in Breast Cancer Treatment Strategy," *Recent Progress in Hormone Research,* Vol. 36, 1980, 135–56.
78. Clark and McGuire, "Progesterone Receptors and Human Breast Cancer," *Breast Cancer Research and Treatment,* Vol. 3, 1983, 157–63.
79. John R. Lee, "Natural Progesterone."
80. Ibid.
81. Lita Lee, "Estrogen."
82. Ibid.
83. Betty Kamen, *Hormone Replacement Therapy: Yes or No?* (Novato, CA: Nutrition Encounter, Inc., 1993).

84. Ibid., 122.

85. Ralph W. Moss, *Cancer Therapy: The Independent Consumer's Guide to Non-Toxic Treatment & Prevention* (New York: Equinox Press, 1992).

86. Ibid.

87. Jeff Nesmith, "Breast Cancer Drug Increases Risk . . . ," *The Atlanta Journal/The Atlanta Constitution*, February 22, 1996.

88. Sherrill Sellman, "Tamoxifen, A Major Medical Mistake?" *Nexus Magazine*, Vol. 5, No. 4, June/July 1998.

89. Early Breast Cancer Trials Collaborative Group, "Systemic treatment of early breast cancer by hormonal, cytotoxic, or immune therapy," *The Lancet*, Vol. 339, No. 8784, 1992, 1–15.

90. Susan Love, M.D., *Dr. Susan Love's Hormone Book* (New York: Random House, 1997), 264.

91. "Studies Spark Tamoxifen Controversy," *Science News*, February 26, 1994, 133.

92. S. Hennessy et al., "Cardiac arrest and ventricular arrhythmia in patients taking antipsychotic drugs: cohort study using administrative data," *British Medical Journal*, Vol. 325, 2002, 1070.

93. L. H. Curtis et al., "Prescription of QT-prolonging drugs in a cohort of about 5 million outpatients," *American Medical Journal*, Vol. 114, 2003, 135–141.

94. Sellman, "Tamoxifen, A Major Medical Mistake?"

95. U. Veronesi et al., "Prevention of Breast Cancer with Tamoxifen: Preliminary Findings from the Italian Randomised Trial Among Hysterectomized Women," *The Lancet*, 1998, Vol. 352, 93–97.

96. "The European Tamoxifen Studies," *The John R. Lee M.D. Medical Letter*, October 1998, 6. See also T. Powles et al., "Interim Analysis of the Incidence of Breast Cancer in the Royal Marsden Hospital Tamoxifen Randomised Chemoprevention Trial," *The Lancet* Vol. 352, 1998, 98–101.

97. U. Veronesi et al., "Prevention of Breast Cancer with Tamoxifen."

98. T. Powles et al., "Interim Analysis of the Incidence of Breast Cancer in the Royal Marsden Hospital Tamoxifen Randomised Chemoprevention Trial," *The Lancet*, Vol. 352, July 11, 1998, 98–101.

99. "That's a Good Question," *The John R. Lee, M.D. Medical Letter*, August 1998, 7. See also U. Veronesi et al., "Prevention of Breast Cancer with Tamoxifen: Preliminary Findings from the Italian Randomized Trial Among Hysterectomized Women"; T. Powles, "Interim Analysis of the Incidence of Breast Cancer in the Royal Marsden Hospital Tamoxifen Randomised Chemoprevention Trial."

100. Liane Clorfene-Casten, *Breast Cancer: Poisons, Profits, and Prevention* (Monroe: ME: Common Courage Press, 1996), 93.

101. Early Breast Cancer Trials Collaborative Group, "Systemic treatment of early breast cancer by hormonal, cytotoxic, or immune therapy."

102. "Studies Spark Tamoxifen Controversy."

103. S. G. Nayfield et al., "Tamoxifen-Associated Eye Disease: A Review," *J Clin Oncol*, Vol. 14, No. 3, 1996, 1018–1026.

104. S. Dessole et al., "Uterine Metastases from Breast Cancer in a Patient Under

Tamoxifen Therapy: A Case Report," *Eur J Gyn Oncol,* Vol. 20, No. 5–6, 1999, 416–417.

105. Marcus Laux, *Naturally Well,* Vol. 2, No. 12, December 1995.

106. John R. Lee, "Natural Progesterone."

107. "Premarin (Conjugated Estrogens Tablets, USP)," Ayerst Laboratories, Inc., Philadelphia, May 1993.

108. Marcus Laux and Christine Conrad, *Natural Woman, Natural Menopause* (New York: HarperCollins, 1997), 23.

109. Ibid, 21.

110. Anne Dickson and Nikki Henriques, *Women on Menopause* (Rochester, VT: Healing Arts Press), 54.

111. Peat, "Estrogen's Mechanisms in Aging and Cancer," *Ray Peat's Newsletter,* March 2003.

112. Ibid.

113. Majid Ali, "Chemical Conflict: The Age of Estrogen Overdrive," *Lifespanner,* December 1994.

114. "Information for Patients," Ayerst Laboratories, Inc., New York, May 1985.

115. Joe Graedon, *The People's Pharmacy* (New York: Avon Books, 1977), 47.

116. "Dangers of Estrogen" (Form P8263-01), Mead Johnson Laboratories, Princeton, NJ, December 1992.

117. Joseph, *My Healing from Breast Cancer,* 17.

118. Marcus Laux, N.D., "Why I Don't Think You Should Trust Mammograms," *Naturally Well,* Vol. 3, No. 5, May 1996.

119. Martin B. Abrams et al., "Early Detection and Monitoring of Cancer With the Anti-Malignin Antibody Test," *Cancer Detection and Prevention,* Vol. 18, No. 1, 1994, 65–78.

120. John R. Lee, "Other Causes of Ovarian Cancer," *The John R. Lee M.D. Medical Letter,* June 1998, 3.

121. Ibid.

122. John Bernard Henry, M.D., *Clinical Diagnosis & Management* (Philadelphia, PA: W. B. Saunders Co.,1991), 298. See also D. E. Pittaway et al., "The Use of Ca-215 in the Diagnosis and Management of Endometriosis," *Fertil. Steril.,* Vol. 46, No. 5, 1986, 790.

123. John R. Lee, "That's a Good Question."

124. Michael Lerner, *Choices in Healing* (Cambridge, MA: The MIT Press, 1994), 4.

125. Ibid., 3.

126. www.agora-inc.com/reports/BUL/W6BUE513/home.cfm

127. The Burton Goldberg Group, *Alternative Medicine* (Puyallup, WA: Future Medicine Publishing, Inc., 1993), 737.

128. Peat, *Nutrition for Women,* 5th ed. (Eugene, OR: Kenogen, 1993), 17, 21.

129. Burton Goldberg Group, *Alternative Medicine,* 733.

130. "Prostate Problems and Hormones," *The John R. Lee, M.D. Medical Letter,* January 1999, 3.

131. John R. Lee, "Prostate disease and hormones," *The John R. Lee, M.D. Medical Letter* February 2002.

132. Ibid.
133. John R. Lee, "That's a Good Question," 7.
134. James South, "Progesterone for Prostate Health," Vol. 18, Number 5, June 2004. [See complete article on Vitamin Research News: www.vrp.com]
135. M. Krieg et al., "Effect of aging on endogenous level of 5 a-dihydrotestosterone, testosterone, estradiol, and estrone in epithelium and stroma of normal and hyperplastic human prostate," *J Clin Endocrinol Metab*, Vol. 77, 1993: 375–81.
136. A. Nakhla et al., "Estradiol causes the rapid accumulation of cAMP in human prostate," *Proc Natl Acad Sci USA*, Vol. 91, 1994: 5402–05.
137. S. Boehm et al., "Estrogen suppression as a pharmacotherapeutic strategy in the medical treatment of benign prostatic hyperplasia: evidence for its efficacy from studies with mepartricin," *Wien Klin Wochenschr*, Vol. 110, 1998: 817–23.
138. Raymond F. Peat, *From PMS to Menopause: Female Hormones in Context*, 65.
139. John R. Lee, "Prostate disease and hormones," *The John R. Lee, M.D. Medical Letter*, February 2002.
140. Elaine Hollingsworth, *Take Control of Your Health and Escape the Sickness Industry*, 6th edition (Australia: Empowerment Press International, 2000), 128.
141. C. Norman Shealy, *DHEA: The Health and Youth Hormone* (New Canaan, CT: Keats Publishing, 1996).
142. Ibid., 45.
143. Ibid. See also B. V. Stadel, "Oral Contraceptives and Cardiovascular Disease," *New England Journal of Medicine*, 1981, 305, 612; M. P. Vessey et al., "Investigation of Relation Between Use of Oral Contraceptives and Thromboembolic Disease," *British Medical Journal* 2, 1968, 199–205; P. W. F. Wilson et al., "Postmenopausal Estrogen Use, Cigarette Smoking, and Cardiovascular Morbidity in Women over 50," *New England Journal of Medicine*, Vol. 313, No. 17, 1985, 1038–43. (Framingham study, 50 percent greater risk with estrogen use.); L. A. Noris et al., "Effect of Oestrogen Dose on Whole Blood Platelet Activation in Women Taking New Low Dose Oral Contraceptives, *Thromb. Haemost.* 72(6), 1994, 926–30; S. M. Goodrich et al., "Effect of Estradiol 17b on Peripheral Venous Blood Flow," *American Journal of Obstetrics and Gynecology*, 1966, 96, 407; B. B. Gerstman et al., "Oral Contraceptive Estrogen Dose and the Risk of Deep Venous Thromboembolic Disease," *American Journal of Epidemiology*, Vol. 133, 1991, 32–36; M. Thorogood, "The Epidemiology of Cardiovascular Disease in Relation to the Estrogen Dose of Oral Contraceptives: A Historical Perspective," *Adv. Contracep.*, 7 (Suppl. 3) 1991, 11–21.
144. Ibid., 21, 23, 45.
145. B. B. Gerstman et al., "Oral Contraceptive Estrogen Dose and the Risk of Deep Venous Thromboembolic Disease," *Amererican Journal of Epidemiology*, Vol. 113, 1991, 32–36.
146. B. V. Stadel, "Oral Contraceptives and Cardiovascular Disease," *New England Journal of Medicine* 1981, 305, 612; M. P. Vessey et al., "Investigation of Relation Between Use of Oral Contraceptives and Thromboembolic Disease," *British Medical Journal*, 2, 1968, 199–205; P. W. F. Wilson et al., "Postmenopausal

Estrogen Use, Cigarette Smoking, and Cardiovascular Morbidity in Women over 50," *New England Journal of Medicine*, 313 (17), 1985, 1038–43. (Framingham study, 50 percent greater risk with estrogen use.)

147. G. N. Rao, "Influence of diet on tumors of hormonal tissues," *Prog Clin Biol Res,* Vol. 394, 1996, 41–56.

148. P. K. Pandalai et al., "The Effects of Omega-3 and Omega-6 Fatty Acids on In Vitro Prostate Cancer Growth," *Anticancer Res,* Vol. 16, No. 2, March/April 1996, 815–20.

149. Walter Pierpaoli et al., *The Melatonin Miracle: Nature's Age-Reversing, Disease-Fighting, Sex-Enhancing Hormone* (New York: Simon & Schuster, 1995), 119.

150. Steven J. Bock and Michael Boyette, *Stay Young the Melatonin Way* (New York: Penguin Books, 1995), 61.

151. Pierpaoli et al., *The Melatonin Miracle,* 27.

152. Ibid., 117.

153. Alan E. Lewis, "Melatonin: Part 2," *Consumer Bulletin, Whole Foods,* March 1996, 102.

154. Stuart M. Berger, *What Your Doctor Didn't Learn in Medical School* (New York: William Morrow, 1988).

155. Day, *Cancer Doesn't Scare Me Anymore!*

156. Ibid.

Chapter 6: Hormonal Support from Our Foods

1. Emanuel Swedenborg, *Arcana Coelestia,* Vol. 8, No. 5949:2, 115.

2. Katharina Dalton, "Premenstrual Syndrome and Postnatal Depression," *Health and Hygiene,* Vol. 11, 1990, 199–201.

3. Raymond Peat, "Diabetes, Scleroderma, Oils and Hormones," *Ray Peat's Newsletter,* Issue 131, July 1995.

4. Egil Ramstad, *Modern Pharmacognosy* (New York: McGraw-Hill, 1959), 119.

5. John R. Lee, "Is Natural Progesterone the Missing Link in Osteoporosis Prevention and Treatment?" *Medical Hypotheses,* 1991.

6. Alan R. Gaby, *Preventing and Reversing Osteoporosis* (Rocklin, CA: Prima Publishing, 1994), xiii.

7. Betty Kamen, *Hormone Replacement Therapy: Yes or No?* (Novato, CA: Nutrition Encounter, Inc., 1993).

8. F. Balmir et al., "An Extract of Soy Flour Influences Serum Cholesterol and Thyroid Hormones in Rats and Hamsters," *J Nutr,* Vol. 126, 1996, 3046–53.

9. Mike Fitzpatrick, Ph.D., "Soy Isoflavones: Panacea or Poison?," *Price-Pottenger Nutrition Foundation Journal,* Vol. 22, No. 3, Fall 1998; also his "Soy Formulas and their Effect on the Thyroid," *The New Zealand Medical Journal,* February 2000.

10. R. D. Walton et al., "Adverse Reactions to Aspartame: Double-blind Challenge in Patients from a Vulnerable Population," *Biol Psychiatry,* Vol. 34, 1993, 13–17; H. L. Roberts, "Does Aspartame Cause Human Brain Cancer?," *Journal of Advancement in Medicine,* Vol. 4, No. 4, Winter 1991, 231–241; P. R. Camfield et

al., "Aspartame Exacerbates EEG Spike-Wave Discharge in Children with Generalized Absence Epilepsy: A Double-Blind Controlled Study," *Neurology,* Vol. 42, May 1992, 1000–1003; Dennis W. Remington, *The Bitter Truth About Artificial Sweeteners* (Provo, UT: Vitality House International Inc., 1987); Russell L. Blaylock, *Excitotoxins: The Taste That Kills* (Sante Fe, NM: Health Press, 1996).

11. "Fake-fat Olestra Sickens Thousands: 15,000 Cases Makes Olestra Most-Complained-About Additive Ever," *CSPI News Release,* December 22, 1998.

12. R. Martin and K. Romano, *Preventing and Reversing Arthritis Naturally: The Untold Story* (Rochester, VT: Healing Arts Press, 2000).

13. David Zava, Ph.D., "Don't Go Overboard with the Soy Foods, *The John Lee M.D. Medical Letter,* May 1998, 5. See also N. L. Petrakis et al., "Stimulatory Influence of Soy Protein Isolate on Breast Secretion in Pre- and Postmenopausal Women," *Cancer Epidemiol Blomarkers Prev.,* Vol. 5, 1996, 785–794; R. C. Santell et al., "Dietary Genistein Exerts Estrogenic Effects Upon the Uterus, Mammary Gland and the Hypothalamic/Pituitary Axis in Rats," *Journal Nutr.,* Vol. 127, No. 2, February 1997, 263–69.

14. Patricia L. Whitten et al., "Influence of Phytoestrogen Diets on Estradiol Action in the Rat Uterus," *Steroids,* Vol. 59, July 1994, 443–49.

15. Kevin L. Medlock et al., "Effects of Coumestrol and Equol on the Developing Reproductive Tract of the Rat," *Proceedings of the Society for Experimental Biology and Medicine,* Vol. 208, 1995, 67–71.

16. E. D. Lephart et al., "Phytoestrogens decrease brain calcium-binding proteins," *Brain Reearch,* Vol. 859, No. 1, March 17, 2000, 123–31.

17. L. Hilakivi-Clarke et al., "Maternal Genistein Exposure Mimics the Effects of Estrogen on Mammary Gland Development in Female Mouse Offspring," *Oncol Rep,* Vol. 5, No. 3, May/June 1998, 609–16.

18. Retha R. Newbold et al., "Uterine Adenocarcinoma in Mice Treated Neonatally with Genistein," *Cancer Research,* Vol. 61, No. 1, June 1, 2001, 4325–28.

19. K. D. R. Setchell et al., "Dietary oestrogens—a probable cause of infertility and liver disease in captive cheetahs," *Gastroenterology,* Vol. 93, 1987, 225–33; A. S. Leopold "Phytoestrogens: Adverse effects on reproduction in California Quail," *Science,* Vol. 191, 1976, 98–100; H. M. Drane et al., "Oestrogenic Activity of Soya-Bean Products," *Food, Cosmetics, and Technology,* Vol. 18, 1980, 425–27; S. Kimura et al., "Development of Malignant Goiter by Defatted Soybean with Iodine-free Diet in Rats," *Gann,* Vol. 67, 1976, 763–65; C. Pelissero et al., "Oestrogenic Effect of Dietary Soybean Meal on Vitellogenesis in Cultured Siberian Sturgeon Acipenser baeri," *Gen Comp End,* Vol. 83, 1991, 447–57; Braden et al., "The Oestrogenic Activity and Metabolism of Certain Isoflavones in Sheep," *Australian J Agricultural Research,* Vol. 18, 1967, 335–48; Extracts from *Nexus Magazine,* Vol. 7, No. 3, April-May 2000.

20. N. L. Petrakis et al., "Stimulatory Influence of Soy Protein Isolate on Breast Secretion in Pre- and Post-Menopausal Women," *Cancer Epid Bio Prev,* Vol. 5, 1996, 785–94.

21. C. Dees et al., "Dietary estrogens stimulate human breast cells to enter the cell cycle," *Environmental Health Perspectives,* Vol. 105, Suppl. 3, 1997, 633–36.

22. L. Hilakivi-Clarke et al., "Maternal Genistein Exposure Mimics the Effects of Estrogen on Mammary Gland Development in Female Mouse Offspring."

23. Mark J. Messina et al., "Soy Intake and Cancer Risk: A Review of the In Vitro and In Vivo Data," *Nutrition and Cancer,* Vol. 21, No. 2, 1994, 113–31.

24. D. R. Doerge and D. M. Sheehan, "Goitrogenic and estrogenic activity of soy isoflavones," *Environ Health Perspect,* Vol. 110, Suppl. 3, June 2002, 349–53.

25. *Cancer Rates and Risks,* 4th edition, edited by Angela Harras (National Institutes of Health, National Cancer Institute, 1996); Joseph J. Rackis et al., "The USDA trypsin inhibitor study. I. Background, Objectives and Procedural Details," *Qualification of Plant Foods in Human Nutrition,* Vol. 35, 1985.

26. N. L. Petrakis et al., "Stimulatory Influence of Soy Protein Isolate on Breast Secretion in Pre- and Post-Menopausal Women," *Cancer Epid Bio Prev,* Vol. 5, 1996, 785–79.

27. *Cancer Forum,* Vol. 14, No. 11/12, Winter 1996.

28. B. Lohrke, "Activation of skeletal muscle protein breakdown following consumption of soybean protein in pigs," *Br J Nutr,* Vol. 85, No.4, April 2001, 447–57.

29. A. D. Ologhobo et al., "Distribution of phosphorus and phytate in some Nigerian varieties of legumes and some effects of processing," *Journal of Food Science,* Vol. 49, No. 1, January/February 1984, 199–201.

30. Sally W. Fallon and Mary G. Enig, "Soy Products for Dairy Products? Not So Fast . . . ," *Health Freedom News,* Vol. 14, No. 5, September 1995.

31. Edward Mellanby, "Experimental rickets: The effect of cereals and their interaction with other factors of diet and environment in producing rickets," *Journal of the Medical Research Council,* Vol. 93, March 1925, 265; M. R. Wills et al., "Phytic Acid and Nutritional Rickets in Immigrants," *The Lancet,* April 8,1972, 771–73.

32. Fallon and Enig, "Soy Products."

33. Rackis et al., "The USDA trypsin inhibitor study. I. Background, Objectives and Procedural Details," 22; Rackis et al., "Evaluation of the Health Aspects of Soy Protein Isolates as Food Ingredients," prepared for FDA by Life Sciences Research Office, Federation of American Societies for Experimental Biology, Contract No. FDA 223-75-2004, 1979.

34. G. M. Wallace, "Studies on the Processing and Properties of Soymilk," *Journal of Science and Food Agriculture,* Vol. 22, October 1971, 526–35.

35. Rackis et al., "The USDA trypsin inhibitor study. I. Background, Objectives and Procedural Details."

36. Joseph J. Rackis, "Biological and Physiological Factors in Soybeans," *Journal of the American Oil Chemists' Society,* Vol. 51, January 1974, 161A–170A.

37. "Food Labeling: Health Claims; Soy Protein and Coronary Heart Disease," Food and Drug Administration, 21 CFR Part 101 (Docket No. 98P-0683).

38. Raymond F. Peat, *Nutrition for Women,* 5th ed. (Eugene, OR: Kenogen, 1993), 18, 67, 68, 92.

39. R. L. Divi et al., "Anti-thyroid Isoflavones from Soybean: Isolation, Characterization, and Mechanisms of Action," *Biochem Pharmacol,* Vol. 54, No. 10, November 15, 1997, 1087–96.

40. Y. Ishizuki et al., "The Effects on the Thyroid Gland of Soybeans Administered Experimentally in Healthy Subjects," *Nippon Naibunpi Gakkai Zasshi*, Vol. 67, No. 5, May 20, 1991, 622–29.

41.

42. Daniel R. Doerge, "Inactivation of Thyroid Peroxidase by Genistein and Daidzein in Vitro and in Vivo; Mechanism for Anti-Thyroid Activity of Soy," presented at the November 1999 Soy Symposium in Washington, DC.

43. Rackis et al., "The USDA trypsin inhibitor study. I. Background, objectives and procedural details."

44. Divi et al., "Anti-thyroid Isoflavones from Soybean: Isolation, Characterization, and Mechanisms of Action."

45. Lohrke, "Activation of Skeletal Muscle Protein Breakdown Following Consumption of Soybean Protein in Pigs."

46. Ibid.

47. Elaine Hollingsworth, *Take Control of Your Health and Escape the Sickness Industry* (Mudgeeraba, Queensland, Australia: Empowerment Press International, 2000).

48. Peat, *Nutrition for Women*, 18, 67, 68, 92.

49. Setchell, "Naturally Occurring Non-Steroidal Estrogens of Dietary Origin," *Estrogens in the Environment* (New York: Elsevier Science, 1985), 79–80.

50. Venus Catherine Andrecht, *The Herb Lady's Notebook* (Ramona, CA: Ransom Hill, 1992), 73–76.

51. Marcus Laux, "Why I Want Women to Choose Natural Hormone Replacement," *Naturally Well*, Vol. 2, No. 12, December 1995, 3.

52. Andrecht, *The Herb Lady's Notebook*.

53. C. Norman Shealy, *DHEA: The Health and Youth Hormone* (New Canaan, CT: Keats Publishing, 1996).

54. Laux, "Why I Want Women to Choose Natural Hormone Replacement."

55. John R. Lee, *Natural Progesterone: The Multiple Roles of a Remarkable Hormone* (Sebastopol, CA: BLL Publishing, 1993), 37.

56. Sari Harrar and Sara Altshul O'Donnell, *The Woman's Book of Healing Herbs* (Emmaus, PA: Rodale Press, Inc., 1999), 228.

57. Julian Whitaker, *Health and Healing*, Vol. 2, No. 7, July 1992.

58. J. Cinatl et al., "Glycyrrhizin, an active component of liquorice roots, and replication of SARS-associated coronavirus," *The Lancet*, Vol. 361, No. 9374, June 14, 2003, 2045–46.

59. M. T. Murray, *The Healing Power of Herbs: The Enlightened Person's Guide to the Wonders of Medicinal Plants* (Rocklin, CA: Prima Publishing 1995), 43–49.

60. Todd Mangum, M.D., "The Dangers of Hormone replacement," Independent Media Institution, November 21, 2002.

61. Marcus Laux, N.D., and Christine Conrad, *Natural Woman, Natural Menopause* (HarperCollins Publishers, Inc., 1997), 110.

62. Murray, *The Healing Power of Herbs*, 375.

63. Jesse Hanley, "PMS and Menopause Without Pain," *Alternative Medicine Digest*, Issue 10, 1996, 35.

64. Daniel M. Sheehan, "The Case for Expanded Phytoestrogen," *Biology and Medicine*, Vol. 108, 1995, 3–4.

65. Whitten et al., "Influence of Phytoestrogen Diets on Estradiol Action in the Rat Uterus."

66. P. L. Whitten, "Potential Adverse Effects of Phytoestrogens," *J. Nutr.*, Vol. 125, No. 3, March 1995, 7715–65.

67. Susan Conova, "Estrogen's Role in Cancer," *In Vivo*, Vol. 2, No. 10, May 26, 2003.

68. Hari K. Bhat et al., "Critical Role of Oxidative Stress in Estrogen-Induced Carcinogenesis," *PNAS*, Vol. 100, No. 7, April 1, 2003, 3913–18.

69. Viana Muller, M.D., "Maca: Discover How This New Phytonutrient Can Ease Menopausal Symptoms," *Nature & Health Magazine*, December 1999/January 2000.

70. Hugo Malaspina, M.D., "Maca regulates sexual functions for both males and females," Notes on Hormone Replacement (Therapy) Properties of Maca Root from www.macaroot.com/science/nurse.

71. Muller, "Maca."

72. Chris Kilham, "Maca: Discover How this New Phytonutrient Can Ease Menopausal Symptoms," *PREVENTION*, January 2000.

73. Elaine Hollingsworth, *Take Control of Your Health and Escape the Sickness Industry*, Australia, Empowerment Press International (6th edition), 2000: 75, 96.

74. Malaspina, Notes on Hormone Replacement (Therapy) Properties of Maca Root from www.macaroot.com/science/nurse.

75. Richard A. Passwater, *Cancer and Its Nutritional Therapies* (New Canaan, CT: Keats Publishing, 1983), 25.

76. Carlton Fredericks, *Breast Cancer: A Nutritional Approach* (New York: Grosset & Dunlap, 1977).

77. Carlton Fredericks, *Guide to Women's Nutrition* (New York: The Putnam Publishing Group, 1989), 42.

78. Ibid., 30, 31.

79. S. J. Lewis et al., "Lower Serum Oestrogen Concentrations Associated with Faster Intestinal Transit," *Br. J. Cancer*, Vol. 76, No. 3, 1997, 395–400.

80. Fredericks, *Guide to Women's Nutrition*.

81. Ibid.

82. Gail Sheehy, *The Silent Passage: Menopause* (New York: Pocket Books, 1993).

83. Fredericks, *Guide to Women's Nutrition*.

84. Peat, *Nutrition for Women*.

85. Peat, "Diabetics."

86. Peat, "Menopause and Its Causes," *Ray Peat's Newsletter*, Summer 1995.

87. Fredericks, *Guide to Women's Nutrition*.

88. Ibid.

89. Peat, *Nutrition for Women*.

90. Ibid.

91. Peat, "Progesterone: Essential to Your Well-Being," *Let's Live*, April 1982.

92. Passwater, *Cancer.*

93. Ibid.

94. Passwater, *Cancer.*

95. Raymond F. Peat, "Estrogen: Simply Dangerous," *Ray Peat's Newsletter,* July 1995.

96. Fredericks, *Guide to Women's Nutrition.*

97. F. Batmanghelidj, *Your Body's Many Cries for Water* (Falls Church, VA: Global Health Solutions, Inc., 1992).

98. Ibid.

99. Ibid.

100. Ibid.

101. Sam Biser, *Using Water to Cure: The Untold Story* (Charlottesville, VA: The University of Natural Healing, 1994), 28, and Jacques de Langre, *Seasalt's Hidden Powers* (Magalia, CA: Happiness Press, 1993).

102. Dr. Norman W. Walker, *Water Can Undermine Your Health* (Prescott, AZ: Norwalk Press 1974).

103. George H. Malkmus, *God's Way to Ultimate Health* (Eidson, TN: Hallelujah Acres Publishing, 1997), 174.

104. Ibid.

105. Paul C. Bragg, N.D., Ph.D., *Water: The Shocking Truth that Can Save Your Life!* (Santa Barbara, CA: Health Science, 1998).

106. Jacques de Langre, *Seasalt's Hidden Powers* (Magalia, CA: Happiness Press, 1993).

107. Ibid., 56.

108. Ibid.

109. Ibid., 28, 56–58, 85–86.

110. Ibid., 76.

111. M. G. Venkatesh Mannar et al., "Double fortification of salt with iron and iodine," *Proceedings of the Sixth International Nutrition Congress,* Seoul, Korea, 1989.

112. R. Martin, K. Romano, *Preventing and Reversing Arthritis Naturally: The Untold Story* (Rochester, VT: Healing Arts Press, 2000).

113. Betty Kamen, Ph.D., *Hormone Replacement Therapy: YES or NO?* (Novato, CA: Nutrition Encounter, Inc., 1993) citing: A. G. March et al., "Vegetarian Lifestyle and Bone Mineral Density," *American Journal of Clinical Nutrition,* Vol. 48, No. 837, 1988.

114. Elaine Newkirk, N.D., L.P.N., M.H., C.N.H.P., "ADHD or Allergy?," *Health Keepers Magazine,* Vol. 11, No. 11, Summer 1999.

115. A. M. Rossignol and H. Bonnlander, "Prevalence and Severity of the Premenstrual Syndrome. Effects of Foods and Beverages That Are Sweet or High in Sugar Content," *Journal of Reproductive Medicine,* Vol. 3, February 1991, 131–136.

116 Nancy Appleton, Ph.D., *Healthy Bones: What You Should Do About Osteoporosis* (Garden City Park, NY: Avery Publishing Group Inc., 1991), 80–87.

117. W. Crook, *The Yeast Connection* (Jackson, TN: Professional Books, 1984).

118. R. Martin and K. Romano, *Preventing and Reversing Arthritis Naturally* citing A. M. Rossignol and H. Bonnlander, "Prevalence and Severity of the Premenstrual

Syndrome. Effects of Foods and Beverages That Are Sweet or High in Sugar Content," *Journal of Reproductive Medicine*, Vol. 3, February 1991, 131–136.

119. Annette T. Lee and Anthony Cermai, "The Role of Glycation in Aging," *Annals of the New York Academy of Science*, Vol. 663, 63–70.

120. Nancy Appleton, Ph.D., *Lick the Sugar Habit* (Garden City Park, NY: Avery Publishing Group, Inc., 1988), 55, 56.

121. R. Pamplona et al., "Mechanisms of Glycation in Atherogenesis," *Medical Hypotheses*, Vol. 40, 1990, 174–181.

122. M. Doren and H. P. Schneider, "Identification and Treatment of Postmenopausal Women at Risk for Development of Osteoporosis," *International Journal of Clinical Pharmacology, Therapy, and Toxicology*, Vol. 30, No. 11, November 1992, 431.

123. A. G. March et al., "Vegetarian Lifestyle and Bone Mineral Density," *American Journal of Clinical Nutrition*, Vol. 48, No. 837, 1988; A. P. Clark and J. A. Schuttinga, "Targeted estrogen/progesterone replacement therapy for osteoporosis: calculation of health care cost savings," *Osteoporosis International*, Vol. 2, No. 4, July 1992, 195–200.

124. Appleton, *Lick the Sugar Habit*; Appleton, *Healthy Bones: What You Should Do About Osteoporosis*.

125. Ibid.

126. K. Heaton, "The Sweet Road to Gallstones," *British Medical Journal*, Vol. 288, April 14, 1984, 1103–1104.

127. Appleton, *Lick the Sugar Habit*, 81–82.

128. Ibid.

129. John Udkin, "Metabolic Changes Induced by Sugar in Relation to Cornonary Heart Disease and Diabetes," *Nutrition and Health*, Vol. 5, No. 1/2, 1987, 5–8.

130. Frances Sheridan Goulart, "Are You Sugar Smart?," *American Fitness*, March/April 1991, 34–38.

131. George A. Ulett, "Food Allergy—Cytotoxic Testing and the Central Nervous System," *Psychiatric Journal of the University of Ottawa*, No. 2, June 1980, 100–108.

132. William Rea et al., "Food and Chemical Susceptibility After Environmental Chemical Overexposure: Case Histories," *Annals of Allergy*, Vol. 41, August 1978, 101–110.

133. Joel Wallach, "Metabolic Therapy for Heart Disease, Cancer, Allergies, and Multiple Sclerosis," Paper presented at the National Health Federation Meeting, Long Beach, CA, January, 1983, Audio tape.

134. R. M. Bostick, et al., "Sugar, Meat and Fat Intake, and Non-dietary Risk Factors for Colon Cancer Incidence in Iowa Women," *Cancer Causes and Controls*, Vol. 5, 1994, 38–52.

135. Clara Morman et al., "Dietary Sugar Intake in the Etiology of Biliary Tract Cancer," *International Journal of Epidemiology*, Vol. 22, No. 2, 1993, 207–214.

136. J Kelsay et al. "Diets High in Glucose or Sucrose and Young Women," *American Journal of Clinical Nutrition*, Vol. 27, 1974, 926–936.

137. Appleton, *Lick the Sugar Habit*, 68–72 citing: Theron G. Randolph and Leona B.

Yeager, "Corn Sugar as an Allergen," *Annals of Allergy,* September/October 1949, 650–661.

138. D. D. Soejarto et al., "Potential sweetening agents of plant origin. II. Field search for sweet-tasting *Stevia* species," *Econ Bot,* Vol. 37, 1983, 74.

139. *Magic and Medicine of Plants* (Pleasantville, NY: The Reader's Digest Association, Inc., 1986): 390; see also A. D. Kinghorn and D. D. Soejarto, "Current Status of Stevioside as a Sweetening Agent for Human Use," in *Economic and Medicinal Plant Research,* Vol. 1, edited by H. Wagner et al. (New York, NY: Academic Press, 1985), 1–51.

140. H. Suzuki et al., "Influence of Oral Administration of Stevioside on Levels of Blood Glucose and Liver Glycogen of Intact Rats," *Nippon Nopei Kagaku Kaishi,* Vol. 51, No. 3, 1977, 171–173.

141. Daniel B. Mowrey, Ph.D., *Scientific Validation of Herbal Medicine* (New Canaan, Conn.: Keats Publishing, 1990).

142. D.D. Soejarto et al., "Potential sweetening agents of plant origin."

143. A. D. Kinghorn and D. D. Soejarto, "Stevioside," in *Economic and Medical Plant Research,* Vol. 7, edited by H. Wagner et al. (New York: Academic Press, 1991), 157–171.

144. Joel Robbins, D.C., N.D., M.D., *Nutrition and Its Relation to Health* (educational cassette) (Tulsa, OK: Health Dynamics Corporation, 1999).

145. A. S. Zino et al., "Randomized Controlled Trial of Effect of Fruit and Vegetable Consumption on Plasma Concentrations of Lipids and Antioxidants," *BMJ,* Vol. 314, 1997, 1787–91.

146. R. Martin, K. Romano, *Preventing and Reversing Arthritis Naturally: The Untold Story.*

147. Earl L. Mindell, "Eggs Have Gotten a Raw Deal," *Let's Live,* September 1994, 8.

148. Peat, *Nutrition for Women.*

149. Sally W. Fallon and Mary G. Enig, "Why Butter is Better," *Health Freedom News,* Vol. 14, No. 6, November/December 1995.

150. Ibid.

151. Fallon and Enig, "Why Butter is Better."

152. Ibid.

153. Deborah Kesten, "The Enlightened Diet: You Become What You Eat," *Spirituality and Health,* May/June 2004, 84.

154. Joseph, *My Healing from Breast Cancer,* 1996, 6–7.

155. John Finnegan, N.D., "Our Need for Essential Fatty Acids," *Health Freedom News,* January-February 1997, 35.

156. William G. Crook, M.D., *The Yeast Connection* (New York: Random House, 1986).

157. E. A. Mascioli et al., "Unsaturated Fats Directly Kill White Blood Cells," *Lipids,* Vol. 22, No. 6, 1987, 421.

158. C. J. Meade and J. Mertin, "Fatty Acids and Immunity," *Adv Lipid Res,* Vol. 16, 1978, 127–65.

159. Eustace Mullins, *Murder by Injection: The Story of the Medical Conspiracy Against America* (Staunton, VA: The National Council for Medical Research, 1988), 214.

160. Bruce Fife, *The Healing Miracles of Coconut Oil* (Colorado Springs, CO: HealthWise, 2000), 19.

161. Joseph, *My Healing from Breast Cancer*, 1996, 143.

162. M. J. Reed et al., "Free Fatty Acids: A Possible Regulator of the Available Oestradiol Fractions in Plasma," *J. Steroid Biochem.*, Vol. 24, No. 2, 1986, 657–59.

163. *Ray Peat's Newsletter*, March 2002, 7.

164. Peat, *Nutrition for Women.*

165. Peat, "Menopause and Its Causes," *Ray Peat's Newsletter*, Summer 1995.

166. Andrew Nicholson, M.D., "Diet and the Prevention and Treatment of Breast Cancer," *Alternative Therapies*, Vol. 2, No. 6, November 1996, 36.

167. Daniel Yee, "Weight, Breast Cancer Tied," *Denver Post*, February 26, 2004, 5A.

168. Peat, *Nutrition for Women*. See also E. A. Mascioli et al., "Unsaturated Fats Directly Kill White Blood Cells," *Lipids*, Vol. 22, No. 6, 1987, 421; C. J. Meade and J. Martin, *Adv. Lipid Res.*, Vol. 127, 1978; B. A. Houssay et al., "Accion de la Administracion Prolongada de Glucosa Sobre la Diabetes de la Rata, "*Rev. Soc. Argent de Biol.*, Vol. 23, 1994, 288–93.

169. Peat, "Estrogen: Simply Dangerous."

170. *Ray Peat's Newsletter*, March 2002, 5.

171. M. L. Pearce and S. Dayton, "Incidence of Cancer in Men on a Diet High in Polyunsaturated Fat," *The Lancet*, Vol. 1, No. 7697, 1971, 464–467; C. V. Felton et al., "Dietary Polyunsaturated Fatty Acids and Composition of Human Aortic Plaques," *The Lancet* Vol. 344, No. 8931, 1994, 1195–1196.

172. Email from Raymond Peat on 9/22/2004 citing H. G. P. Swarts et al., "Binding of Unsaturated Fatty Acids to Na+,K+-ATPase Leading to Inhibition and Inactivation," *Biochem Biophys Acta*, Vol. 1024, 1990, 32–40.

173. M. Guichardant et al., "Specific Markers of Lipid Peroxidation Issued from n-3 and n-6 Fatty Acids,"*Biochem Soc Trans*, Vol. 32, Part 1, February 2004, 139–40.

174. S. Parchmann and M. J. Mueller, "Evidence for the Formation of Dinor Isoprostanes E1 from Alpha-Linolenic Acid in Plants," *J Biol Chem*, Vol. 273, No. 49, December 4, 1998, 32650–5.

175. E. A. Mascioli et al., "Unsaturated Fats Directly Kill White Blood Cells," *Lipids*, Vol. 22, No. 6, 1987, 421.

176. Fife, *The Healing Miracles of Coconut Oil*, 118.

177. Ibid., 107, citing B. A. Watkins et al., "Importance of Vitamin E in Bone Formation and in Chondroncyte Protein Diets Cause Osteoporosis?," *Wise Traditions*, Vol. 1, No. 4, 38.

178. Udo Erasmus, *Fats that Heal, Fats that Kill* (Burnaby, B.C., Canada: Alive Books, 1997), 103.

179. Ibid; Ray Peat citing C. W. Welsch, "Review of the Effects of Dietary Fat on Experimental Mammary Gland Tumorigenesis: Role of Lipid Peroxidation," *Free Radical Biol Med*, Vol. 18, No. 4, 1995, 757–73.

180. P. S. Tappia et al., "Influence of Unsaturated Fatty Acids on the Production of Tumor Necrosis Factor and Interleukin-6 By Rat Peritoneal Macrophages," *Mol Cell Biochem*, Vol. 143, No. 2, 1995, 89–98.

181. Fife, The *Healing Miracles of Coconut Oil,* 118, citing B. S. Reddy, "Dietary Fat and Colon Cancer: Animal Model Studies," *Lipids,* Vol. 27, No. 10, 1992, 807.

182. L. A. Cohen, "Medium Chain Triglycerides Lack Tumor-Promoting Effects in the N-Methylnitrosourea-Induced Mammary Tumor Model," *The Pharmacological Effects of Lipids,* Vol. 111, 1988.

183. L. A. Cohen and D.O. Thompson, "The Influence of Dietary Medium Chain Triglycerides on Rat Mammary Tumor Development," *Lipids,* Vol. 22, No. 6, 1987, 455.

184. G. J. Hopkins et al., "Polyunsaturated Fatty Acids as Promoters of Mammary Carcinogenesis Induced in Sprague-Dawley Rats by 7, 12-Dimethylbenzanthracene," *J Natl Cancer Inst,* Vol. 66, No. 3, 1981, 517.

185. Fife, The *Healing Miracles of Coconut Oil,* 118 citing Reddy, "Dietary Fat and Colon Cancer."

186. Ibid.

187. B. S. Reddy, "Dietary Fat and Colon Cancer: Animal Model Studies," *Lipids,* Vol. 27, No. 10, 1992, 807.

188. Cohen and Thompson, "The Influence of Dietary Medium Chain Triglycerides on Rat Mammary Tumor Development."

189. H. Kaumitz, "Medium Chain Triglycerides (MCT) in Aging and Arteriosclerosis," *J Environ Pathol Toxicol Oncol,* Vol. 6, No. 3-4, 1986, 115.

190. Fife, *The Healing Miracles of Coconut Oil,* 77.

191. Ibid., 48.

192. S. Mendis and R. Kaumarasunderam, "The Effect of Daily Consumption of Coconut Fat and Soya-bean Fat on Plasma Lipids and Lipoproteins of Young Normolipidaemic Men," *British Journal of Nutrition,* Vol. 63, 1990, 547.

193. Fife, The *Healing Miracles of Coconut Oil,* 118 citing Reddy, "Dietary Fat and Colon Cancer."

194. Fife, *The Healing Miracles of Coconut Oil,* 107.

195. William Regelson, M.D., and Carol Colman, *The Super-Hormone Promise* (New York: Simon & Schuster, 1996).

196. Ray Sahelian, M.D., *Pregnenolone* (Garden City Park, NY: Avery Penguin Putnam, October 1997).

197. Ibid; Fife, *The Healing Miracles of Coconut Oil,* 45

198. C. E. Isaacs et al., "Inactivation of Enveloped Viruses in Human Bodily Fluids by Purified Lipid," *Annals of the New York Academy of Sciences,* Vol. 724, 1994, 457

199. H. Thomar et al, "Inactivation Enveloped Viruses and Killing of Cells by Fatty Acids and Monoglycerides," *Antimicrobial Agents and Chemotherapy,* Vol. 31, 1987, 27.

200. J. C. Hierholzer et al., "In vitro Effects of Monolaurin Compounds on Enveloped RNA and DNA viruses," *Journal of Food Safety,* Vol. 4, 1982, 1.

201. K. T. Holland et al., "The Effect of Glycerol Monolaurate on Growth of and Production of Toxic Shock Syndrome Toxin-1 and Lipase By Staphylococcus Aureau," *Journal of Anti-Microbial Chemotherapy,* Vol. 33, 1994, 41.

202. G. Bergsson et al., "In Vitro Inactivation of Chlamydia Trachmatis by Fatty Acids and Monoglycerides," *Antimicrobial Agents and Chemotherapy,* Vol. 42, 1998, 2290.

203. B. W. Petschow et al., "Susceptibility of Helicobacter Pylori to Bactericidal Properties of Medium-Chain Monoglycerides and Free Fatty Acids," *Antimicrobial Agents and Chemotherapy*, Vol. 145, 1996, 876.

204. J. M. Wan and R. F. Grimble, "Effect of Dietary Linoleate Content on the Metabolic Response of Rats to Escherichia Coli Endotoxin," *Clinical Science*, Vol. 72, No. 3, 1994, 383–85.

205. J. J. Kabara, "Antimicrobial Agents Derived from Fatty Acids," *Journal of the American Chemists Society*, Vol. 61, 1984, 397.

206. J. J. Kabara, "Fatty Acids and Derivatives as Antimicrobial Agents," Review in *The Pharmacological Effect of Lipids*, 1978, 1–14.

207. P. K. Thampan, *Facts and Fallacies About Coconut Oil* (Jakarta, Indonesia: Asian and Pacific Coconut Community, 1994), 4–5.

208. C. E. Isaacs and H. Thormar, "The Role of Milk-Derived Antimicrobial Lipids as Antiviral and Antibacterial Agents in Immunology of Milk and the Neonate," *Adv Exp Med Biol*, Vol. 310, 1991, 159–65.

209. Fife, *The Healing Miracles of Coconut Oil*, 107, citing J. J. Azain, "Effects of Adding Medium-Chain Triglycerides to Sow Diets During Late Gestation and Early Lactation on Litter Performance," *J Anim Sci*, Vol. 71, No. 11, 1993, 3011 and U. V. Vaidya et al., "Vegetable Oil Fortified Feeds in the Nutrition of Very Low Birthweight Babies," *Indian Pediatr*, Vol. 29, No. 12, 1992, 1519.

210. Ibid., 120, citing D. L. Ross et al., "Early Biochemical and EEG correlates of the Ketogenic Diet in Children with Atypical Absence Epilepsy," *Pediatr Neurol*, Vol. 1, No. 2, March/April 1985, 104–8.

211. Ibid., 82.

212. Ibid., 65.

213. Ibid., 66.

214. Ibid., 119, citing A. J. Monserrat et al., "Protective Effect of Coconut Oil on Renal Necrosis Occurring in Rats Fed a Methyl-Deficient Diet," *Ren Fail*, Vol. 17, No. 5, 1995, 525–37.

215. S. Sadeghi et al., "Dietary Lipids Modify the Cytokine Response to Bacterial Lipopolysaccharide in Mice," *Immunology*, Vol. 96, No. 3, 1999, 404.

216. Fife, *The Healing Miracles of Coconut Oil*, 103.

217. Peat, *Nutrition for Women*. See also R. B. Wolf, *J Am Chem Soc*, Vol. 59, No. 230, 1982; F. Berschauer et al., "Nutritional-Physiological Effects of Dietary Fats in Rations for Growing Pigs"; Effects of Sunflower Oil and Coconut Oil on Protein and Fat Retention, Fatty Acid Pattern and Back Fat and Blood Parameters in Piglets," *Arch Tieremahr*, Vol. 34, No. 2, 1984, 19–33; B. A. Houssay and C. Martinez, "Experimental Diabetes and Diet," *Science*, Vol. 105, 1947, 548–49; C. J. Henry et al., "Protein Utilization, Growth and Survival in Essential Fatty-Acid-Deficient Rats," *Br J Nutri*, Vol. 75, No. 2, February 1996, 237–48.

218. Peat, *Progesterone in Orthomolecular Medicine* (Eugene, OR: Kenogen, 1993).

219. Langre, *Seasalt's Hidden Powers*.

220. Elizabeth Tracey, M.S., "Extra-Virgin Olive Oil Reduces Need for Blood Pressure Medication," WebMD.com Medical News Archive, March 29, 2000.

221. Ibid.
222. R. Martin, K. Romano, *Preventing and Reversing Arthritis Naturally: The Untold Story.*
223. Peat, *Nutrition for Women.*
224. Fife, *The Healing Miracles of Coconut Oil,* 19, citing S. A. Hashim et al., "Effect of Mixed Fat Formula Feeding on Serum Cholesterol Level in Man," *Am J Clin Nutr,* Vol. 7, No.1, 1959, 30–34 and N. J. Greenberger and T. G. Skillman, "Medium-Chain Triglycerides: Physiologic Considerations and Clinical Implications," *N Engl J Med,* Vol. 180, 1969, 1045–58.
225. A. Geliebter, "Overfeeding with Medium-Chain Triglycerides Diet Results in Diminished Deposition of Fat," *Am J Clin Nutr,* Vol. 37, 1983, 104.
226. N. Baba, "Enhanced Thermogenesis and Diminished Deposition of Fat in Response to Overfeeding with a Diet containing Medium Chain Triglycerides," *Am J Clin Nutri,* Vol. 35, 1982, 678.
227. G. A. Bray et al., "Weight Gain of Rats Fed Medium-Chain Triglycerides is Less Than Rats Fed Long-Chain Triglycerides," *Int J Obes,* Vol. 4, 1980, 27–32.
228. Fife, *The Healing Miracles of Coconut Oil,* 92.
229. Ibid., 90.
230. Ibid., 91, citing T. Fishiki and K. Matsumoto, "Swimming Endurance Capacity of Mice is Increased by Chronic Consumption of Medium-Chain Triglycerides," *Journal of Nutrition,* Vol. 125, 1995, 531. And Applegate, L. "Nutrition," 1996 *Runner's World* 31:26.
231. Tappia et al., "Influence of Unsaturated Fatty Acids on the Production of Tumor Necrosis Factor and Interleukin-6 By Rat Peritoneal Macrophages."
232. C. W. Welsch, "Review of the Effects of Dietary Fat on Experimental Mammary Gland Tumorigenesis: Role of Lipid Peroxidation," *Free Radical Biol Med,* Vol. 18, No. 4, 1995, 757–73.
233. Mary G. Enig, Ph.D., "Health and Nutritional Benefits from Coconut Oil," *Price-Pottenger Nutrition Foundation Health Journal,* Vol. 20, 1998, 1–6.
234. Monserrat et al., "Protective Effect of Coconut Oil on Renal Necrosis Occurring in Rats Fed a Methyl-Deficient Diet," *Ren Fail,* Vol. 17, No. 5, 1995, 525–37.
235. Fife, *The Healing Miracles of Coconut Oil,* 45–48.
236. E. A. Mascioli et al., "Unsaturated Fats Directly Kill White Blood Cells," *Lipids,* Vol. 22, No. 6, 1987, 421.
237. C. V. Felton et al., "Dietary Polyunsaturated Fatty Acids and Composition of Human Aortic Plaques," *The Lancet,* Vol. 344, No. 8931, 1994, 1195–96.
238. Fife, *The Healing Miracles of Coconut Oil,* 100, citing E. V. Macalalag et al., "Buko Water of Immature Coconut is a Universal Urinary Stone Solvent," Padivid Coconut Community Conference, Metro Manila, August 14–18, 1997 and F. E. Anzaldo et al., "Coconut Water as Intravenous Fluid," *Philippine J Pediatrics,* Vol. 24, 1975, 143.
239. Ibid., 109.
240. Erasmus, *Fats That Heal, Fats That Kill,* 259, 260.
241. Ibid.

242. John R. Lee, M.D., et al., *What Your Doctor May Not Tell You About Premenopause* (New York: Warner Books, Inc., 1999), 139–40.

243. Erasmus, *Fats That Heal, Fats That Kill*, 260.

244. James F. Balch and Phyllis A. Balch, *Prescription for Nutritional Healing* (Garden City Park, NY: Avery Publishing Group Inc., 1990), 14, 15, 69.

245. The Burton Goldberg Group, *Alternative Medicine* (Puyallup, WA: Future Medicine Publishing, Inc., 1993), 181–82.

246. Carol H. Munson and Diane K. Gilroy, *The Good Fats* (Emmaus, PA: Rodale Press, 1988), and Udo Erasmus, *Fats & Oils* (Burnaby, BC: Alive Books, 1991).

247. Adelle Davis, *Let's Get Well* (New York: Harcourt Brace Jovanovich, Inc., 1972), 76.

248. Jason Theodosakis, M.D., M.S., M.P.H., Brenda Adderly, M.H.A., and Barry Fox, Ph.D., *The Arthritis Cure* (New York: St. Martin's Press, 1997), 120.

249. Susan Smith Jones, Ph.D., *The Main Ingredients of Health & Happiness* (Nevada City, CA: Dawn Publications, October 1995).

250. Paavo Airola, *Are You Confused?* (Sherwood, OR: Health Plus Publishers, 1971), 76.

251. Raymond H. Peat, Ph.D., *From PMS to Menopause: Female Hormones in Context* (Eugene, OR, 1997), 157.

252. M. Jenab and L. U. Thompson, "The influence of flaxseed and lignans on colon carcinogenesis and beta-glucuronidase activity," *Carcinogenesis*, Vol. 17, No. 6, June 1996, 1343–48.

253. Sahelian, *Pregnenolone*, 18; Betty Kamen, *Hormone Replacement Therapy: Yes or No?* (Novato, CA: Nutrition Encounter Inc., 1993), 34, 41; John R. Lee, *Natural Progesterone: The Multiple Roles of a Remarkable Hormone* (Sebastopol, CA: BLL Pub., 1993), 12.

Chapter 7: Planning a Personal Approach

1. Christiane Northrup, *Health Wisdom for Women*, Vol. 1, No. 2, February 1995.

2. Gail Sheehy, *The Silent Passage: Menopause* (New York: Pocket Books, 1993).

3. Raquel Martin, *Today's Health Alternative* (Bozeman, MT: America West Publishers, 1992).

4. Sheehy, *The Silent Passage,*

5. John R. Lee, "Significance of Molecular Configuration Specificity—The Case of Progesterone and Osteoporosis," *Townsend Letter for Doctors*, June 1993, 558.

6. John R. Lee, *Natural Progesterone: The Multiple Roles of a Remarkable Hormone* (Sebastopol, CA: BLL Publishing, 1993), 76.

7. John R. Lee, "Significance of Molecular Configuration Specificity."

8. John R. Lee, *Natural Progesterone.*

9. Katharina Dalton, "Ante-natal Progesterone and Intelligence," *British Journal of Psychiatry*, Vol. 114, 1968.

10. Joel T. Hargrove et al., "Menopausal Hormone Replacement Therapy with Continuous Daily Oral Micronized Estradiol and Progesterone," *Obstetrics & Gynecology*, Vol. 73. No. 4, April 1989, 606–12.

11. John R. Lee, "Is Natural Progesterone the Missing Link in Osteoporosis Prevention and Treatment?" *Medical Hypotheses*, 1991.
12. J. C. Prior, Y. Vigna, and N. Alojada, "Progesterone and the Prevention of Osteoporosis," *Canadian Journal of OB/GYN & Women's Health Care*, Vol. 3, No. 4, 1991, 181.
13. C. M. Dolibaum and G. P. Dowe, "Absorption of Progesterone after Topical Applications: Serum and Saliva Levels," Evidence Presented at the 7th Annual Meeting of the American Menopause Society, 1997.
14. Debbie Moskowitz, "New Test Offers Information About Hormone Levels," *Natural Solutions*, Vol. 4, Issue 1, Winter 1996.
15. John R. Lee, "David Zava's New Lab and New Formula for Assessing Hormone Balance," *The John R. Lee, M.D. Medical Letter*, November 1998.
16. Nan Kathryn Fuchs, Ph.D., *The Newest Breakthrough in Detecting and Preventing Breast Cancer* (Atlanta: Soundview Publications, Inc., 2002).
17. Nan Kathryn Fuchs, Ph.D., *Women's Health Letter*, August 2004, 9.
18. John R. Lee, "David Zava's New Lab and New Formula for Assessing Hormone Balance."
19. Raymond F. Peat, Ph.D., "Estrogen: Simply Dangerous," *Ray Peat's Newsletter*, July 1995.
20. Marcus Laux and Christine Conrad, *Natural Woman, Natural Menopause* (New York: HarperCollins, 1997), 106, 107.
21. Sherrill Sellman, *Hormone Heresy* (Honolulu: Get Well International, 1998), 68.
22. Ibid.
23. Jan Bresnick and Toby Hanlon, "Custom Tailored Hormone Therapy," *Prevention,* July 1995, 65.
24. Alvin H. Follingstad, "Estriol, the Forgotten Estrogen?" *Journal of the American Medical Association*, Vol. 239, No. 1, January 2, 1978.
25. John R. Lee, "Is Natural Progesterone the Missing Link?"
26. Stuart M. Berger, *What Your Doctor Didn't Learn in Medical School* (New York: William Morrow, 1988).

Appendix A: Ways and Means of Hormone Application

1. Marcus Laux and Christine Conrad, *Natural Woman, Natural Menopause* (New York: HarperCollins, 1997), 74; and John R. Lee, *What Your Doctor May Not Tell You About Menopause* (New York: Warner Books, 1996).
2. Norman Shealy, *Natural Progesterone Cream: Safe and Natural Hormone Replacement* (Los Angeles: Keats Publishing, 1999), 9.
3. Todd Mangum, "The Dangers of Hormone Replacement," Independent Media Institute, November 21, 2002.
4. John R. Lee, *What Your Doctor May Not Tell You About Menopause* (New York: Warner Books, 1996), 322.
5. John R. Lee, *Natural Progesterone: The Multiple Roles of a Remarkable Hormone* (Sebastopol, CA: BLL Publishing, 1993), 78, 264, 265, 267.

6. Katharina Dalton, M.D., *Once a Month* (Pomona, CA: Hunter House, 1979), 145.
7. Ibid.
8. Raymond Peat, Ph.D., *From PMS to Menopause: Female Hormones in Context* (Eugene, OR: International University, 1997), 74.
9. Dalton, *Once a Month,* 182; William Regelson, M.D., and Carol Colman, *The Super-Hormone Promise* (New York, Simon & Schuster, 1996), 103, 108.
10. Alan R. Gaby, M.D., *Preventing and Reversing Osteoporosis* (Rocklin, CA: Prima Publishing, 1994), 164.
11. Ibid., 167.
12. "Scientific Verdict Still Out on DHEA," *Medical News & Perspectives,* November 6, 1996: 5.
13. W. R. Regelson et al., "Hormonal Intervention: 'Buffer Hormones' or 'State Dependency,' The Role of Dehydroepiandrosterone (DHEA), Thyroid Hormone, Estrogen, and Hypophysectomy in Aging," *Acad Sci* 521: 260–273.
14. Peat, *From PMS to Menopause,* 74.
15. Bruce Fife, *The Healing Miracles of Coconut Oil* (Colorado Springs, CO: HealthWise, 2000), 107.
16. H. Aldercreutz, "Dietary Phyto-estrogens and the Menopause in Japan," *The Lancet,* Vol. 339, 1992, 266–267.
17. Katharina Dalton, M.D., *Once a Month* (Pomona, CA, Hunter House, 1979), 145.
18. Anne Dickson and Nikki Henriques, *Women on Menopause* (Rochester, VT: Healing Arts Press, 1988), 59.
19. Raymond F. Peat, "Effectiveness of Progesterone Assimilation for the Relief of Premenstrual Symptoms" (educational brochure), Eugene, OR.
20. Betty Kamen, *Hormone Replacement Therapy: Yes or No?* (Novato, CA: Nutrition Encounter, Inc., 1993), 109–212.

Appendix B: Synthetic Compounds

1. Todd Mangum, M.D., "The Dangers of Hormone Replacement," Independent Media Institute, November 21, 2002.
2. William Boyd, *Textbook of Pathology,* 8th ed., (Philadelphia: Lea & Febiger, 1970), 18.
3. *Physicians' Desk Reference* (Montvale, NJ: Medical Economics Data Production Company, 1995).
4. Alfred Gilman and Louis Goodman, *Goodman & Gilman's The Pharmacological Basis of Therapeutics,* 6th ed., (New York: Macmillan, 1980), 1420–38.
5. *Facts and Comparisons 1994 and 2000* (St. Louis, MO: Facts and Comparisons, Inc.), 96–108 (looseleaf booklet published monthly: 111 West Port Plaza, Suite 400, St. Louis, MO, 63146).
6. Ibid.
7. Ibid.
8. Ibid.
9. Ibid.

10. Ibid.
11. Ibid.

Appendix C: Natural Formulas for Infants

1. P. A. Chorazy et al., "Persistent Hypothyroidism in an Infant Receiving Soy Formula: Case Report Review and Review of the Literature," *Pediatrics* 96, 1995: 148–150.
2. T. H. Shepard, "Soybean Goiter," *New England Journal of Medicine* 262, 1960: 1099–1103.
3. "Soy Infant Formula Could Be Harmful to Infants: Groups Want It Pulled," *Nutrition Week* 29 (46), December 10, 1999: 1–2.
4. New Zealand Ministry of Health, "Soy-based Infant Formula," December 1998.
5. M. A. Jabbar, J. Larrea, R. A. Shaw, "Abnormal thyroid function test in infants with congenital hypothyroidism: the influence of soy-based formula," *Journal of the American College of Nutrition* 16, 1997: 280–282.
6. P. Fort, N. Moses, M. Fasano, T. Goldberg, F. Lifshitz, "Breast and soy-formula feedings in early infancy and the prevalence of autoimmune thyroid disease in children," *Journal of the American College of Nutrition* 9 (2), April 1990: 167–167.
7. P. Fort, R. Lanes, S. Dahlem, B. Recker, M. Weyman-Daum, M. Pugliese, F. J. Lifshitz, "Breast-feeding and insulin-dependent diabetes mellitus in children," *Journal of the American College of Nutrition* 5 (5), 1986: 439–441.
8. Fort et al., "Breast and soy-formula feedings . . ."
9. Bulletin de l'Office Fédéral de la Santé Publique, no. 28, July 20, 1992.
10. "Soy Infant Formula . . ." *Nutrition Week* 29 (46).
11. Soy Nutritive Content, United Soybean Board, in M. G. Enig, S. A. Fallon, "Tragedy and Hype, The Third International Soy Symposium," *Nexus Magazine* 7 (3), April-May 2000.
12. "IEH Assessment on Phytoestrogens in the Human Diet," *Final Report to the Ministry of Agriculture, Fisheries, and Food,* United Kingdom, November 1997, 11.
13. "DC on Line," *Dynamic Chiropractic,* September 1, 2003: 36, 37.
14. A. H. El Tiney, "Proximate Composition and Mineral and Phytate Contents of Legumes Grown in Sudan," *Journal of Food Composition and Analysis* 2, 1989: 6778.
15. A. D. Ologhobo et al., "Distribution of phosphorus and phytate in some Nigerian varieties of legumes and some effects of processing," *Journal of Food Science* 49 (1), January/February 1984: 199–201.
16. C. C. Pfeiffer, E. R. Braverman, "Zinc, the Brain, and Behavior," *Biological Psychiatry* 17 (4), April 1982: 513–532.
17. Sally Fallon, *Nourishing Traditions: The Cookbook that Challenges Politically Correct Nutrition and the Diet Dictocrats,* 2nd edition (Winona Lake, IN: New Trends Publishing, 1999).
18. Soy Nutritive Content, United Soybean Board.
19. Sally W. Fallon and Mary G. Enig, "Soy Products for Dairy Products? Not So Fast. . . ." *Health Freedom News,* Vol. 14, No. 5, September 1995.

20. Sally Fallon, Pat Connolly, and Mary G. Enig, *Nourishing Traditions: The Cookbook That Challenges Politically Correct Nutrition and the Diet Dictocrats* (San Diego: ProMotion Publishing, 1995), 564.
21. Ibid., 561.
22. Joel Robbins, D.C., N.D., M.D., *Pregnancy, Childbirth & Children's Diet*, 18.
23. Ibid.
24. Fallon and Enig, "Soy Products for Dairy Products?"
25. Ibid.

Appendix D: Resources for Cancer Patients

1. Lorraine Day, *Cancer Doesn't Scare Me Anymore!* (videotape) (Rancho Mirage, CA: Rockford Press, 1994).
2. Stanley Englebardt, "Straight Talk About Mammograms," *Reader's Digest*, November 1994.
3. William C. Bryce, "The Truth about Breast Cancer," *Health Freedom News*, May 1993, 11.
4. Bales Scientifics, "How Mammography Causes Cancer," *Alternative Medicine*, Issue 31, September 1999, 32.
5. "Mammograms are Hazardous to Your Health," *Second Opinion*, vol. XI, no. 4, April 2001: 5.
6. Joann G. Elmore et al., "Ten-year Risk of False Positive Screening Mammograms and Clinical Breast Examinations," *N Engl J Med*, vol. 338, no. 16, April 16, 1998: 1089–97.
7. Peter C. Gotzsche et al., "Is Screening for Breast Cancer with Mammography Justifiable?," *The Lancet*, vol. 355, no. 9198, January 8, 2000: 129–134.
8. . M. Liff et al., "Does Increased Detection Account for the Rising Incidence of Breast Cancer?," *American Journal of Public Health*, 81 (4), April 1991: 462–65.
9. J. Law, "Variations in Individual Radiation Dose in a Breast Cancer Screening Programmed and Consequence for the Balance Between Associated Risk and Benefit," *Br J Radiol* 66, 1993: 691-8.
10. W. W. Van de Houven van Oordit et al., "The Genetic Background Modifies the Spontaneous and X-ray-Induced Tumor Spectrum in the Apc 1638N Mouse Model," *Genes Chromosomes and Cancer* 24, 1999: 191-8.
11. A. Miller et al., "Mortality From Breast Cancer After Irradiation during Fluoroscopic Examination in Patients Being Tuberculoses," *N Engl J Med* 321, 1989: 1285-9.
12. "Radiation-induced Breast Cancer," *Br Med J* 1 (6055), 1977 Jan 22: 191–2.
13. V. Ascroft, "Adjuvant Radiotherapy and Risk of Contralateral Breast Cancer," *J Natl Cancer Inst* 84, 1992: 1245–50.
14. N. Hilreth, et al., "The Risk of Breast Cancer after Irradiation of the Thymus in Infancy," *N Engl J Med* 321, 1989: 1281–4.
15. Marcus Laux, "Why I Don't Think You Should Trust Mammograms," *Naturally Well*, Vol. 3, No. 5, 1996, 2.

16. Ibid.; *Archives of Internal Medicine,* Vol. 56, No. 2, 1996, 209–13; W. W. Fletcher, "Why Question Screening Mammography for Women in Their Forties?" *Radiol. Clin. North America,* Vol. 33, No. 6, 1995, 1259–71; Karla Kerlikowski, "Efficacy of Screening Mammography: A Meta-analysis," *Journal of the American Medical Association,* Vol. 273, No. 2, 1995; K. Lockwood, S. Moesgard, and K. Folders, "Partial and Complete Regression of Breast Cancer in Patients in Relation to Dosage of Coenzyme Q10," *Biochem. Biophys. Res. Commun.,* Vol. 199, No. 3, 1994, 1504–08.

17. Day, *Cancer Doesn't Scare Me Anymore!*

18. Bales Scientifics, "Breast Cancer Detection Years Earlier," *Alternative Medicine,* Issue 31, September 1999, 32.

19. Ibid.

20. Norma Peterson, "Mammograms May Rupture In Situ Cysts, Causing Invasive Cancer," *Breast Cancer Action Newsletter,* Vol. 38, October/November 1996, 9.

21. Maureen Roberts, "Breast Screening: Time for a Rethink?" *British Medical Journal,* Vol. 299, 1989, 1153–55.

22. C. J. Wright and C. B. Mueller, "Screening Mammography and Public Health Policy: The Need for Perspective," *The Lancet,* 346, July 1995, 29–32.

23. Bales Scientifics, "Breast Cancer Detection Years Earlier," 30.

24. Ibid.

25. P. Skrabanek, *The Lancet,* August 10, 1985, 316–20.

26. Ibid.

27. Samuel S. Epstein, "New Drug Poses Risk of Ovarian Cancer," *Chicago Tribune,* April 19, 1998; *Cancer Watch,* People Against Cancer, Winter/Summer 1993.

28. John W. Gofman, M.D., *Preventing Breast Cancer* (San Francisco: Committee for Nuclear Responsibility, 1995).

29. Bales Scientifics, "Breast Cancer Detection Years Earlier," 32.

30. John W. Gofman, M.D., Ph.D., "Preventing Breast Cancer: The Story of a Major, Proven, Preventable Cause of This Disease," 1996.

31. *Ray Peat's Newsletter,* March 2002: 4.

32. "Estrogen's Mechanisms in Aging and Cancer," *Ray Peat's Newsletter,* March 2003: 7.

33. Linda Rector-Paige, Healthy Healing: An Alternative Reference (Soquel, CA: Healthy Healing Publications, 1992), 166, 329.

34. Ibid., 167.

35. Dee Ito, Without Estrogen: Natural Remedies for Menopause and Beyond (New York: Carol Southern Books, 1994), 14.

36. Bales Scientifics, "Breast Cancer Detection Years Earlier," 31.

37. "Estrogen's Mechanisms in Aging and Cancer."

38. Ibid. citing J. L. Kipp and V. D. Ramirez, "Effect of estradiol, diethylstilbestrol, and resveratrol on F0F1-ATPase activity from mitochondrial preparations of rat heart, liver, and brain," *Endocrine* 15 (2), July 2001:165–75; K. S. Russell et al., "Estrogen stimulates heat shock protein 90 binding to endothelial nitric oxide synthase in human vascular endothelial cells," *J Biol Chem* 275 (7), February 18, 2000: 5026–30.;

S. Jain et al., "Effect of estradiol and selected antiestrogens on Pro- and Antioxidant Pathways in Mammalian Uterus," *Contraception* 60 (2), August 1999: 111–8.

39. C. J. Huber et al., "Breast Fibrocystic Disease and Thermography," from the American Thermographic Symposium, Toronto, March 31–April 1, 1979, published in *Journal of Thermology*.

40. "Estrogenic Activity: US Meat Industry," Breast Cancer Research and Treatment, 12/26/2001, www.annieappleseedproject.org/esacusmeatin.html.

41. Dr. E. T. Krebs Jr., "The Extraction, Identification, and Packaging of Therapeutically Effective Amygdalin," The Robert Cathey Research Source, www.navi.net/~rsc/isomyg.htm.

Appendix F: Clinical Studies and Research Reports

1. John R. Lee, "Is Natural Progesterone the Missing Link in Osteoporosis Prevention and Treatment?" *Medical Hypotheses*, 1991, 35, 316, 318.

2. J. C. Prior, Y. Vigna, and N. Alojada, "Progesterone and the Prevention of Osteoporosis," *Canadian Journal of OB/GYN & Women's Health Care*, Vol. 3, No. 4, 1991, 181.

3. Carlton Fredericks, *Guide to Women's Nutrition* (New York: Putnam, 1989).

4. Alvin Follingstad, M.D., "Estriol, the Forgotten Estrogen?" *Journal of the American Medical Association* 239, no.1, January 2, 1978.

5. Fredericks, *Guide to Women's Nutrition*.

6. Raymond F. Peat, Ph.D., *From PMS to Menopause: Female Hormones in Context* (Eugene, OR: Kenogen, 1997), 122, 123.

7. T. I. Belova, "Structural Damage to the Mesencephalic Reticular Formation Induced by Immobilization Stress," *Bull Ep Biol & Med* 1108, No. 7, 1989, 126030.

8. Raymond F. Peat, Ph.D., "Estrogen: Simply Dangerous," *Ray Peat's Newsletter*, July 1995.

9. B. L. Weiss, "Failure of Nalmefene and Estrogen to Improve Memory in Alzheimer's Disease," *American Journal of Psychiatry* 144, 1987, 386–87.

10. H. C. Liu et al., "Performance on a Dementia Screening Test in Relation to Demographic Variables: Study of 5,297 Community Residents in Taiwan," *Arch Neurol* 51, No. 9, 1994, 910–15.

11. D. E. Brenner et al., "Postmenopausal Estrogen Replacement Therapy and the Risk of Alzheimer's Disease: A Population-Based Case-Control Study," *American Journal of Epidemiology* 140, 1994, 262–67.

12. Weiss, "Failure of Nalmefene."

13. Barbara Joseph, M.D. *My Healing from Breast Cancer* (New Canaan, CT: Keats Publishing, Inc., 1996), 12. See also Malone, K., et al. "Oral Contraceptives in Relation to Breast Cancer," *Epidemiologic Reviews* 15, No. 1, 1993, 80–97.

14. Virginia Soffa, *The Journey Beyond Breast Cancer* (Rochester, VT: Healing Arts Press, 1994), 33.

15. Rose Kushner, *Alternatives: New Developments in the War on Breast Cancer* (New York: Warner Books, 1984), 128–50.

Appendix G: Sources of Natural Progesterone

1. Marcus Laux and Christine Conrad, *Natural Woman, Natural Menopause* (New York: HarperCollins, 1997), 70.
2. Jane E. Brody, *New York Times National Section,* November 28, 1994.
3. John R. Lee, *Natural Progesterone: The Multiple Roles of a Remarkable Hormone* (Sebastopol, CA: BLL Publishing, 1993), 76.
4. Ibid.
5. John R. Lee, *What Your Doctor May Not Tell You About Menopause* (New York: Warner Books, 1996), 270, 305.
6. Reader's Digest Editors, *Magic and Medicine of Plants* (New York: Reader's Digest Association, Inc., 1993), 71.
7. Sam Biser, *The Last Chance Health Report,* Vol. 6, Nos. 2–4, 12.
8. Barbara Griggs, *Green Pharmacy: The History and Evolution of Western Herbal Medicine* (New York: Viking Press, 1981), 332, 361.

Index